DreamsAlive

COMPREHENSIVE REVIEW FOR
NCLEX-RN

NKECHINYERE AGU

Editorial and Communications Consultant
Dr. MarkAnthony Nze
People & Polity Inc.
New York

AuthorHouse™
1663 Liberty Drive
Bloomington, IN 47403
www.authorhouse.com
Phone: 833-262-8899

This book is printed on acid-free paper.

ISBN: 978-1-6655-4917-2 (sc)
ISBN: 978-1-6655-4918-9 (e)

Library of Congress Control Number: 2022900504

Print information available on the last page.

Published by AuthorHouse 01/27/2022

authorHOUSE

CONTENTS

Chapter 16 Answer with Explanation

INTRODUCTION

Dreamsalive NCLEX-RN Comprehensive Review is ideal for registered nurses to take preparation to pass their National Council Licensure Examination. This test preparation is essential to getting success. I have developed the NCLEX-RN Exam preparation Guide to support you to pass the exam. I will provide you with the documents, resources, and strategies to make you successful. Besides, to help you make your exam preparation as confident as possible. If you have already developed your NCLEX-EN study plan, you should review this guide and the suggested resources and documents.

To become an RN called Registered Nurse in Nova Scotia, you must pass the NCLEX-RN exam. At the end of the guide, I will provide you with the checklist to help you develop your exam plan. All the concepts are described, and not a single point I passed in this guide. Here are the critical sections of the exam:

Basic Care and Comfort
Health Promotion and Maintenance
Management of Care
Pharmacological and Parenteral Therapies
Physiological Adaptation
Psychosocial Integrity
Reduction of Risk Potential
Safety and Infection Control

All sections detail you will get into the Book. Most of the practice guides have only questions and solutions. In this Book, you will find the strategies to make the preparation confident and tips to get good results. The Dreamsalive test preparation guide will provide you with all the NCLEX questions and their answers. Also, the explanation of the responses as well. To make your concept depth, you will get each answer in detail.

CHAPTER 1:
What Is The NCLEX-RN?

The National Council Licensure Examination, known as NCLEX. It is a mandatory exam needed by the nursing association to assess a candidate's eligibility for working entry-level nursing.

Nursing candidates must have an accredited nursing degree and pass either the NCLEX-RN or NCLEX-PN to become licensed. This step is significant because it provides you with a method to validate your nursing knowledge and assess your ability to practice as a nurse. Think, Would you want to treat a nurse who hasn't proved that they've followed these guidelines? Most definitely not!

There has a purpose for the NCLEX exam. This exam will decide which nurses are eligible for entry-level nurse jobs. In your educational background, you will not give any similar tests. It's different. You learn information-based information and NCLEX test analysis and their applications in your academic background. This assessment will check your ability to figure out the critical problems. Before you can even consider scheduling or arranging where you want to take the NCLEX, you need to make your application to a Province or Territory. This exam is open for students who hold an accredited nursing degree.

Why is the NCLEX so important?

The National Council Licensure Examination is constructed to assess the capability and competencies required to perform as an entry-level nurse who is newly licensed. There are two types of exams available. Candidates who wish to become registered nurses will attend the NCLEX-RN exam, and those who want to become practical nurses will take the NCLEX-PN exam.

After completing their school, nurses must advance to the next level before starting a job. To obtain a nursing license, all nurses must pass the NCLEX exam.

The NCLEX is necessary since it removes any barriers between being a graduate or nursing student, and if this is your aim for your healthcare professional, you must pass the NCLEX test.

The curriculum developed for Lincoln Technical Institute's nursing preparation programs, for example, is intended to prepare students to take NCLEX exams. As a result, direct practical experience training is provided, including simulations of laboratories and hospitals and real scenarios.

Both practical nurses (PN) and registered nurses (RN) are given the necessary training to pass the exams. Qualified educators provide students with the tools they need to succeed. After passing the exam, these nurses are ready to work in public health organizations, hospitals, schools, doctor's offices, nursing homes, and wherever nurses are required.

If you want a nursing license in the United States and are already a nursing graduate, you will be able to attend the NCLEX-RN test and give you a permit. Then, you can work as a nurse in the United States with this license!

Every test lasts about 2 to 3 hours, and candidates who do not pass must wait 45 to 90 days before retaking it.

If you consider a nursing career, keep the NCLEX exam in mind while deciding where to attend school. A few colleges place a premium on preparing students for this exam because the license granted for passing is essential if you wish to work as a nurse.

When it comes to taking the NCLEX exam, all students face tension and nervousness. However, you will understand how worthy your complex works are when you finish your exam. When you pass the NCLEX test and become a licensed registered or practical nurse, you should cherish the confidence you've gained and be proud of your success.

Who must take the NCLEX?

Every NCLEX candidate interested in working as a nurse must take and pass the NCLEX test. The NCLEX test is divided into two types based on level of education.

Candidates with a Practical Nursing diploma who want to become a LICENSED PRACTICAL NURSE should take the NCLEX-PN. Those with an associate's or bachelor's degree who wish to become registered nurses (RNs) should take the NCLEX-RN exam.

How to Register For the NCLEX-RN

Your initial step is to apply to the National Council of State Boards of Nursing (NCSBN). You will need to follow the techniques established by the individual State Boards of Nursing. A few states have combined registration for the NCLEX-RN exam with licensure applications. You need to send your application for your license, and that's how you will get a permit for all the states. You will contact a Candidate Bulletin to register for the NCLEX-RN exam whenever you have applied.

Your nursing school will send you two applications about six weeks before graduation: one for licensure and one for the NCLEX-RN exam.

On a predetermined date, you must submit the completed structures and the licensure fees to your nursing school. After receiving authorization to test, you should schedule your test date and time. Testing is available year-round, 15 hours per day, six days per week, in 6-hour time slots.

To take the NCLEX, you must first get a nursing license from your state's governing nursing agency. If they conclude that you match the exam eligibility standards, you will be able to register to take the exam at that time. In your mail, you will notice that it will include another Authorization to Take the Test (ATT).

NCLEX-RN Exam and Licensure Fees

The expense to take the NCLEX-RN exam is $200. The individual State Boards of Nursing are determining more licensure fees. Telephone registrants are needed to pay by VISA or Master Card. In addition, there is a $9.50 administration expense for the telephone enlistment. If you like, you might send an individual check, cashier's check or cash order to the National Council of State Boards of Nursing.

You'll get a postcard acknowledging receipt of registration. But you cannot plan an appointment to take the exam until your State Board of Nursing announces you are eligible and you get an Authorization to Test (ATT) via the mail.

Send your finished test application and fee to the National Council of State Boards of Nursing. In addition, you can enlist by telephone by calling: 1-866-496-2539 in the USA (1-952-681-3815 for outside the USA) between 8 a.m. and 8 p.m. (Eastern), Monday through Friday.

C H A P T E R   2 :
Preparation for NCLEX

Passing the NCLEX is attainable for each nursing school graduate with the proper planning. That being said, the test ought to be viewed. Earning a straight A's or 4.0 GPA in nursing school doesn't foresee success on the NCLEX.

Perfect time of starting preparation for NCLEX

We're sharing a few hints on when you should begin preparing for the NCLEX and how to get everything rolling.

How early is Too Early?

Even though you may not begin studying until nearer to the time you take the exam, it is never too right on time to start preparing for the NCLEX! Regardless of where you are on the nursing school timeline, everything you can manage to prepare is to familiarize yourself with NCLEX-style test questions. The more agreeable you are with the questions and testing styles you will see on exam day, the more it will assist you with being successful since quite a while ago.

In most expresses, the earliest you can take the exam is roughly 45 days later than your graduation date. As I stated before, it's essential to take the Nursing Regulatory Board (NRB) license. Otherwise, you need to take a licensed state by state. Also, it will be a time-wasting if you need to take a licensed shape by state.

Decide for test timing when you want to take it.

Various individual factors determine when a graduating student wants to enter the workforce, but this question — when would I like to begin my career? —decides when you'll want to take your NCLEX. When you should start preparing for the NCLEX depends on when you take it. First, you need to know about NCSBN, the National Council of State Boards of Nursing.

If you do not intend to take the exam within a few months or even a year, you need not be hurried. Indeed, it could be a valuable time of study with a top-notch test prep resource, so you are sure and ready on exam day.

But most students are anxious to begin their life as practicing clinicians immediately. If you're looking to get everything rolling without a moment's delay, that 45-day mark is something to keep your eye on.

It's vital to note that you can't simply show up to a testing community on an exam day and take the NCLEX. Before going for an exam, you need to follow a few steps.

- Pay the registration fees and Register with Pearson VUE
- Accept your Authorization to Test (ATT)

- for licensure, you need to Apply the nursing regulatory body (NRB)
- Plan your exam date with Pearson VUE

Start Preparing About 6 Months Out

This is a great time to start studying again. You may not remember all your school study preparation, so you need to learn and review topics you may not recognize or recall now. To allow sufficient opportunity to audit the broad measure of information that will be covered on the NCLEX, successful candidates usually begin studying around five or a half years before they are planned to step through the exam, which is presumably around the beginning of your final semester in nursing school.

It's vital to note that the 5 to 6-month window for preparing is an idea, but every candidate is different. You realize you're learning habits and study skills the best, so make sure to give yourself ample time to overcome all of the information. In addition, you need to make a timetable for the exam if you are slow in reading or writing. Time slots will help you give you confidence for the exam.

How long can you remember learning from your school?

You need to spend lots of time studying if you do not have a plan to take an exam in the next three months. One of the benefits of taking the NCLEX quickly upon graduation is that the information you have learned in nursing school is moderately new in your mind. Maintaining pertinent information might be a challenge for students who put off taking their exams.

The challenging NCLEX-style questions, point-by-point reasoning, specific delineation, and precise execution tracking will assist with reinforcing the information you have gained in your nursing system and increase your odds of NCLEX success.

Do You Feel Confident That You Have Prepared?

If you are ready enough, that is something worth being thankful for— you're going to do effectively! You risk getting a good result if you are not planning your time. So do you need to ask yourself if you are ready for this high-value exam? Whenever you take the exam one year after graduating or 30 days after graduation, this question will be huge for every candidate.

The NCLEX is an adaptive computer test that measures your skill with each question asked. Each new question is more enthusiastically or easier based on your past answers. There is no issue with getting fortunate or anything on the exam day. Your insight level will be uncovered.

The most fitting answer to "How long should you wait to require for the NCLEX later you graduate?" is presumably this. It depends on you, but you need to make sure that you are fully prepared for the exam when you are taking the exam.

Along these lines, how would you "prepare sure you're?" Here are some essential steps:

1. Utilize flashcards with dispersed repetition innovation
2. Track your progress and take self-assessments to check your readiness
3. Build a study plan and begin studying well ahead of your exam day.
4. Use superior grade, industry-leading practice questions
5. Choose a test prep resource written by experienced nurse educators and practicing clinicians

I will give you 900 questions and their answers to make your preparation healthy for getting preparation. If you check all 900 questions in my book, you will surely get a good result in your NCLEX exam because all the questions are from the previous NCLEX exam.

How would I be able to get ready for the NCLEX?

Feeling confident and ready for the NCLEX is significant, so knowing how to read up appropriately for the exam is fundamental. You will be facing a challenge in taking the exam of NCLEX. First of all: Don't pack without a second to spare. Put in the legitimate energy, concentrate on the exam itself and how it works and make a point to take heaps of practice tests. If you get all questions together, then it will be helpful for anyone. That's why in the last part of my guide, I added lots of questions.

How to Study for the NCLEX?

Like any test, the critical component to success is planning, so you should foster a study strategy that works for you. Here are some study tips:

1. Study consistently, even in short five to ten minutes bursts.
2. Maximize your time and study materials you are less familiar with first.
3. Review all of your nursing textbooks. Then, take the chapter test alongside reading the chapter summaries.
4. Maintain a decent attitude and challenge yourself; be determined that you CAN pass the NCLEX!
5. Purchase comprehensive NCLEX study materials that include practice tests.

A few online websites with various resources accessible to nursing students studying for the NCLEX. You can download different materials for nothing that experienced nurses have written. The study materials usually include four comprehensive practice exams like what you will find in the National Council Licensure Examination itself and section tests.

Which Subjects Are Covered on the Exam?

There is no chance to skipping the questions and you need to go forward after answering the previous questions. This means you should spend some of your study time developing strategies for determining the best answer, even if the question is vague.

The exam will have between 75 and 265 questions. Discover the explanation of how the exam is graded below to see why there is such a large range. Regardless of how many questions you answer, the following is the rate split of requests by content region:

- ✓ 17-23% questions will be about Management of Care
- ✓ 9-15% questions will be about Security and Infection Control
- ✓ 6-12% questions will be about Health Promotion and Maintenance
- ✓ 6-12% questions will be about Psychosocial Integrity
- ✓ 6-12% questions will be about Basic Care and Comfort
- ✓ 12-18% questions will be about Pharmacological and Parenteral Therapies
- ✓ 9-15% questions will be about Decrease of Risk Potential
- ✓ 11-17% questions will be about Physiological Adaptation

The exam could take up to six hours to complete. You have the option of skipping two quick breaks within that period. The amount of time it takes to answer each question is determined on the number of questions you must answer.

For attending the test How much I need to study?

You ought to spend no less than several weeks reviewing all the material and working on your ability to recall realities rapidly. To do that, get the "Dreamsalive NCLEX-RN Comprehensive Review" which gives an intensive breakdown of each content region, including all the essential terms and ideas you should know.

To work on your outstanding ability on all that material, get a book of "Dreamsalive NCLEX-RN Comprehensive Review". Repetition is probably the most effective way to retain a ton of information. Tragically, repetition can get, well, repetitive. You can prepare yourself within your expected way. It will help you to guide you from preparation to the exam end time.

CHAPTER 3:
NCLEX-RN Test Format

The NCLEX-RN exam is coordinated according to the framework, "Meeting Client Needs." In this NCLEX exam there are practical questions, and this will consists 4 main category and 8 subcategory. There have other nursing exam also but they all are about caring, mental, pediatric, this types.

Sample question

A 23-year-elderly person with insulin subordinate diabetes mellitus (IDDM) is gotten back to the recuperation room one hour later a standard delivery of a nine lb., eight oz., and child kid. The nurse would expect the lady's glucose to

1. Rise
2. Fall
3. Remain Stationary
4. Fluctuate

To choose the correct answer, you must consider the pathophysiology of diabetes alongside the principles of work and delivery.

Taking the NCLEX-RN CAT

CAT is an abbreviation for "adaptive computer test," an interactive testing design based on your reaction to the questions. Based on your ability level, the CAT guarantees that the questions are not "too hard" or "too easy."

Your first question will be generally easy—beneath the degree of minimum capability. Next, the PC chooses a slightly more complicated question if you answer it effectively. If answered incorrectly, the computer selects a little easier question. By doing this all through the test, the PC can determine your degree of ability.

What kinds of questions are included on the NCLEX?

According to Kelly Beischel, a licensed nurse and NCLEX success mentor, "NCLEX questions are prepared at the application or more important levels of cognitive capacity to assess the candidate's puzzling thought processing." "There are many decision, fill-in-the-blank, issue area, different reaction, and ordered reaction items that can be used."

You will get multiple answers for making the correct answer. Choosing the "most right" answer for the situation, on the other hand, can demonstrate that you'll think critically and make competent decisions as a nurse.

RN Esfira Shakhmurova explains, "The NCLEX encourages you to think through every issue presented." "It confuses the reader by presenting four or five scenarios, but as a nurse, you need to prioritize your work and work within your limitation." Some inquiries throw you off, but you're simply prepared to respond to the inquiry." Shakhmurova proposes that you break down each question to understand what is being requested and how you should accommodate the patient first.

Other NCLEX questions demand the same vital memory and knowledge of reality as any other test, so you'll need to commit a large amount of time to learning and memorizing important nursing concepts.

Questions are primarily different decisions with four possible answers; however, there are other question forms as well. Multiple-response, fill-in-the-blank, problem areas, diagram/exhibit, and intuitive questions are examples of alternative question kinds. All of the questions include nursing content that has been integrated.

CHAPTER 4:
Dos and Don'ts for Passing the NCLEX

The exam contains questions from a few substance classes, making it necessary for graduate nurses to study consistently between the time they register and the date the exam happens. People who want to pass NCLEX-RN they will get the registered nurse certificate. It's a most valuable certification for registered nurse.

Do: Take a few practices exam

NCLEX study materials and practice tests are available from Kaplan and other educational publishers, allowing you to get a feel for the test. Take the test numerous times in the months leading up to your exam day for the best results. Solving the practice questions will help you to make your time schedule that how you can answer all the questions. It will increase your capability to answer all questions with confidence. Taking the practice test again a few weeks before your scheduled exam can help you identify areas where you are still weak, allowing you to catch up on complex ideas. Act as if the practice test is the real exam to see how you'll perform. Set aside your study materials, sit in a quiet area, and time yourself while you complete the exam items.

Don't: Panic

Because the NCLEX is a high-stakes exam, it's natural to be concerned about how much you know and how well you'll perform. However, worrying about the exam will make it harder to recall what you studied, resulting in a poor performance. If passing the NCLEX is a must for you, strive to have a level head. Before entering the test community, eat a decent breakfast, avoid caffeine, and take a few deep breaths.

Because the NCLEX is a high-stakes exam, it's natural to be concerned about how much you know and how well you'll perform. However, worrying about the exam will make it harder to recall what you studied, resulting in a poor performance. If passing the NCLEX is a must for you, try to have a calm head. Before entering the test community, eat a decent breakfast, avoid caffeine, and take a few deep breaths.

Do: Need to study with a group

Group study will give you befits from the other candidate's preparation. You will get much knowledge attending the group study. For example, in a study published in the Journal of Nursing and Education, Ashley and O'Neil report that in danger students who joined personnel drove concentrate on improved on the NCLEX than in danger students who were examined all alone. This shows that joining a study group can help you achieve your goal of passing the NCLEX.

Don't: Cram for the test

The NCLEX covers a few substance classes, some more difficult than others, making reliable reviews the ideal way to master the material. However, if you wait for as long as possible to begin reviewing, you're likely to forget important information upon the arrival of the test, making it more outlandish that you'll pass. Besides, cramming doesn't work because your brain tricks you into thinking that you have memorized the material. In reality, your brain is only familiar with the material; when the time comes to step through the examination, you're likely to fail to remember much of what you reviewed during a last-minute cramming session, explains psychologist Tom Stafford.

Do: Understand the NCLEX test plan

The National Council of State Boards of Nursing will help you to give you guideline that when you need to go for exam. If you read this book then it will also help you to make decision. According to the NCSB, the arrangement includes nursing activity statements, sample test items, solid substance examples and a summary of the extent of the exam. Reading the test questions and solution will help you to achieve your goal.

Don't: Procrastinate

NCLEX test will valid only for 90 days after completing registration for NCLEX. This implies you should begin studying well before your registration; otherwise, you may not be ready in time for your test date. The NCLEX is a thorough exam, so a few weeks of intensive concentrate presumably will not be enough to help you pass. Furthermore, first-time test-takers had a passing rate underneath 90% in 2019; this addresses the difficulty of the test and the significance of planning when creating your study plan.

CHAPTER 5:
NCLEX-RN Four Major Categories

Safe And Effective Care Environment

The primary Client Needs Category, Safe and Effective Care Environment, includes two ideas:

Security and Infection Control represents 9-15% of exam questions. Nursing activities include Accident Prevention, Error Prevention, Hazardous Materials, Surgical Asepsis, Standard Precautions, and Use of Restraints.

Management of Care represents 17-23% of questions on the NCLEX-RN exam. A portion of the nursing activities included in this subcategory is Advanced Directives, Client Rights, Concepts of Management, Confidentiality, Continuity of Care, Advocacy, Case Management, Quality Improvement, Delegation, Establishing Priorities, Ethical Practice, Informed Consent, Legal Responsibilities, Referrals, and Supervision.

Physiological Integrity

The final Client Needs Category is Physiological Integrity. It includes four ideas:

Decrease of Potential Risk records for 9-15% of the exam. Its tested nursing activities include Diagnostic Tests, Laboratory Values, and Potential for Complications from Surgical Procedures and Health Alterations, and Therapeutic Procedures.

Pharmacological and Parenteral Therapies represent 12-18% of the exam. Tested nursing activities include Adverse Effects, Contraindications, Blood and Blood Products, Central Venous Access Devices, Chemotherapy, Expected Effects, Intravenous Therapy, Medication Administration, Pharmacological Pain Management, Total Parenteral Nutrition, and Dosage Calculations.

Basic Care and Comfort represent 6-12% of questions on the NCLEX-RN exam. Nursing activities included in this subcategory are Assistive Devices, Elimination, Mobility, Nonpharmacological Comfort Interventions, Nutrition and Oral Hydration, Personal Hygiene, and Rest and Sleep.

Physiological Adaptation represents 11-17% of the exam. Its tested nursing activities include Alterations in the Body Systems, Fluid and Electrolyte Imbalances, Hemodynamics, Medical Emergencies, Pathophysiology, and Unexpected Response to Therapies.

Health Promotion and Maintenance

The subsequent Client Needs Category is Health Promotion and Maintenance. These questions represent 6-12% of the exam. Nursing activities tested include the Aging Process, Ante/Intra/Postpartum and Newborn Care, Disease Prevention, Health Screening, Self-Care, Lifestyle Choices, Physical Assessment Techniques, Developmental Stages and Transitions, Health Promotion Programs, and High-Risk Behaviors.

Psychosocial Integrity

Psychosocial Integrity is the third Client Needs Category. Stress Management, Support Systems, Grief and Loss, Coping Mechanisms, Mental Health Concepts, Coping Mechanisms, End-of-Life Care, Sensory/Perceptual Alterations, Therapeutic Communication, Chemical Dependency, Spiritual Influence on Health, Behavioral Interventions, Crisis Intervention, and Family Dynamics are among the nursing activities tested.

C H A P T E R   6 :
How is the NCLEX administered?

The NCLEX exams are given utilizing updated versatile testing, which is a type of testing (CAT). This means that the PC will re-evaluate your nursing competence based on your responses and the difficulty of the questions each time you answer one. This technique is designed to present you with questions that are sufficiently challenging based on your previous responses to give you a 50% chance of answering correctly.

When you get to the test place upon the arrival of your exam, you'll need to introduce a correct type of identification, read and sign the paperwork, store individual belongings and continue to the testing room. Here you'll have as long as six hours to finish the exam. If that appears like an inordinately long measure of time for a test, you can have confidence knowing that you'll have ample time to think through each question. There are no less than two predetermined breaks presented during the exam.

This testing approach also means that the duration of the test may vary from one candidate to the next. If you're on the verge of passing, you'll be quizzed until you either run out of time or gain enough confidence by correctly answering enough questions.

While this may appear complicated, there are valid justifications for this configuration. For one's purposes, a high-ability candidate passing based exclusively on their ability to answer the "easy" questions accurately is anything but an incredible impression of their ability to work in a natural setting. Additionally, providing a progression of high-difficulty questions to a marginal candidate frequently prompts guessing. A suitable series of guesses leading to a passing outcome isn't great, either. This responsive organization fosters a superior check of a nurses' overall ability.

How Is the NCLEX-RN Exam Scored?

The NCLEX-RN is graded using an impressive system. This exam's pointing will show based on "Logit", it will not making pointing with the correct answer.

If it isn't 95% certain of your outcomes, you will continue to see questions until it is inevitable or until you arrive at the limit of 265 questions. Then, if you reach the greatest, it will do a final assessment to determine whether or not you have fulfilled the passing standard.

Think of it along these lines – there is an even line on a pivot, and I will call it the "pass line." Anything above it is passing, and anything beneath it isn't passing. So, you start precisely on the line at question zero, and with each right and incorrect answer, you get knocked up an indent and down a score, separately. The PC will give dynamically more complex questions to determine your pinnacle information with each correct answer.

This may all solid a little complicated, but basically: the better you do, the fewer questions you have to answer. But even if you wind up having to answer 265 questions, you may, in any case, pass the exam.

If you have fulfilled the passing guideline, you will essentially be informed that you passed the exam. However, you will just see a definite report of how you performed on each test segment if you fizzled.

A logit is a measurement unit that indicates the general difference between your assessed ability level (based on your education, training, and experience) and your actual ability level (based on how you performed on the test). At regular periods, the board reexamines the passing standard. You'll need a logit of 0.00 or above right now.

This Logit varied depending on your number of answers and it always changing. The test will terminate when you have completed 75 questions and the computer software can decide whether you have passed or failed with 95 percent accuracy.

There will be a minimum of 75 questions and a maximum of 265 questions on the test. When the tester answers enough questions correctly to stay over the pass line with a 95 percent confidence interval, the candidate passes the test. In contrast, if the candidate does not rise above the pass line with 95 percent certainty, they will fail the test.

To pass, you must, at last, transcend the pass line that demonstrates competency with marginal uncertainty. The test can end anytime this determination is made, between questions 75 – 265 or at the maximum time allowance (6 hours).

After failing the NCLEX exam what should you do?

If any candidate fails to their exam, then it will take few days to take the retake exam. Every exam attempt costs $200, so it's in the best interests of nursing grads to make the most of their time and money by passing the first time.

Which Percentage Do You Have to Get on the NCLEX to Pass?

There is certainly not a specific number or rate that you need to answer accurately to pass the NCEX. Instead, the exam's computational algorithm assesses the correct answers within the context of their difficulty and an assortment of topic information. The versatile test will determine that you are at an adequate level to pass in each branch of knowledge using a 95% confidence rule, or a choice will be made at the most extreme time (6-hour imprint) or maximum question allowance (265).

Comparing NCLEX-PN versus NCLEX-RN

What are the real distinctions between the NCLEX-PN and NCLEX-RN exams? When it comes to the overall organization, there are more parallels than differences. However, there are minor variances in the number of questions and time limit on the tests; the majority of the variation is due to the content of the questions.

However, LPNs and RNs both give care to patients; RNs have an increased extent of the practice, and the NCLEX-RN questions mirror that. Since registered nurses can supervise LPNs, the NCLEX-RN contains more questions on managing others while the NCLEX-PN focuses on coordinating consideration between health professionals. RNs can also oversee total parenteral nutrition and the administration of blood and blood items to patients, so questions on the two topics are included on the NCLEX-RN.

However, the tests cover different material; the two-give a thorough assessment of a nurse's critical abilities for practicing at their qualification level.

How the Next Generation NCLEX Exam Works?

The NCSBN has made a model that addresses the few phases of specialized ability and information that nurses must show skill in to pass the NCELX. An exceptional exploration segment was added to the furthest limit of NCLEX exams that was intended to gather information on new item types that could expand or improve the measurement of entry-level nursing ability that includes clinical judgment. Accordingly, the Clinical Judgment Model was made to enhance the NCLEX exam and guarantee that all nursing students working toward an ADN or BSN are ready for their choices in certifiable medical situations.

CHAPTER 7:
Basic Information for NCLEX exam

The NCLEX is not like the other examinations you'll take as a nursing student, so it's important to know what to expect on test day.

Many first-time test takers pass the NCLEX, but it takes a lot of preparation to do so. Because the NCLEX is different from the other examinations you'll take as a nursing student, it's important to know what to expect on test day. Many nursing students and graduates are concerned about passing the NCLEX examination.

So, you've decided to pursue an ADN or BSN degree because you understand the differences between the two nursing programs, or you've opted to pursue an LPN degree. You're probably wondering if this is another abbreviation you should have been aware of before enrolling in your classes.

The NCLEX is the final step in acquiring your nursing license and is one of the most important milestones you will attain as a nursing student. It's not only a huge accomplishment to pass the NCLEX, but it also means you're ready to start your nursing career!

The National Council Licensure Exam (NCLEX) has been a rite of passage for nursing students for decades. It was originally known as "the sheets," or the State Board Test Pool Examination, until The National Council of Nurses took it in 1982 and renamed it the National Council Licensure Exam (NCLEX). The conversion to an automated test design in 1994, which is still used today, was another notable development in the exam's history.

You need to understand the basics before start. The NCLEX is a series of exams that you must pass in order to become a nurse in the United States. To administer the test, you must learn a variety of skills, which may be challenging for someone who is just beginning their career as a nurse. Furthermore, how you can completely rely on the outcome of a single exam is a terrifying potential that you never asked for in the first place.

However, because many of Grade Hacker's clients work in healthcare, I've created this guide to help you grasp the 7 Most Important Things You Should Know About the NCLEX.

When you've finished reading, you should recognize that this exam is a logical next step after you've completed your initial scholastic journey into nursing. The NCLEX, rather than looking like a Goliath waiting for you at the finish line, is more like the last jump before you win the reward you've been working so hard for.

As a result, I'll start with the fundamentals:

How Is The NCLEX Set Up?

The NCLEX is a computer-adaptive test. First, this implies that you will initially take the exam on the PC set in a testing focus of your decision. Second, according to your initial presentation in the exam, the difficulty of the following questions will.

For example, if you miss the past question, the following one will be a bit easier. Then again, if you get one question right, the following one will be slightly more challenging. This configuration is made to get a more precise outcome wherein you are better at or need improvement.

Versatile testing also influences the length of the exam. Depending on your exhibition, you get between 75 to 265 questions. However, you will forever have 6 hours to finish the cycle with breaks included. Around 90% of the questions are numerous decisions, while the rest is split between fill-in-the-clear, diagram-reading, good listening, or comparable sorts of questions.

You will need approval to take the exam

An Authorization to Test, commonly known as an ATT letter, is required to take the NCLEX. To obtain this approval, you must contact your nursing regulatory body (NRB) and submit an application. From NRB you will get an ATT through email. This clearance will expire in around 90 days; if you do not complete the test within that timeframe, you should.

Remember the ABCs

Recollect your ABCs—Airway, Breathing, Circulation. Make your determinations in that order. For example, answers should zero in on stabilizing the patient and prioritizing their needs based on the situation given in the question. The ABCs is an excellent method for running through test questions and determining what steps ought to be taken first.

It's critical to evaluate information from other sources, including as study guides and practice tests, as well as the educational plan basics taught in your nursing school lectures, when studying for the NCLEX exam.

Know your learning and study style

Understanding what method helps you with learning best is a significant aspect of preparing for the NCLEX. While some may like using flashcards or studying alone, others may improve more interactive practices or in a social environment. Try out different studying techniques and see what works best for you.

- Ask professors or different students for input on answers to questions – you may get new insight on something you didn't realize.
- Talk to other students about their favored studying strategies or study with them!
- Pick a study space with minimal interruptions to remain focused.
- Studying too much on the double can be as terrible as not learning enough. Remember to sit down from time to time to recharge your mind.

Understand the test design

The NCLEX is available in two versions, and your nursing degree will determine which one you need to take. One is the NCLEX-PN, which is designed for LPNs or those with a functional or professional nursing diploma. The NCLEX-RN, on the other hand, is for registered nurses or those with an associate's (ASN) or bachelor's (BSN) degree in nursing.

The NCLEX is divided into four major knowledge categories. These are some of the areas:

- Safe and effective care management
- Health promotion and maintenance

- Psychological integrity
- Physiological integrity (the largest section)

You should be entirely learning in every one of these areas to finish the exam successfully.

What Will Your NCLEX Exam Day Be Like?

Be asked which variation of the test you will be taking, and you will get a sheet with information. Once you are finished with that, you will be asked to give a Government Issued ID that includes a photo, a mark in a digital cushion, fingerprint, and palm vein scanning, which sounds threatening but is only a method for checking that you are, indeed, you. Then, at that point, a digital photo will be taken, and you are all set!

You have the option of storing your stuff (since telephones and different gadgets are not allowed). After that, you'll meet your test administrator and go through another quick identification process; they'll offer you a calculator and an erasable note board if you need them. Finally, you will be escorted to your testing station, where you will be given access to a computer and your exam. Keep in mind that these tests are proctored, which means that your voice and video will be recorded.

Expect a variety of question types

To access students critical thinking ability there are 3 types of NCLEX questions. The first are general information inquiries, which are frequently presented in a variety of choice formats. Following that, there are a number of analysis and application problems, which may incorporate diagrams, tables, or realistic pictures. The most challenging level three problems require students to apply realities, cycles, and rules to obtain the answers. They're frequently provided in an unfinished state. You should expect the majority of your inquiries to fall under categories two and three.

The test consists of 75 to 265 questions, however the number of questions you must complete is determined by how you answered each previous question. As a result, there are no two examinations that are alike. In addition, 15 questions are classified as "trial questions" and will not be factored into your final score.

You will receive your nursing license after passing the exam, which is valid in the state where you took it. There is a cycle through which you can move your license if you wind up being used in another capacity.

Finally, if you're intending on taking the NCLEX soon, be sure to check out these NCLEX study recommendations so you can feel prepared for the exam. I hope everything goes well for you in terms of karma and remember to relax — you've got this!

When you need a break or are finished, raise your hand toward the administrator so they can assist you. All of the focuses are ADA (Americans with Disabilities Act) compliant, so you'll get any help you need.

C H A P T E R 8 :
Study Tips and Strategies
for Passing the NCLEX

When you plan your review methods, you are most of the way there headed for success. With the proper planning, NCLEX can be cleared in one go. Each nursing graduate must ideally write this exam as soon as they graduate because, at that time, you are accustomed to devoting 'concentrate on hours.' To remember, scoring A's, or a 4.0 GPA in nursing school doesn't foresee success on the NCLEX.

You must commit a minimum of two months to study the course material and get familiar with the organization of the exam. Also, before you choose to take the exam casually, recall that every one of your endeavors costs you CAD 470 (around). Therefore, it's wiser to make your time and money worthwhile by studying dedicatedly for it. Further, I have a few hints that can help you prepare better for the examination.

Passing the NCLEX-RN exam is the last significant milestone standing between you and your definitive prize—a Registered Nurse license. It's difficult to stop the frenzy from setting in, but you have been preparing for this test for a long time! You are more prepared than you feel.

Many nurses have preceded you and realize precisely how nerve-wracking this time can be. So have confidence; I will assist you with passing the NCLEX-RN (National Council Licensure Examination—Registered Nurse) at the initial time.

Following quite a while of dreary studying and long clinical days, you have procured the ability to require a little bit off from the grind of education. So, offer yourself a reprieve to unwind and make time to treat yourself.

How would you be able to manage all of your freshly discovered time? First, rest! Snooze past dawn or interface with loved ones that you've missed during your nursing school venture—zero in on wellness activities like yoga, meditation, long strolls, massages, or steam showers. Next, sustain your spirit, so you are loose and open to focusing on the NCLEX.

Try not to put a hold on nursing material. Staying new will allow you to retain the information you gained in school. However, the NCLEX will require additional training.

When you're ready, submit an application to your leading nursing/regulatory body (BON/RB) and register for an Authorization to Test with Pearson VUE (ATT). Plan for the NCLEX a few months ahead of time so that you can meet this deadline. Plan on studying for the NCLEX-RN for approximately two months. **Take Time**

It's incredibly essential to take on a steady speed when taking the NCLEX-RN. You will have as long as four hours to finish the exam in its aggregate. Usually, with many timed exams, the best practice is to answer the easy questions first, then, at that point, return to the harder ones. This interaction is unimaginable with the

NCLEX-RN. Because of its computer-adaptive nature, you can't move on to the next question until you have finished the last one. Furthermore, there is no natural method of knowing how many more questions you need to answer to finish the exam while taking it. Along these lines, you should spend as much time as you need to carefully break down each question (more correct answers equal fewer questions) but maintain a steady pace so that you may finish within the allocated time.

Test-Taking Skills

It's critical to mentally prepare yourself for a wide range of possible NCLEX questions. The NCLEX employs flexible electronic testing to ensure that each exam is unique. The machine is smart enough to choose an issue based on your performance in a question bank with a variety of themes and question kinds (around 90 percent are numerous decisions). When you've responded correctly enough to stay one point above the "pass line," you've passed the test.

Anything over this mark is a pass, while anything below it is a failure. You are on the pass line when you begin the test. You will be knocked up as you explore the test and select the correct answers. You will be knocked down if you choose incorrect answers. Each time you correctly answer a question, the test will logically progress to progressively difficult questions. To pass the test, you must cross the pass line at a location that has been statistically proven to determine your nursing skill. The exam will be completed at a later time. It's the longest exam you'll ever take – 6 hours. Remember that 15 practice test questions are not graded and are used to determine how well candidates perform. They are questions that might show up on a future NCLEX exam. Try not to try to measure where you are difficulty-wise during the test. If you got a couple of easy questions, it doesn't imply that you are below the pass line.

Because of the random samples, you can get simple questions. Concentrate on each question. Don't worry about the questions you've already sent; they'll be answered eventually. Don't be concerned about the level of difficulty. Consider it a long-distance race. When you have proved the ability to complete a minimum skill (or lack thereof) and answered no less than 75 questions, or when you have answered all 265 questions, the test will end.

Preparing for the NCLEX

You need to gather enough nursing knowledge to pass the exam without frying your brain. To begin, make a schedule that specifies which days of the week you want to focus on and how long you want to work. While each student's ability to accomplish a certain amount in one day varies, historical success stories demonstrate that three to four hours of studying every day is ideal.

Your study schedule should include when you will take practice examinations. As long as you are deliberate, you can set any objective that works with your strengths and weaknesses.

Try not to pack! It's proper to go home every week, as long as you make the days that you work beneficial. For example, put out an objective to finish a specific number of questions a day or complete a certain number of practice tests.

Participate in dynamic studying rather than passively staring at pages of notes or rewriting information from NCLEX prep books.

Study with Mnemonics

Memory helpers are a retention strategy that allows you to recall complex ideas quickly. These are typically short phrases or abbreviations that you can call on.

Day before the exam you need to be relax

Day before the exam you need to wake up early and make it relaxed with enjoying the morning. Instead, practice or meditate, have a comfortable breakfast and scrub down. Zero in on the present, and don't allow your mind to wander into dread.

The NCLEX is proof-based, and all questions come from diaries, reading material, and scientific information. Disregard recounted information from the forefronts of nursing. As difficult as it might be, don't draw from your history as a nurse's helper or nursing student!

Regularly, having experience furnishes you with invaluable abilities when caring for your patients. It might cloud your ability to answer exam questions effectively in this specific case. Nurses give care differently, and occasionally, you might be observing negative propensities.

Positivity is Key

The exam is challenging and will require studying! You might have minutes during the exam when you question everything from your insight to your future as a nurse. It's to be expected to be baffled—it's a challenging exam. But, if it wasn't difficult, anyone could be a nurse. So, trust your abilities and imagine yourself as a Registered Nurse. Passing this test is only the last advance.

Go beyond the Practice Questions

Practice exams are fantastic, and the most effective method for preparing – HOWEVER – essentially taking the practice exam questions is just 50% of the cycle.

It is similarly as vital to:

- Write down notes of which ideas you want to revisit, so with your next concentrate on meeting; you can zero in on pain points.
- Look into questions that you answered incorrectly. Practice question banks give clarifications as to why each answer decision is right or wrong and outline the specific substance topic it falls under.
- Practice, practice, practice. It is beneficial to take something like 1 or 2 complete online fake NCLEX exams, so you are used to the experience of PC testing. You'll be miles ahead if you go through as much of the question bank as possible before the exam.

Give Yourself Plenty of Time to Prepare

Passing the NCLEX-RN exam is a significant milestone in your nursing career, which implies that it should not be messed with. Giving yourself much time to study and plan—weeks or even months—is one method for ensuring that you are prepared to expert the exam when your test day shows up.

Deal with Your Anxiety

It's natural to grow nervous or restless about passing the NCLEX-RN exam because it's such a significant milestone. Some stress is beneficial since it shows that you are committed to succeeding. If you are becoming stressful then you will not get good output. Pre-exam anxiety is best managed by ensuring that you are prepared by studying and practicing the exam. And it's always a good idea to think about yourself, including getting enough sleep, exercise, and diet in the weeks coming up to the test. Self-care is essential for stress and tension management.

Prepare for Exam Day

- Bring garments you can layer in case you will more often than not get cold. If you try to control your current circumstance as much as conceivable, it will assist you with feeling great and ready for the exam itself.
- Plan your exam time with your typical inclination for testing. If you are a morning individual, plan a morning test. If you appreciate slow mornings and sleeping in, then, at that point, schedule an evening exam.
- Make sure to rest the week soundly before the exam.
- Bring snacks to the middle to keep in your storage if you decide to enjoy some time off during the exam.
- Show up sooner than expected to the testing community, ready with vital records for testing.
- Put gas in your vehicle the previous night.
- Set a reliable caution.

Take Break time

Ensure your break time. Try not to keep test-taking if your bladder is complete, your stomach rumbling, or you feel overpowered. You won't focus as expected on the questions at hand. Instead, go to the bathroom or splash your face if needed. Alternatively, go to your storage and obstacle a drink or eat a tidbit. There will be a testing administrator which called TA. TA will give you 2-hour flexible time and then again 3 and half hour. But within that time if you need to go outside then you will need to raise your hand and getting permission from the TA, you may go. Remember that the exam clock doesn't stop while you are on a break and combine it with your exam time. You can get to your pack, food, drink, and lip ointment during holidays, so plan accordingly. Try not to get to your mobile phone during the test, nor bring anything into the testing region with you. Candidates need to Follow the National Council of State Boards of Nursing (NCSBN) rules. Disregard them and risk invalidating your exam, losing the expense, and your nursing board potentially pursuing further discipline.

Study by Teaching

Respond concentrate on meetings with your friends by teaching examples to one another and quizzing one another. If there is no classmates are capable to tech you. If you can show your businesswoman mother about cytokines and the inflammatory cycle, you're killing it!

Continue practicing

Plan somewhere around two online fake NCLEX exams into your arrangement to assist you with becoming accustomed to long stints of PC testing. Being ready to sit and consider nursing questions for significant stretches will reenact the perseverance you need for the NCLEX.

Dealing with Low Practice Test Scores

Are you worried about your low practice test scores? Preliminary exams are not the authority NCLEX, so don't take the outcomes so brutally. Instead, use them as a tool to assist with developing your qualities and tease out your weaknesses.

Go through every single one of our free NCLEX practice tests. If you feel sure about the information, you are miles ahead. If you missed a question or were uncertain of the answer, survey the bank reasoning's. Also, with the assistance of our challenge bank, the questions you miss are prepared for you to study at a minute's notice. Finally, if you don't completely understand, use your nursing school material to plunge into that specific material and make an additional arrangement for audit.

When in Doubt

There are a couple of attempted but obvious NCLEX stunts. Recollect these tips when you're uncertain of the right decision.

Calling your doctor is not a best approach for a nurse. At first you need to examine the patient and use your medical brain and then if you don't find any result then you will call your doctor. Try not to shoot in obscurity—use your nursing information and rationale to settle on a good choice, regardless of whether you feel confused.

You've been developing your clinical reasoning all through your program. Trust you're growing "nurse intuition." You will experience the "select all that apply" questions.

Cautiously take a gander at every decision and eliminate incorrect answer decisions.

Thoroughly understand the exam design

The NCLEX exam follows an electronic versatile testing design, implying that no exam is indistinguishable. Based on the presentation of the last question, the next question is delivered. A candidate should remain over the pass line with a 95% confidence interval to pass the examination.

"There is a flat line on a pivot, and I will call it the "pass line." Anything above it is passing, and anything underneath it isn't passing. You start precisely on the line at question zero, and with each right and incorrect answer, you get knocked up an indent and down a score, separately. The PC will give dynamically harder questions to determine your pinnacle information with each right answer. To pass, you must, at last, transcend the pass line that exhibits ability with marginal uncertainty. The test can end anytime when this determination is made, between questions 75 – 265, or at the most extreme time allowance (6 hours)."

Keep the stressing components away

Right off the bat, it's typical to be apprehensive and restless. But, also, you can generally remind yourself to be distinct and sans stress in certain situations. For example, appearing for an exam simply can make you stressed, but you must shove that transitory feeling aside and spotlight the master plan. Keep in mind; you endured nursing school to take the exam.

- Maintain an equilibrium. Give some time to studying and some time to rejuvenating
- Try not to train your mind to pack current realities
- Exam day morning you need to reach earlier as I said before. And then you can walk around the ground, and you can listen some music also. It will make you relaxed and stress relived.

Test nervousness is a real thing, but you endured nursing school, so continue to get ready in the way that worked for you in the past. Even if you typically have test nervousness, there is a possibility that you will be apprehensive just from the pressure of such a significant test.

There are a couple of keyways of keeping stress at a minimum.

In the first place, plan for the exam genuinely but don't make studying your life. It's essential to, in any case, keep an equilibrium in the weeks and months leading up to the exam.

Allot time in your days for work out, appropriate rest, and whatever you accomplish for the sake of entertainment! By keeping an equilibrium, your mind won't develop the test second to anything more significant than it is.

Also, when it comes time to take the NCLEX, don't study or pack information the day of. Instead, take the morning before the test to quiet your mind. Listening music or go for a walk whatever you like to comfortable do that in the ground it will help you a lot.

Eventually, the most effective way to subside your nerves is to concentrate fittingly. Then, when you feel confident and ready, the NCLEX doesn't appear to be all that terrifying.

Make a study plan

Everyone has their own way of learning and they will plan their preparation in their own way. Here I will only help you to give some ideas. So that it will help you to make a decision in your own way. Some need a hypothetical way to understand things; some need sound tutorials, while others find functional execution easy. So, assess your way of learning, and based upon that, chalk out a study plan for yourself. Then, when an arrangement is set up, you must settle when you want to devote studying.

Set a timetable, orchestrate a few days off and get set rolling. Another significant thing you must consider is that once you have an arrangement, you also need to define your goals. Like, set the number of topics/questions you expect to finish within the given time frame. Doing this will additionally help your confidence to accomplish more work in a limited ability to focus time.

If you're not convinced that making an arrangement is important, consider how studying carelessly and without order might lead to inadvertent time waste. You have to utilize your time in a productive way. Don't need to spend lots of time but you need to use a productive time which may give you good result.

Invest in reference books

If you have some reference material for NCLEX then it will be helpful for you to take preparation. Your learning will be more extensive if you have more study materials. Check the customer surveys and the substance structure before purchasing a book or reading material to see if it delivers something new. You might also ask your friends and companions whether they are using a different source of information. To summarize, the more money you put into reference books, the better.

Solve practice questions

It's great to practice a most disproportionate number of questions a week before the examination. This is the most effective way to amend what you've been studying in all these long periods of arrangement. You can benefit from answering practice questions in a variety of ways. You can then work on solidifying your thoughts by identifying the questions that were answered wrong. Another significant reason presented with the practice questions is that you also become accustomed to the experience of computer testing.

Going on from exam preparation advice, the most important piece of advice is to believe in your own abilities, as this is the first step toward moving forward. It's ordinary to feel diverted and uninterested initially, but when you clear the NCLEX, you inch nearer to being eligible for the nursing registration.

Don't Self-Evaluate During the Test

There's no use trying to self-assess while you test. Try not to assume that you are beneath pass level because you got a couple of "easy" questions in succession. Simply center on the questions at hand. What appears easy to you may be challenging to another person. Each question is as significant as the following.

This exam is all with regards to perseverance. So, plan to sit the whole time, and then, at that point, you won't stress the possibility that you need to.

Know Your NLCEX Study Style

I have slightly different learning styles, and you presumably know yours at this point. Make sure you study in a way that works for you!

Draw out severe representations of heart chambers, shading coded medicinal classes, and so on if you comprehend things well with images. If you are an auditory student, there are a lot of YouTube addresses online and podcasts that cover NCLEX.

If you learn best through conversation, make sure to make a study group talk through ideas together.

As a general rule, using mental aides assist most students with harder-to-learn ideas. Don't simply rehash, rewrite, and duplicate old notes. Try connecting ideas. Consider how it applies to your clinical experiences in school and what you're learning from a holistic perspective.

Make a Study Plan

Commit to the arrangement that the test merits. Go into studying with an account, here is an example:

- Make study days a priority. Make a schedule that includes which days of the week you'll study, which days you'll take off, and which days you'll take practice examinations.
- Before each study session, set a goal for yourself. Perhaps it's to complete a certain number of practice questions or to master a specific substance topic but make it a point to be deliberate.

Studying without an arrangement is a waste of your time and will not decisively assist you with passing the NCLEX. It's not with regards to the hours you put in; it's with regards to how you use them.

This is one exam you can by no means pack for – the NCLEX is a holistic test model that expects to test information gained throughout the span of years, not days.

Do not rely on previous clinical or work experiences.

Unfortunately, those of you who have worked in hospitals as nursing specialists or assistants may find that your ability to answer test questions has been clouded by your experience. Indeed, it is typically evident that many themes or clinical skills are different between course readings and real-world healthcare, even from what you witnessed as a student nurse in clinical.

The NCLEX is based on demonstrated, explored-based, proof-based practice. Even if your past facility something in a different manner that is comparably protected or similarly as right, don't assume that this applies to the NCLEX.

Answering NCLEX questions as though you don't have any real constraints as a nurse is critical. Assume you have plenty of time and resources to think through each response option.

Hone Your Test-Taking Skills

The NCLEX is similar as much with regards to knowing how the test is written as it learns the correct answers. Utilize test-taking techniques to eliminate wrong answers, stay away from "limits" like ALL or NONE answers, and make sure to put patient security first consistently.

With practice, you will see a few subjects in answers:

- Continuously assess the patient first; calling the doctor immediately isn't usually the best initial step
- Use the Airway-Breathing-Circulation approach, and so on
- Use insightful reasoning even if you have not thought regarding the ideas driving the topic
- If all else comes up short, it depends on that budding feeling that I like to call "nurse intuition."

You will presumably experience the feared select-all-that-apply questions. Use something similar, efficient way to deal with eliminate incorrect answer decisions based on information and wording of answers.

Believe in Yourself

In particular, believe in yourself. You have the right to pass, and you have, as of now, demonstrated your potential as a nurse by graduating from nursing school. This is just the final advance on your exciting and new excursion to being a Registered Nurse – so congrats!

You've been studying for the second to become a certified nurse from the beginning of nursing school. All that is left is to stroll into this exam with the confidence to realize that you are intended to be an RN. Positive thinking can represent the moment of truth you on the NCLEX. The more you develop this test in your mind, the higher your tension will climb. Try not to see this exam as an obstacle because this test is an opportunity to show off what you have achieved. You can profit from reviewing nursing curriculum in more ways than just passing the NCLEX. Every second you spend studying helps you become a better nurse. Above all, believe in yourself! You have overcome much and demonstrated your value by completing nursing school. Try not to allow any in your method of achieving your fantasy! What is the direst outcome imaginable? Well, 45 days and $200 later, you can retake it. You have a nursing school degree on your wall. Get yourself, dry your tears, and hit the books. When you stroll into the NCLEX, tell yourself, "I will be a nurse today!"

C H A P T E R   9 :

Knowledge you need to gather before taking EXAM

The NCLEX (National Council Licensure Examination) will be different from any exam you have taken up to this point. So, relax; however, "Dreamsalive NCLEX-RN Comprehensive Review"

Has you covered! The purpose of the NCLEX is to assess if you are qualified to practice as a nurse after completing nursing school. The NCLEX will test you on application, inquiry, and how to use your insight to make key decisions, despite the fact that you will use the material you gained in nursing school. Underneath, we'll make a plunge on the top questions nursing students have about the NCLEX so you can be ready for what is to come!

How many questions do you have to get right to pass the NCLEX?

On the NCLEX examination, test takers will see a minimum of 75 questions and a limit of 265 (145 most extreme due to new COVID-19 policies). The NCLEX examination is taken through Computer Adaptive Testing (CAT). During the five-hour examination, test takers will be offered two discretionary breaks. Please note, setting a speed for yourself during this examination is critical. When you submit an answer to a question, you can't get to that question again. CAT can provide food for the exam specifically to the test takers' abilities. Your score isn't based on the level of questions answered effectively. Your score is based on the PC's gauge of your ability. To pass the NCLEX-RN, the PC uses one of 3 guidelines:

1. the most extreme length of the exam rule is used if you have arrived at the most significant number of questions (145) and the PC has not determined if you have performed over the passing standard. In this case, the PC will use the latest ability gauge to determine your score. If your most late meter is above passing, you will pass. If not, your score will be accounted for as failing to satisfy the passing guideline.
2. The computer determines with 95% confidence that you are over the passing standard. This means the computer estimates with 95% confidence that you can answer medium-difficulty questions accurately, basically half of the time.
3. The use up all available time rule applies if the PC has not determined with 95% confidence that you can satisfy the passing guideline when the most extreme allowed time has passed. If you use up all available time, the PC will check out your last 60 ability evaluations to determine if you have given."

What is the best way to pass the NCLEX-RN in 75 questions?

You can do many things to be as ready as feasible for the NCLEX examination. Here are our top tips on passing the NCLEX-RN in 75 questions!

1. Use plenty of study resources. "Dreamsalive NCLEX-RN Comprehensive Review" is an extraordinary asset, to begin with! Most importantly, Dreamsalive has a specific question set only for the NCLEX. I prescribe utilizing the 4 Weeks to NCLEX Workbook and Study Planner to go with this playlist!

2. Manage your test stress. Keeping yourself in a decent mood has a significant effect on studying for a major exam. Zero in on taking breaks when you need to and not letting yourself feel too overpowered.

3. Start studying at once and use survey guides. The more pre-arranged you are, the more successful you will be. "Dreamsalive NCLEX-RN Comprehensive Review" has a 4 Weeks to NCLEX Workbook and Study Planner to help you launch your examinations! This workbook and study organizer is a definitive report to Dreamsalive for Nursing! This workbook is jam-loaded with study tips and information to remove all the stress from studying. Then, when you finish the review plan, you'll be prepared to stroll into your NCLEX exam with confidence.

4. Stay practical. Try not to hope to pass the NCLEX in the minimum measure of questions. Prepare for the most extreme instead to keep away from any disappointment that happens when you hit question 76. If you pass at 75, that is fantastic! If not, that's perfectly ok as well. The most important thing is to retain your focus and pass the examination.

5. Maintain an optimistic attitude! This is, of course, easier said than done. However, after countless hours of studying and preparing for the NCLEX, you know the content better than anyone. You've got this!

6. Question types similar to those found on a board should be practiced. You can gain a solid understanding of how to read up and plan for the exam by practicing board-style questions. The NCLEX covers text-based, numerous decisions, and four-option questions. Be ready for some questions to accompany diagrams, outlines, and tables. There are countless incredible assets to practice NCLEX board-style questions.

CHAPTER 10:
Key Sections of the NCLEX Exam

The exam was initially evolved in the 1940s but has gone through many changes since then, at that point. The NCLEX-RN is now a computer-adaptive test, which means that the difficulty of each question is determined by previous responses. Therefore, examinees will continue to receive questions until the exam has decided to have adequate information.

In this way, nursing school is behind you, and all that is left is to pass the NCLEX-RN, and you're set for the perfect career. Try not to allow this test to stand in your manner—do all you can to plan, including taking benefit of our Free Practice Questions for the NCLEX-RN exam and other study materials. We'll assist you with finding out what you do know and what areas you need some practice.

Test takers should expect to receive between 75 and 265 questions due to the computer-adaptive nature of the test. Most of the questions are standard numerous decision questions, even though there are also some questions in different configurations, including various decisions with more than one answer, fill-in-the-clear estimations, ordered reaction, and problem area questions where the examinee must click on a screen area to answer the question.

NCLEX RN program is for testing nurses' ability. The NCLEX-RN exam tests an expected nurse's information and job abilities to guarantee that they can give protected and powerful client care.

Topics shrouded in the exam include Safe and Effective Care Environment, Health Promotion and Maintenance, Psychosocial Integrity, and Physiological Integrity.

Basic Care and Comfort

The content in this part, Basic Care and Comfort fall under the more extensive umbrella of topics identified with Physiological Integrity, one of the four significant classifications of questions on this test. Questions regarding this subcategory make up around 6% to 12% of the test and are identified with tasks that increase the client's solace during day-by-day living. A question might cover such things as assistive gadgets, assistance with cleanliness, or monitoring normal physical processes.

Health Promotion and Maintenance

Questions regarding this topic possess between 6% and 12% of the whole test. Questions in this space of nursing address issues in many classifications, including the phases of life, health screening, and lifestyle decisions. The substance typically identifies with the nurse's job in client education and direction toward a healthy lifestyle.

Management of Care

lies within the larger umbrella of issues associated with Safe and Effective Care Environment, one of the four major groupings of questions on this test. Items assessing your insight in this space will involve 17% and 23% of the test. The questions will concern different aspects of healthcare management, including client freedoms, legal aspects of care, and quality improvement.

Pharmacological and Parenteral Therapies

lies within the larger umbrella of themes associated with Physiological Integrity, one of the test's four major categories of questions. You can hope to see issues from this subcategory in around 12% to 18% of the test questions. These questions usually identify with medicine management and delivery, including drug interaction and aftereffects. They can also assess your insight into the use of blood and blood items, as well as pain management.

Physiological Adaptation

Physiological Integrity, one of the four important questions in this test, lies under a larger, more expansive canopy of topics. The level of test questions regarding this subcategory is between 11% and 17%. Past routine healthcare, these questions deal with providing administrations for clients with natural, long-haul health conditions. The substance contains different techniques for managing constant sickness and medical crises with these clients.

Psychosocial Integrity

Around 6% to 12% of the whole test comprises questions from this space of nursing. Much of this space is dedicated to mental health ideas and how the healthcare expert can promote excellent emotional health. This should be possible through such methodologies as emergency intervention, sensitivity to stressful occasions in life, and the arrangement of solid practices during client care.

Reduction of Risk Potential

Physiological Integrity, one of the four important questions on this test, is part of a larger, more expansive umbrella of topics referred to as Physiological Integrity. This test subcategory will identify from 9% to 15% of the test questions. A main pressing issue in healthcare is anticipating the additional problems caused by treatment and strategies. Medical tests can flag potential unfriendly impacts, enabling experts to reduce the risk. Questions of this sort expect you to be familiar with many of these tests and use the results during treatment.

Safety and Infection Control

Physiological Integrity, one of the four important questions in this test, comes under a larger, more comprehensive canopy of topics. Around 9% to 15% of the test items will address this nursing space. These healthcare questions rotate about dealing with crises, using hardware securely, and working with dangerous materials.

CHAPTER 11:
What to Expect on the NCLEX

It will be a great plan if you can reach a bit early in the exam hall. So that you can get some time to prepare yourself and it will give your nerve a rest which will help you to make the calm exam. The testing site will also gather biometric information when you show up, including a signature, a photograph, and a palm vein check. And if you show up more than 30 minutes late, you must forfeit your NCLEX appointment and expenses paid. You should re-register to take the exam, so having additional time is brilliant.

Taking the NCLEX-RN exam can be extremely nerve-wracking but understanding what's in store is the ideal way to lessen tension and perform well on exam day. The exam is timed, albeit the sections are not. Examinees will have as long as four hours to finish all areas, including two discretionary breaks. Because the test is pretty long, it's critical to guarantee that you've had a decent night's rest and a nutritious dinner before arriving. You should also dress serenely but professionally.

Rules of Test-taking

1. Read all instructions given thoroughly and cautiously.
2. Need to be more careful during the question reading because you need to identify that what is the answer is asking here.
3. Try to answer in a brief that specific answer wanted in the exam question.
4. Find a steady speed. Try not to take too long on any question but give yourself time.
5. Answer all exam questions, even if it requires instructed guessing.

What to Bring

It's essential that you bring a valid type of lawful identification, like a driver's license or passport. In addition, the first and last names on your ID must precisely match the first and last names on your Authorization to Test email. If the names don't coordinate, you will be needed to reregister and pay additional exam fees.

What Not to Bring

Individual items—including gadgets, frills, and outerwear—are not permitted in the testing room. Some test habitats have small storage spaces that might be accessible for you to use for individual belongings, even though you should check beforehand whether your test site has this element. If you don't have the foggiest idea or can't determine whether there is storage for individual belongings, leaving these items at home or in your vehicle is ideal.

You also don't have to bring any testing helps, for example, a calculator or scratch paper. Instead, you will have admittance to these items on-screen within the test itself.

CHAPTER 12:
Techniques to Identify the Correct Answer

Since you are more knowledgeable about the parts of numerous decision test questions, I should discuss specific techniques that you can use to issue address your way to correct answers on the NCLEX-RN exam.

The NCLEX-RN exam isn't a test about recognizing realities. You must have the option to identify what the question is posing effectively. Try not to focus on foundation information that isn't needed to answer the question. Instead, the NCLEX-RN exam focuses on thinking through an issue or situation.

I will teach you a bit-by-bit technique to pick the fitting way. You need to keep calm during reading the questions and try to make your nerve strong. The Kaplan Nursing group has fostered a choice tree that shows you how to move toward each NCLEX-RN exam question.

There are a few systems that you must follow on each NCLEX-RN exam test question. First, you must consistently sort out the question you are asking, permanently eliminating answer decisions. Choosing the correct answer regularly involves selecting the best of a few solutions that have the correct information. This might affect your proper investigation and interpretation of what the question is asking. So, I should discuss how to sort out the question is posing. If you find yourself "dumbfounded" later you painstakingly read a question, follow these means:

1. In the wake of reading the answer decisions, revamp the question using the signs you have obtained.
2. Oppose the motivation to peruse and rehash the question. Read the question only once. Identify the topic of the question. It is regularly implicit.
3. Peruse the answer decisions, not to choose the correct answer but to sort out, "What is the topic of the question?" or "What should I think?" You are looking for pieces of information from the answer decisions.
4. Then, at that point, use the procedures recently examined to answer the question you have figured.

Strategies for Making Educated Guesses

When you're uncertain which is the right or "best" answer choice, make a reasonable deduction. The following are techniques for improving your shot at selecting the correct answer when making a ballpark estimation.

- Use the course of elimination.
- Eliminate any answer decision that doesn't react to the question posed in the stem, even if it gives the correct answer.
- Outright terms, for example, never, consistently, all, must, each, and none regularly indicate an incorrect answer you can eliminate.
- When you are uncertain between two answers, try to communicate each in your own words, and then, at that point, look at the two. Then, finally, try to determine which of the two most suitable answers to the posed question.
- Eliminate unmistakably incorrect answers, including solutions that are duplicates, irrelevant to the question, etc.
- Each time you eliminate an answer choice, you increase your odds of selecting the correct right answer by 25%.

C H A P T E R   1 3 :
Reduce Test Taking Anxiety

Here are a few procedures that might assist with reducing your test tension:

- Establish a steady pretest routine. Realize what works for you and follow similar advances each time you prepare to take a test. This will ease your stress level and assist with ensuring that you're well-ready.
- Get some physical activity. Regular aerobic activity, as well as exercise on exam day, can help relieve stress.
- Get plenty of rest. Rest is inextricably linked to scholastic accomplishment. Adolescents and children, in particular, require regular, uninterrupted sleep. If you want good productive result you need to sleep well.
- Learn how to concentrate effectively. Amass resources that will aid you in learning procedures and test-taking systems. If you study and practice the subject that will be on the test in a systematic manner, you will feel more at ease.
- Don't ignore a learning disability. Test uneasiness might improve by addressing an underlying condition that interferes with the ability to learn, concentration or concentrate — for example, consideration deficit/hyperactivity disorder (ADHD) or dyslexia. In many cases, a student determined to have a learning disability is entitled to assistance with test-taking, for example, additional time to finish a test, testing in a less distracting room or having questions perused resoundingly.
- Prioritize ahead of schedule and in comparable locations. It's far better to learn a little bit over time rather than cramming everything into one sitting. Moreover, need to spend more in the same chapters, again and again, to recall your memories in the exam time.
- Converse with your educator. Ensure you understand what will be on each test and your ability to plan. In addition, let your instructor in that you feel restless when you step through exams. The individual in question might have ideas to assist you with succeeding.
- Become familiar with relaxation techniques. You need to follow some relaxation techniques, like deep breathing and relaxing your muscle sometimes. It will help you to make stress relief and keep you calm during the exam. It will remove your nervousness.
- Remember to eat and drink. Your brain needs fuel to work. So, eat the day of the test and drink a lot of water. Stay away from sweet drinks, for example, soft drinks, which can cause your glucose to top and then, at that point, drop, or caffeinated refreshments, for example, energy drinks or espresso, which can increase nervousness.
- See an expert advisor, if fundamental. Talk treatment (psychotherapy) with a therapist or other mental health expert can assist you with working through feelings, contemplations and practices that cause or demolish nervousness. Ask if your school has counseling administrations or if your boss offers counseling through a worker assistance program.

CHAPTER 14:
Common NCLEX Mistakes to Avoid

Taking the NCLEX exam is the most stressful and challenging second in their nursing education for many nursing students. Your dedication will truly test, as will your critical thinking skills, and even your commitment to your chosen nursing career.

It's for good reason that the NCLEX may be the most challenging test you'll at any point take. Nurses save the lives of patients consistently. They're so great at saving lives that nursing has been viewed as the most confided in calling in the United States for a long time. You didn't consume long stretches of your time on earth studying for a cakewalk, so prepare.

Thankfully, 1.3 million people have passed the NCLEX and are now working as nurses, and you can too. So, study hard, avoid these six common blunders, and use our helpful tips and tools to ensure that you pass the exam.

Mistake Number 1: Cramming just before the test

The NCLEX is hard. You may have gotten past a nursing school with long-distance race all-nighters, but last-minute cramming won't be sufficient to pass the NCLEX.

Cramming before a test regularly has the opposite impact, leading to:

- Preventing the association of old and new information, which is essential to input ideas into memory
- Reading exhaustion during study time, causing low energy during testing
- Nervousness and disappointment
- Mixing up the realities you've as of now scholarly
- Put away somewhere around a month, and plan to concentrate on a few hours consistently for that month. No cramming needed!

Mistake Number 2: Thinking your notes are good enough

Your notes are not good enough. A study app is not good enough. In addition to a review application, even your messages are presumably not sufficient.

This is due to the fact that the NCLEX does not test you on the same questions you were asked in nursing school. Instead, you'll be judged on your critical thinking skills, so look for new content to help you overcome the NCLEX's various obstacles.

To conquer the mother, you'll need high-quality study resources to pass the NCLEX. It can be beneficial to study more than one source, regardless of whether you have a favorite study guide.

While I can't listen for a minute specific questions, you'll see on your NCLEX exam, I can let you know this: Always pick the answer that keeps the patient protected and alive.

Mistake Number 3: Assuming the NCLEX is the same as the tests you did in nursing school.

If you remember the success of your nursing school's exam, then it sounds good. for a different level of success now, because the NCLEX is a completely different ballgame.

Because you excelled on tests in nursing school doesn't mean you'll expert this one. Unlike nursing school exams, which test for information, the NCLEX tests your ability to apply and dissect situations using the nursing information you gained in school. In addition, rationale and critical thinking, rather than repetition retention, are emphasized in this test—making it much more complex and far-reaching.

Mistake Number 4: Avoiding considerations about test day

Go on, think about it. Sometimes I keep away from considerations about things that stress me to put it off or get away from tension. But significant occasions like taking the NCLEX require some thought, and you'll presumably feel more ready if you think about it more. So go on, think about things like:

- Where will I stop?
- Would I be able to bring snacks and a water bottle?
- What will parking be like?

What time would it be a good idea to set my caution? (And would it be a good idea for me to put a backup alert?)

Think about each point that is on your mind, write it down, and then, at that point, stop worrying with regards to the things you can anticipate now!

Mistake Number 5: Reading rapidly like you know the answer

If you've at any point been told to "dial back," you should keep up that mantra when taking the NCLEX. A few of us are calculated and mindful, but when it comes to taking the most critical test of our lives against the clock, I all have a propensity to fly through the questions that look familiar. For the people who instinctively rush, the NCLEX is an executioner and will challenge you if you move too fast.

That is because it doesn't simply test for information and ability; the NCLEX tests critical thinking, judgment, reasoning, and insightful reflection. There are no other options for these skills.

Peruse the questions twice. Assume you don't have a clue about the answer.

Mistake Number 6: Believing disappointment implies you'll flop again

Many extraordinary nurses take the NCLEX more than once. If you've bombed previously, you know what's in store. You know what to zero in on, how much time you'll need, and what areas are especially hard for you.

Those current nurses may have been having an awful day. They may have found anxious and flubbed solutions, or they probably won't have concentrated on enough. Unfortunately, none of these reasons keeps 14.6 percent of nurses from retaking the NCLEX.

It's OK to be frightened of failing. So, take a full breath, hit the books with a vengeance, and try again.

CHAPTER 15:
Practice Question Set

Will get all answers with explanation in the next chapter. Arranged the question set and answer set separately so that Candidates can prepare themselves accurately.

Practice Question Set-1

QUESTION NUMBER 01.01

After cardiac surgery, a client's blood pressure measures 126/80 mm Hg. Nurse Katrina determines that mean arterial pressure (MAP) is which of the following?

A. 46 mm Hg

B. 80 mm Hg

C. 95 mm Hg

D. 90 mm Hg

QUESTION NUMBER 01.02

Question is about - chest pain
Category of the Question - Physiological Integrity, Reduction of Risk Potential

A female client arrives at the emergency department with chest and stomach pain and a report of black tarry stool for several months. Which of the following orders should the nurse Oliver anticipate?

A. Cardiac monitor, oxygen, creatine kinase and lactate dehydrogenase levels
B. Prothrombin time, partial thromboplastin time, fibrinogen and fibrin split product values
C. Electrocardiogram, complete blood count, testing for occult blood, comprehensive serum metabolic panel
D. Electroencephalogram, alkaline phosphatase, and aspartate aminotransferase levels, basic serum metabolic panel

QUESTION NUMBER 01.03

Question is about - coronary artery bypass graft
Category of the Question - Physiological Integrity, Physiological Adaptation

Olivia had coronary artery bypass graft (CABG) surgery 3 days ago. Which of the following conditions is suspected by the nurse when a decrease in platelet count from 230,000 ul to 5,000 ul is noted?

A. Pancytopenia
B. Idiopathic thrombocytopenic purpura (ITP)
C. Disseminated intravascular coagulation (DIC)
D. Heparin-associated thrombosis and thrombocytopenia (HATT)

QUESTION NUMBER 01.04
Question is about - idiopathic thrombocytopenic purpura
Category of the Question - Physiological Integrity, Pharmacological and Parenteral Therapies

Which of the following drugs would be ordered by the physician to improve the platelet count in a male client with idiopathic thrombocytopenic purpura (ITP)?

A. Acetylsalicylic acid (ASA)
B. Corticosteroids

C. Methotrexate
D. Vitamin K

QUESTION NUMBER 01.05
Question is about - heart valve replacement
Category of the Question - Physiological Integrity, Reduction of Risk Potential

A female client is scheduled to receive a heart valve replacement with a porcine valve. Which of the following types of transplant is this?

A. Allogeneic
B. Autologous

C. Syngeneic
D. Xenogeneic

QUESTION NUMBER 01.06
Question is about - ankle injury
Category of the Question - Physiological Integrity,Physiological Adaptation

Marco falls off his bicycle and injures his ankle. Which of the following actions shows the initial response to the injury in the extrinsic pathway?

A. Release of Calcium
B. Release of tissue thromboplastin

C. Conversion of factors XII to factor XIIa
D. Conversion of factor VIII to factor VIIIa

QUESTION NUMBER 01.07
Question is about - systemic lupus erythematosus
Category of the Question - Physiological Integrity, Physiological Adaptation

Instructions for a client with systemic lupus erythematosus (SLE) would include information about which of the following blood dyscrasias?

A. Dressler's syndrome
B. Polycythemia

C. Essential thrombocytopenia
D. Von Willebrand's disease

QUESTION NUMBER 01.08
Question is about - Hodgkin's disease
Category of the Question - Physiological Integrity, Physiological Adaptation

The nurse is aware that the following symptom is most commonly an early indication of stage 1 Hodgkin's disease?

A. Pericarditis
B. Night sweat

C. Splenomegaly
D. Persistent hypothermia

QUESTION NUMBER 01.09
Question is about - leukemia, neutropenia
Category of the Question - Physiological Integrity, Reduction of Risk Potential

Francis with leukemia has neutropenia. Which of the following functions must be frequently assessed?

A. Blood pressure

B. Bowel sounds

C. Heart sounds

D. Breath sounds

QUESTION NUMBER 01.10
Question is about - multiple myeloma
Category of the Question - Physiological Integrity, Physiological Adaptation

The nurse knows that neurologic complications of multiple myeloma (MM) usually involve which of the following body systems?

A. Brain

B. Muscle spasm

C. Renal dysfunction

D. Myocardial irritability

QUESTION NUMBER 01.11
Question is about - HIV, AIDS
Category of the Question - Physiological Integrity, Physiological Adaptation

Nurse Patricia is aware that the average length of time from human immunodeficiency virus (HIV) infection to the development of acquired immunodeficiency syndrome (AIDS)?

A. Less than 5 years

B. 5 to 7 years

C. 10 years

D. More than 10 years

QUESTION NUMBER 01.12
Question is about - disseminated intravascular coagulation
Category of the Question - Physiological Integrity, Reduction of Risk Potential

An 18-year-old male client admitted with heat stroke begins to show signs of disseminated intravascular coagulation (DIC). Which of the following laboratory findings is most consistent with DIC?

A. Low platelet count

B. Elevated fibrinogen levels

C. Low levels of fibrin degradation products

D. Reduced prothrombin time

QUESTION NUMBER 01.13
Question is about - Hodgkin's disease
Category of the Question - Physiological Integrity, Physiological Adaptation

Mario comes to the clinic complaining of fever, drenching night sweats, and unexplained weight loss over the past 3 months. Physical examination reveals a single enlarged supraclavicular lymph node. Which of the following is the most probable diagnosis?

A. Influenza

B. Sickle cell anemia

C. Leukemia

D. Hodgkin's disease

QUESTION NUMBER 01.14
Question is about - blood transfusion
Category of the Question - Physiological Integrity, Physiological Adaptation

A male client with a gunshot wound requires an emergency blood transfusion. His blood type is AB negative. Which blood type would be the safest for him to receive?

A. AB Rh-positive

B. A Rh-positive

C. A Rh-negative

D. O Rh-positive

QUESTION NUMBER 01.15
Question is about - acute lymphoid leukemia
Category of the Question - Health Promotion and Maintenance

Stacy was diagnosed with acute lymphoid leukemia (ALL). She was discharged from the hospital following her chemotherapy treatments. Which statement of Stacy's mother indicated that she understands when she will contact the physician?

A. "I should contact the physician if Stacy has difficulty in sleeping".

B. "I will call my doctor if Stacy has persistent vomiting and diarrhea".

C. "My physician should be called if Stacy is irritable and unhappy".

D. "Should Stacy have continued hair loss, I need to call the doctor".

QUESTION NUMBER 01.16
Question is about - acute lymphoid leukemia
Category of the Question - Psychosocial Integrity

Molly Sue is diagnosed with acute lymphoid leukemia (ALL) and beginning chemotherapy. Her mother states to the nurse that it is hard to see Molly Sue with no hair. The best response for the nurse is:

A. "Molly Sue looks very nice wearing a hat".

B. "You should not worry about her hair, just be glad that she is alive".

C. "Yes, it is upsetting. But try to cover up your feelings when you are with her or else she may be upset".

D. "This is only temporary; Molly Sue will re-grow new hair in 3-6 months but may be different in texture".

QUESTION NUMBER 01.17
Question is about - stomatitis
Category of the Question - Physiological Integrity, Basic Care and Comfort

Brittany who is undergoing chemotherapy for her throat cancer is experiencing stomatitis. To promote oral hygiene and comfort, the nurse-in-charge should:

A. Provide frequent mouthwash with normal saline.

B. Apply viscous Lidocaine to oral ulcers as needed.

C. Use lemon glycerine swabs every 2 hours.

D. Rinse mouth with Hydrogen Peroxide.

QUESTION NUMBER 01.18
Question is about - chemotherapy
Category of the Question - Safe and Effective Care Environment, Management of Care

During the administration of chemotherapy agents, Nurse Oliver observed that the IV site is red and swollen when the IV is touched Stacy shouts in pain. The first nursing action to take is:

A. Notify the physician.

B. Flush the IV line with saline solution.

C. Immediately discontinue the infusion.

D. Apply an ice pack to the site, followed by warm compress.

QUESTION NUMBER 01.19
Question is about - blue bloater
Category of the Question - Physiological Integrity, Physiological Adaptation

The term "blue bloater" refers to a male client under which of the following conditions?

A. Adult respiratory distress syndrome (ARDS)

B. Asthma

C. Chronic obstructive bronchitis

D. Emphysema

QUESTION NUMBER 01.20
Question is about - pink puffer
Category of the Question - Physiological Integrity, Physiological Adaptation

The term "pink puffer" refers to the female client with which of the following conditions?

A. Adult respiratory distress syndrome (ARDS)

B. Asthma

C. Chronic obstructive bronchitis

D. Emphysema

QUESTION NUMBER 01.21
Question is about - ABG
Category of the Question - Physiological Integrity, Reduction of Risk Potential

Jose is in danger of respiratory arrest following the administration of a narcotic analgesic. An arterial blood gas value is obtained. Nurse Oliver would expect the paco2 to be which of the following values?

A. 15 mm Hg

B. 30 mm Hg

C. 40 mm Hg

D. 80 mm Hg

QUESTION NUMBER 01.22
Question is about - ABG
Category of the Question - Physiological Integrity, Reduction of Risk Potential

Timothy's arterial blood gas (ABG) results are as follows; pH 7.16; Paco2 80 mm Hg; Pao2 46 mm Hg; HCO3- 24 mEq/L; Sao2 81%. This ABG result represents which of the following conditions?

A. Metabolic acidosis

B. Metabolic alkalosis

C. Respiratory acidosis

D. Respiratory alkalosis

QUESTION NUMBER 01.23
Question is about - hypertension
Category of the Question - Physiological Integrity, Physiological Adaptation

Norma has started a new drug for hypertension. Thirty minutes after she takes the drug, she develops chest tightness and becomes short of breath and tachypnea. She has a decreased level of consciousness. These signs indicate which of the following conditions?

A. Asthma attack

B. Pulmonary embolism

C. Respiratory failure

D. Rheumatoid arthritis

QUESTION NUMBER 01.24
Question is about - liver cirrhosis
Category of the Question - Physiological Integrity, Reduction of Risk Potential

Mr. Gonzales was admitted to the hospital with ascites and jaundice. To rule out cirrhosis of the liver which laboratory test indicates liver cirrhosis?

A. Decreased red blood cell count

B. Decreased serum acid phosphatase level

C. Elevated white blood cell count

D. Elevated serum aminotransferase

QUESTION NUMBER 01.25
Question is about - cirrhosis
Category of the Question - Physiological Integrity, Reduction of Risk Potential

The biopsy of Mr. Gonzales confirms the diagnosis of cirrhosis. Mr. Gonzales is at increased risk for excessive bleeding primarily because of:

A. Impaired clotting mechanism

B. Varix formation

C. Inadequate nutrition

D. Trauma of invasive procedure

QUESTION NUMBER 01.26
Question is about - hepatic encephalopathy
Category of the Question - Physiological Integrity, Physiological Adaptation

Mr. Jay develops hepatic encephalopathy. Which clinical manifestation is most common with this condition?

A. Increased urine output

B. Altered level of consciousness

C. Decreased tendon reflex

D. Hypotension

QUESTION NUMBER 01.27
Question is about - lactulose
Category of the Question - Physiological Integrity, Pharmacological and Parenteral Therapies

Patrick who is diagnosed with liver cirrhosis is experiencing symptoms of hepatic encephalopathy. The physician ordered 50 ml of Lactulose p.o. every 2 hours. Patrick suddenly develops diarrhea. The nurse best action would be:

A. "I'll see if your physician is in the hospital".

B. "Maybe you're reacting to the drug; I will withhold the next dose".

C. "I'll lower the dosage as ordered so the drug causes only 2 to 4 stools a day".

D. "Frequently, bowel movements are needed to reduce sodium level".

QUESTION NUMBER 01.28

Question is about - abdominal aortic aneurysm

Category of the Question - Physiological Integrity, Physiological Adaptation

Which of the following groups of symptoms indicates a ruptured abdominal aortic aneurysm?

A. Lower back pain, increased blood pressure, decreased red blood cell (RBC) count, increased white blood (WBC) count.

B. Severe lower back pain, decreased blood pressure, decreased RBC count, increased WBC count.

C. Severe lower back pain, decreased blood pressure, decreased RBC count, decreased RBC count, decreased WBC count.

D. Intermittent lower back pain, decreased blood pressure, decreased RBC count, increased WBC count.

QUESTION NUMBER 01.29

Question is about - cardiac catheterization

Category of the Question - Physiological Integrity, Reduction of Risk Potential

After undergoing a cardiac catheterization, Tracy has a large puddle of blood under his buttocks. Which of the following steps should the nurse take first?

A. Call for help.

B. Obtain vital signs.

C. Ask the client to "lift up".

D. Apply gloves and assess the groin site.

QUESTION NUMBER 01.30

Question is about - unstable angina

Category of the Question - Physiological Integrity, Physiological Adaptation

Which of the following treatments is a suitable surgical intervention for a client with unstable angina?

A. Cardiac catheterization

B. Echocardiogram

C. Nitroglycerin

D. Percutaneous transluminal coronary angioplasty (PTCA)

QUESTION NUMBER 01.31

Question is about - cardiac output

Category of the Question - Physiological Integrity, Physiological Adaptation

The nurse is aware that the following terms used to describe reduced cardiac output and perfusion impairment due to ineffective pumping of the heart is:

A. Anaphylactic shock

B. Cardiogenic shock

C. Distributive shock

D. Myocardial infarction (MI)

QUESTION NUMBER 01.32
Question is about - hypertension
Category of the Question - Physiological Integrity, Physiological Adaptation

A client with hypertension asks the nurse which factors can cause blood pressure to drop to normal levels?

A. Kidneys' excretion to sodium only.
B. Kidneys' retention of sodium and water.
C. Kidneys' excretion of sodium and water.
D. Kidneys' retention of sodium and excretion of water.

QUESTION NUMBER 01.33
Question is about - furosemide
Category of the Question - Physiological Integrity, Pharmacological and Parenteral Therapies

Nurse Rose is aware that the statement that best explains why furosemide (Lasix) is administered to treat hypertension is:

A. It dilates peripheral blood vessels.
B. It decreases sympathetic cardio acceleration.
C. It inhibits the angiotensin-converting enzymes.
D. It inhibits the reabsorption of sodium and water in the loop of Henle.

QUESTION NUMBER 01.34
Question is about - systemic lupus erythematosus
Category of the Question - Physiological Integrity, Reduction of Risk Potential

Nurse Nikki knows that laboratory results supports the diagnosis of systemic lupus erythematosus (SLE) is:

A. Elevated serum complement level
B. Thrombocytosis, elevated sedimentation rate
C. Pancytopenia, elevated antinuclear antibody (ANA) titer
D. Leukocytosis, elevated blood urea nitrogen (BUN) and creatinine levels

QUESTION NUMBER 01.35
Question is about - concussion
Category of the Question - Health Promotion and Maintenance

Arnold, a 19-year-old client with a mild concussion is discharged from the emergency department. Before discharge, he complains of a headache. When offered acetaminophen, his mother tells the nurse the headache is severe and she would like her son to have something stronger. Which of the following responses by the nurse is appropriate?

A. "Your son had a mild concussion, acetaminophen is strong enough."
B. "Aspirin is avoided because of the danger of Reye's syndrome in children or young adults."
C. "Narcotics are avoided after a head injury because they may hide a worsening condition."
D. Stronger medications may lead to vomiting, which increases the intracranial pressure (ICP)."

QUESTION NUMBER 01.36
Question is about - arterial blood gas
Category of the Question - Physiological Integrity, Reduction of Risk Potential

When evaluating an arterial blood gas from a male client with a subdural hematoma, the nurse notes the Paco2 is 30 mm Hg. Which of the following responses best describes the result?

A. Appropriate; lowering carbon dioxide (CO2) reduces intracranial pressure (ICP).
B. Emergent; the client is poorly oxygenated.
C. Normal.
D. Significant; the client has alveolar hypoventilation.

QUESTION NUMBER 01.37
Question is about - prioritization
Category of the Question - Management of Care

When prioritizing care, which of the following clients should the nurse Olivia assess first?

A. A 17-year-old client 24-hours post appendectomy.
B. A 33-year-old client with a recent diagnosis of Guillain-Barre syndrome.
C. A 50-year-old client 3 days post myocardial infarction.
D. A 50-year-old client with diverticulitis.

QUESTION NUMBER 01.38
Question is about - colchicine
Category of the Question - Physiological Integrity, Physiological Adaptation

JP has been diagnosed with gout and wants to know why colchicine is used in the treatment of gout. Which of the following actions of colchicines explains why it's effective for gout?

A. Replaces estrogen.
B. Decreases infection.
C. Decreases inflammation.
D. Decreases bone demineralization.

QUESTION NUMBER 01.39
Question is about - osteoarthritis
Category of the Question - Physiological Integrity, Physiological Adaptation

Norma asks for information about osteoarthritis. Which of the following statements about osteoarthritis is correct?

A. Osteoarthritis is rarely debilitating.
B. Osteoarthritis is a rare form of arthritis.
C. Osteoarthritis is the most common form of arthritis.
D. Osteoarthritis affects people over 60.

QUESTION NUMBER 01.40
Question is about - thyroid therapy
Category of the Question - Physiological Integrity, Pharmacological and Parenteral Therapies

Ruby is receiving thyroid replacement therapy, develops the flu and forgets to take her thyroid replacement medicine. The nurse understands that skipping this medication will put the client at risk for developing which of the following life threatening complications?

A. Exophthalmos

B. Thyroid storm

C. Myxedema coma

D. Tibial myxedema

QUESTION NUMBER 01.41
Question is about - Cushing's syndrome
Category of the Question - Physiological Integrity, Physiological Adaptation

Nurse Sugar is assessing a client with Cushing's syndrome. Which observation should the nurse report to the physician immediately?

A. Pitting edema of the legs

B. An irregular apical pulse

C. Dry mucous membranes

D. Frequent urination

QUESTION NUMBER 01.42
Question is about - diabetes insipidus
Category of the Question - Physiological Integrity, Physiological Adaptation

Cyrill with severe head trauma sustained in a car accident is admitted to the intensive care unit. Thirty-six hours later, the client's urine output suddenly rises above 200 ml/hour, leading the nurse to suspect diabetes insipidus. Which laboratory findings support the nurse's suspicion of diabetes insipidus?

A. Above-normal urine and serum osmolality levels.

B. Below-normal urine and serum osmolality levels.

C. Above-normal urine osmolality level, below-normal serum osmolality level.

D. Below-normal urine osmolality level, above-normal serum osmolality level.

QUESTION NUMBER 01.43
Question is about - hyperosmolar hyperglycemic nonketotic syndrome
Category of the Question - Health Promotion and Maintenance

Jomari is diagnosed with hyperosmolar hyperglycemic nonketotic syndrome (HHNS) and is stabilized and prepared for discharge. When preparing the client for discharge and home management, which of the following statements indicates that the client understands her condition and how to control it?

A. "I can avoid getting sick by not becoming dehydrated and by paying attention to my need to urinate, drink, or eat more than usual."

B. "If I experience trembling, weakness, and headache, I should drink a glass of soda that contains sugar."

C. "I will have to monitor my blood glucose level closely and notify the physician if it's constantly elevated."

D. "If I begin to feel especially hungry and thirsty, I'll eat a snack high in carbohydrates."

QUESTION NUMBER 01.44
Question is about - hyperparathyroidism

Category of the Question - Physiological Integrity, Physiological Adaptation

A 66-year-old client has been complaining of sleeping more, increased urination, anorexia, weakness, irritability, depression, and bone pain that interferes with her going outdoors. Based on these assessment findings, the nurse would suspect which of the following disorders?

A. Diabetes mellitus

B. Diabetes insipidus

C. Hypoparathyroidism

D. Hyperparathyroidism

QUESTION NUMBER 01.45
Question is about - Addisonian crisis
Category of the Question - Health Promotion and Maintenance

Nurse Lourdes is teaching a client recovering from Addisonian crisis about the need to take fludrocortisone acetate and hydrocortisone at home. Which statement by the client indicates an understanding of the instructions?

A. "I'll take my hydrocortisone in the late afternoon, before dinner."
B. "I'll take all of my hydrocortisone in the morning, right after I wake up."
C. "I'll take two-thirds of the dose when I wake up and one-third in the late afternoon."
D. "I'll take the entire dose at bedtime."

QUESTION NUMBER 01.46
Question is about - pituitary adenoma
Category of the Question - Physiological Integrity, Reduction of Risk Potential

Which of the following laboratory test results would suggest to the nurse Len that a client has a corticotropin-secreting pituitary adenoma?

A. High corticotropin and low cortisol levels
B. Low corticotropin and high cortisol levels
C. High corticotropin and high cortisol levels
D. Low corticotropin and low cortisol levels

QUESTION NUMBER 01.47
Question is about - pituitary tumor
Category of the Question - Physiological Integrity, Reduction of Risk Potential

A male client is scheduled for a transsphenoidal hypophysectomy to remove a pituitary tumor. Preoperatively, the nurse should assess for potential complications by doing which of the following?

A. Testing for ketones in the urine.
B. Testing urine specific gravity.
C. Checking temperature every 4 hours.
D. Performing capillary glucose testing every 4 hours.

QUESTION NUMBER 01.48
Question is about - insulin
Category of the Question - Physiological Integrity, Pharmacological and Parenteral Therapies

Capillary glucose monitoring is being performed every 4 hours for a client diagnosed with diabetic ketoacidosis. Insulin is administered using a scale of regular insulin according to glucose results. At 2 p.m., the client has a capillary glucose level of 250 mg/dl for which he receives 8 U of regular insulin. Nurse Mariner should expect the dose's:

A. Onset to be at 2 p.m. and its peak to be at 3 p.m.
B. Onset to be at 2:15 p.m. and its peak to be at 3 p.m.
C. Onset to be at 2:30 p.m. and its peak to be at 4 p.m.
D. Onset to be at 4 p.m. and its peak to be at 6 p.m.

QUESTION NUMBER 01.49
Question is about - hyperthyroidism
Category of the Question - Physiological Integrity, Reduction of Risk Potential

The physician orders laboratory tests to confirm hyperthyroidism in a female client with classic signs and symptoms of this disorder. Which test result would confirm the diagnosis?

A. No increase in the thyroid-stimulating hormone (TSH) level after 30 minutes during the TSH stimulation test.
B. A decreased TSH level.
C. An increase in the TSH level after 30 minutes during the TSH stimulation test.
D. Below-normal levels of serum triiodothyronine (T3) and serum thyroxine (T4) as detected by radioimmunoassay.

QUESTION NUMBER 01.50
Question is about - insulin
Category of the Question - Health Promotion and Maintenance

Rico with diabetes mellitus must learn how to self-administer insulin. The physician has prescribed 10 U of U-100 regular insulin and 35 U of U-100 isophane insulin suspension (NPH) to be taken before breakfast. When teaching the client how to select and rotate insulin injection sites, the nurse should provide which instruction?

A. "Inject insulin into healthy tissue with large blood vessels and nerves."
B. "Rotate injection sites within the same anatomic region, not among different regions."
C. "Administer insulin into areas of scar tissue or hypertrophy whenever possible."
D. "Administer insulin into sites above muscles that you plan to exercise heavily later that day."

QUESTION NUMBER 01.51
Question is about - hyperosmolar hyperglycemic nonketotic syndrome
Category of the Question - Physiological Integrity, Reduction of Risk Potential

Nurse Sarah expects to note an elevated serum glucose level in a client with hyperosmolar hyperglycemic nonketotic syndrome (HHNS). Which other laboratory finding should the nurse anticipate?

A. Elevated serum acetone level.
B. Serum ketone bodies.

C. Serum alkalosis.
D. Below-normal serum potassium level.

QUESTION NUMBER 01.52
Question is about - Grave's disease
Category of the Question - Physiological Integrity, Basic Care and Comfort

For a client with Graves' disease, which nursing intervention promotes comfort?

A. Restricting intake of oral fluids.
B. Placing extra blankets on the client's bed.

C. Limiting intake of high-carbohydrate foods.
D. Maintaining room temperature in the low-normal range.

QUESTION NUMBER 01.53
Question is about - Colles' fracture
Category of the Question - Physiological Integrity, Physiological Adaptation

Patrick is treated in the emergency department for a Colles' fracture sustained during a fall. What is a Colles' fracture?

A. Fracture of the distal radius.
B. Fracture of the olecranon.

C. Fracture of the humerus.
D. Fracture of the carpal scaphoid.

QUESTION NUMBER 01.54
Question is about - osteoporosis
Category of the Question - Physiological Integrity, Physiological Adaptation

Cleo is diagnosed with osteoporosis. Which electrolytes are involved in the development of this disorder?

A. Calcium and sodium
B. Calcium and phosphorous

C. Phosphorus and potassium
D. Potassium and sodium

QUESTION NUMBER 01.55
Question is about - smoke inhalation
Category of the Question - Physiological Integrity, Physiological Adaptation

Johnny, a firefighter, was involved in extinguishing a house fire and is being treated for smoke inhalation. He developed severe hypoxia 48 hours after the incident, requiring intubation and mechanical ventilation. He most likely has developed which of the following conditions?

A. Adult respiratory distress syndrome (ARDS)
B. Atelectasis

C. Bronchitis
D. Pneumonia

QUESTION NUMBER 01.56
Question is about - hypoxia
Category of the Question - Physiological Integrity, Physiological Adaptation

A 67-year-old client develops acute shortness of breath and progressive hypoxia requiring right femur. The hypoxia was probably caused by which of the following conditions?

A. Asthma attack
B. Atelectasis

C. Bronchitis
D. Fat embolism

QUESTION NUMBER 01.57
Question is about - shortness of breath
Category of the Question - Physiological Integrity, Physiological Adaptation

A client with shortness of breath has decreased to absent breath sounds on the right side, from the apex to the base. Which of the following conditions would best explain this?

A. Acute asthma

B. Chronic bronchitis

C. Pneumonia

D. Spontaneous pneumothorax

QUESTION NUMBER 01.58
Question is about - pneumothorax
Category of the Question - Physiological Integrity, Physiological Adaptation

A 62-year-old male client was in a motor vehicle accident as an unrestrained driver. He's now in the emergency department complaining of difficulty of breathing and chest pain. On auscultation of his lung field, no breath sounds are present in the upper lobe. This client may have which of the following conditions?

A. Bronchitis

B. Pneumonia

C. Pneumothorax

D. Tuberculosis (TB)

QUESTION NUMBER 01.59
Question is about - pneumonectomy
Category of the Question - Physiological Integrity, Physiological Adaptation

If a client requires a pneumonectomy, what fills the area of the thoracic cavity?

A. The space remains filled with air only.

B. The surgeon fills the space with a gel.

C. Serous fluids fill the space and consolidate the region.

D. The tissue from the other lung grows over to the other side.

QUESTION NUMBER 01.60
Question is about - pulmonary embolism
Category of the Question - Physiological Integrity, Physiological Adaptation

Hemoptysis may be present in the client with a pulmonary embolism because of which of the following reasons?

A. Alveolar damage in the infarcted area.

B. Involvement of major blood vessels in the occluded area.

C. Loss of lung parenchyma.

D. Loss of lung tissue.

QUESTION NUMBER 01.61
Question is about - pulmonary embolism
Category of the Question - Physiological Integrity, Reduction of Risk Potential

Alvin with a massive pulmonary embolism will have an arterial blood gas analysis performed to determine the extent of hypoxia. The acid-base disorder that may be present is?

A. Metabolic acidosis

B. Metabolic alkalosis

C. Respiratory acidosis

D. Respiratory alkalosis

QUESTION NUMBER 01.62

Question is about - pneumothorax

Category of the Question - Physiological Integrity, Reduction of Risk Potential

After a motor vehicle accident, Armand, a 22-year-old client, is admitted with a pneumothorax. The surgeon inserts a chest tube and attaches it to a chest drainage system. Bubbling soon appears in the water seal chamber. Which of the following is the most likely cause of the bubbling?

A. Air leak

B. Adequate suction

C. Inadequate suction

D. Kinked chest tube

QUESTION NUMBER 01.63

Question is about - IV flow rate

Category of the Question - Physiological Integrity, Pharmacological and Parenteral Therapies

Nurse Michelle calculates the IV flow rate for a postoperative client. The client receives 3,000 ml of Ringer's lactate solution IV to run over 24 hours. The IV infusion set has a drop factor of 10 drops per milliliter. The nurse should regulate the client's IV to deliver how many drops per minute?

A. 18

B. 21

C. 35

D. 40

QUESTION NUMBER 01.64

Question is about - congenital heart disorder

Category of the Question - Physiological Integrity, Pharmacological and Parenteral Therapies

Mickey, a 6-year-old child with a congenital heart disorder is admitted with congestive heart failure. Digoxin (lanoxin) 0.12 mg is ordered for the child. The bottle of Lanoxin contains .05 mg of Lanoxin in 1 ml of solution. What amount should the nurse administer to the child?

A. 1.2 ml

B. 2.4 ml

C. 3.5 ml

D. 4.2 ml

QUESTION NUMBER 01.65

Question is about - elastic stockings

Category of the Question - Health Promotion and Maintenance

Nurse Alexandra teaches a client about elastic stockings. Which of the following statements, if made by the client, indicates to the nurse that the teaching was successful?

A. "I will wear the stockings until the physician tells me to remove them."

B. "I should wear the stockings even when I am asleep."

C. "Every four hours I should remove the stockings for a half hour."

D. "I should put on the stockings before getting out of bed in the morning."

QUESTION NUMBER 01.66

Question is about - frostbite

Category of the Question - Physiological Integrity, Physiological Adaptation

The primary reason for rapid continuous rewarming of the area affected by frostbite is to:

A. Lessen the amount of cellular damage

B. Prevent the formation of blisters

C. Promote movement

D. Prevent pain and discomfort

QUESTION NUMBER 01.67

Question is about - hemodialysis

Category of the Question - Reduction of Risk Potential

A client recently started on hemodialysis wants to know how the dialysis will take the place of his kidneys. The nurse's response is based on the knowledge that hemodialysis works by:

A. Passing water through a dialyzing membrane

B. Eliminating plasma proteins from the blood

C. Lowering the pH by removing nonvolatile acids

D. Filtering waste through a dialyzing membrane

QUESTION NUMBER 01.68

Question is about - AIDS, measles

Category of the Question - Health Promotion and Maintenance

During a home visit, a client with AIDS tells the nurse that he has been exposed to measles. Which action by the nurse is most appropriate?

A. Administer an antibiotic

B. Contact the physician for an order for immune globulin

C. Administer an antiviral

D. Tell the client that he should remain in isolation for 2 weeks

QUESTION NUMBER 01.69

Question is about - methicillin-resistant staphylococcus aureus

Category of the Question - Safe and Effective Care Environment, Safety and Infection Control

A client hospitalized with MRSA (methicillin-resistant staph aureus) is placed on contact precautions. Which statement is true regarding precautions for infections spread by contact?

A. The client should be placed in a room with negative pressure.

B. Infection requires close contact; therefore, the door may remain open.

C. Transmission is highly likely, so the client should wear a mask at all times.

D. Infection requires skin-to-skin contact and is prevented by hand washing, gloves, and a gown.

QUESTION NUMBER 01.70
Question is about - above-the-knee amputation, phantom limb pain
Category of the Question - Physiological Integrity, Physiological Adaptation

A client who is admitted with an above-the-knee amputation tells the nurse that his foot hurts and itches. Which response by the nurse indicates an understanding of phantom limb pain?

    A. "The pain will go away in a few days."
    B. "The pain is due to peripheral nervous system interruptions. I will get you some pain medication."
    C. "The pain is psychological because your foot is no longer there."
    D. "The pain and itching are due to the infection you had before the surgery."

QUESTION NUMBER 01.71
Question is about - Whipple procedure
Category of the Question - Physiological Integrity, Reduction of Risk Potential

A client with cancer of the pancreas has undergone a Whipple procedure. The nurse is aware that during the Whipple procedure, the doctor will remove the:

    A. Head of the pancreas
    B. Proximal third section of the small intestines
    C. Stomach and duodenum
    D. Esophagus and jejunum

QUESTION NUMBER 01.72
Question is about - neutropenia, minimum-bacteria diet
Category of the Question - Health Promotion and Maintenance

The physician has ordered a minimal-bacteria diet for a client with neutropenia. The client should be taught to avoid eating:

    A. Packed fruits
    B. Salt
    C. Fresh raw pepper
    D. Ketchup

QUESTION NUMBER 01.73
Question is about - Coumadin (sodium warfarin)
Category of the Question - Health Promotion and Maintenance

A client is discharged home with a prescription for Coumadin (sodium warfarin). The client should be instructed to:

    A. Have a Protime done monthly
    B. Eat more fruits and vegetables
    C. Drink more liquids
    D. Avoid crowds

QUESTION NUMBER 01.74
Question is about - central venous catheter
Category of the Question - Physiological Integrity, Reduction of Risk Potential

The nurse is assisting the physician with removal of a central venous catheter. To facilitate removal, the nurse should instruct the client to:

    A. Perform the Valsalva maneuver as the catheter is advanced
    B. Turn his head to the left side and hyperextend the neck
    C. Take slow, deep breaths as the catheter is removed
    D. Turn his head to the right while maintaining a sniffing position

QUESTION NUMBER 01.75
Question is about - streptokinase
Category of the Question - Physiological Integrity, Pharmacological and Parenteral Therapies

A client has an order for streptokinase. Before administering the medication, the nurse should assess the client for:

    A. Allergies to pineapples and bananas
    B. A history of streptococcal infections
    C. Prior therapy with phenytoin
    D. A history of alcohol abuse

Practice Question Set-2

QUESTION NUMBER 02.01
Question is about - leukemia
Category of the Question - Health Promotion and Maintenance

The nurse is providing discharge teaching for the client with leukemia. The client should be told to avoid:

    A. Using oil- or cream-based soaps   C. The intake of salt
    B. Flossing between the teeth   D. Using an electric razor

QUESTION NUMBER 02.02
Question is about - tracheostomy
Category of the Question - Reduction of Risk Potential

The nurse is changing the ties of the client with a tracheostomy. The safest method of changing the tracheostomy ties is to:

    A. Apply the new tie before removing the old one.
    B. Have a helper present.
    C. Hold the tracheostomy with the nondominant hand while removing the old tie.
    D. Ask the doctor to suture the tracheostomy in place.

QUESTION NUMBER 02.03
Question is about - lung resection
Category of the Question - Physiological Integrity, Reduction of Risk Potential

The nurse is monitoring a client following a lung resection. The hourly output from the chest tube was 300mL. The nurse should give priority to:

A. Turning the client to the left side
B. Milking the tube to ensure patency

C. Slowing the intravenous infusion
D. Notifying the physician

QUESTION NUMBER 02.04
Question is about - Tetralogy of Fallot
Category of the Question - Physiological Integrity, Pharmacological and Parenteral Therapies

The infant is admitted to the unit with tetralogy of fallot. The nurse would anticipate an order for which medication?

A. Digoxin
B. Epinephrine

C. Aminophylline
D. Atropine

QUESTION NUMBER 02.05
Question is about - Self-breast exam
Category of the Question - Health Promotion and Maintenance

The nurse is educating the lady's club in a self-breast exam. The nurse is aware that most malignant breast masses occur in the Tail of Spence. On the diagram below, select where the Tail of Spence is.

QUESTION NUMBER 02.06
Question is about - ventricular septal defect
Category of the Question - Physiological Integrity, Physiological Adaptation

The toddler is admitted with a cardiac anomaly. The nurse is aware that the infant with a ventricular septal defect will:

A. Tire easily
B. Grow normally

C. Need more calories
D. Be more susceptible to viral infections

QUESTION NUMBER 02.07
Question is about - nonstress test
Category of the Question - Physiological Integrity, Reduction of Risk Potential

The nurse is monitoring a client with a history of stillborn infants. The nurse is aware that a nonstress test can be ordered for this client to:

A. Determine lung maturity
B. Measure the fetal activity
C. Show the effect of contractions on fetal heart rate
D. Measure the wellbeing of the fetus

QUESTION NUMBER 02.08
Question is about - labor
Category of the Question - Health Promotion and Maintenance

The nurse is evaluating the client who was admitted 8 hours ago for induction of labor. The following graph is noted on the monitor. Which action should be taken first by the nurse?

A. Instruct the client to push
B. Perform a vaginal exam
C. Turn off the Pitocin infusion
D. Place the client in a semi-Fowler's position

QUESTION NUMBER 02.09
Question is about - ECG, cardiac arrhythmia
Category of the Question - Physiological Integrity, Reduction of Risk Potential

The nurse notes the following on the ECG monitor. The nurse would evaluate the cardiac arrhythmia as:

A. Atrial flutter
B. A sinus rhythm
C. Ventricular tachycardia
D. Atrial fibrillation

QUESTION NUMBER 02.10
Question is about - lovenox (Enoxaparin)
Category of the Question - Physiological Integrity, Pharmacological and Parenteral Therapies

A client with clotting disorder has an order to continue lovenox (Enoxaparin) injections after discharge. The nurse should teach the client that lovenox injections should:

A. Be injected into the deltoid muscle
B. Be injected into the abdomen
C. Aspirate after the injection
D. Clear the air from the syringe before injections

QUESTION NUMBER 02.11
Question is about - valium (Diazepam), phenergan (Promethazine)
Category of the Question - Physiological Integrity, Pharmacological and Parenteral Therapies

The nurse has a preop order to administer valium (Diazepam) 10mg and phenergan (Promethazine) 25mg. The correct method of administering these medications is to:

A. Administer the medications together in one syringe
B. Administer the medication separately
C. Administer the Valium, wait 5 minutes, and then inject the Phenergan
D. Question the order because they cannot be given at the same time

QUESTION NUMBER 02.12
Question is about - urinary tract infection
Category of the Question - Health Promotion and Maintenance

A client with frequent urinary tract infections asks the nurse how she can prevent the recurrence. The nurse should teach the client to:

A. Douche after intercourse

B. Void every 3 hours

C. Obtain a urinalysis monthly

D. Wipe from back to front after voiding

QUESTION NUMBER 02.13
Question is about - nursing assistant
Category of the Question - Safe and Effective Care Environment, Management of Care

Which task should be assigned to the nursing assistant?

A. Placing the client in seclusion

B. Emptying the Foley catheter of the preeclamptic client

C. Feeding the client with dementia

D. Ambulating the client with a fractured hip

QUESTION NUMBER 02.14
Question is about - thyroidectomy
Category of the Question - Physiological Integrity, Reduction of Risk Potential

The client has recently returned from having a thyroidectomy. The nurse should keep which of the following at the bedside?

A. A tracheostomy set

B. A padded tongue blade

C. An endotracheal tube

D. An airway

QUESTION NUMBER 02.15
Question is about - histoplasmosis
Category of the Question - Physiological Integrity, Physiological Adaptation

The physician has ordered a histoplasmosis test for the elderly client. The nurse is aware that histoplasmosis is transmitted to humans by:

A. Cats

B. Dogs

C. Turtles

D. Birds

QUESTION NUMBER 02.16
Question is about - chest pain
Category of the Question - Physiological Integrity, Physiological Adaptation

What's the first intervention for a patient experiencing chest pain and an p02 of 89%?

A. Administer morphine

B. Administer oxygen

C. Administer sublingual nitroglycerin

D. Obtain an electrocardiogram (ECC)

QUESTION NUMBER 02.17
Question is about - abdominal aortic aneurysm
Category of the Question - Physiological Integrity, Physiological Adaptation

Which of the following signs and symptoms usually signifies rapid expansion and impending rupture of an abdominal aortic aneurysm?

A. Abdominal pain

B. Absent pedal pulses

C. Chest pain

D. Lower back pain

QUESTION NUMBER 02.18
Question is about - cardiomyopathy
Category of the Question - Physiological Integrity, Physiological Adaptation

In which of the following types of cardiomyopathy does cardiac output remain normal?

A. Obliterative

B. Restrictive

C. Dilated

D. Hypertrophic

QUESTION NUMBER 02.19
Question is about - chest pain
Category of the Question - Physiological Integrity, Physiological Adaptation

Which of the following interventions should be your first priority when treating a patient experiencing chest pain while walking?

A. Have the patient sit down.

B. Get the patient back to bed.

C. Obtain an ECG.

D. Administer sublingual nitroglycerin.

QUESTION NUMBER 02.20
Question is about - acute pulmonary edema
Category of the Question - Physiological Integrity, Physiological Adaptation

Which of the following positions would best aid breathing for a patient with acute pulmonary edema?

A. Lying flat in bed

B. Left side-lying position

C. High Fowler's position

D. Semi-Fowler's position

QUESTION NUMBER 02.21
Question is about - abruptio placentae

Category of the Question - Physiological Integrity, Reduction of Risk Potential

A pregnant woman arrives at the emergency department (ED) with abruptio placentae at 34 weeks' gestation. She's at risk for which of the following blood dyscrasias?

A. Heparin-associated thrombosis and thrombocytopenia (HATT)

B. Idiopathic thrombocytopenic purpura (ITP)
C. Thrombocytopenia
D. Disseminated intravascular coagulation (DIC)

QUESTION NUMBER 02.22
Question is about - vehicle accident, fracture
Category of the Question - Physiological Integrity, Physiological Adaptation

A 16-year-old patient involved in a motor vehicle accident arrives in the ED unconscious and severely hypotensive. He's suspected to have several fractures of his pelvis and legs. Which of the following parenteral fluids is the best choice for his current condition?

A. Packed red blood cells
B. 0.9% sodium chloride solution

C. Lactated Ringer's solution
D. Fresh frozen plasma

QUESTION NUMBER 02.23
Question is about - corticosteroids
Category of the Question - Physiological Integrity, Pharmacological and Parenteral Therapies

Corticosteroids are potent suppressors of the body's inflammatory response. Which of the following conditions or actions do they suppress?

A. Cushing syndrome
B. Pain receptors

C. Immune response
D. Neural transmission

QUESTION NUMBER 02.24
Question is about - HIV, zidovudine
Category of the Question - Physiological Integrity, Pharmacological and Parenteral Therapies

A patient infected with human immunodeficiency virus (HIV) begins zidovudine therapy. Which of the following statements best describes this drug's action?

A. It stimulates the immune system.
B. It destroys the outer wall of the virus and kills it.

C. It interferes with viral replication
D. It promotes excretion of viral antibodies.

QUESTION NUMBER 02.25
Question is about - pneumonia
Category of the Question - Physiological Integrity, Basic Care and Comfort

A 20-year-old patient is being treated for pneumonia. He has a persistent cough and complains of severe pain on coughing. What could you tell him to help him reduce his discomfort?

A. "Hold your cough as much as possible."
B. "Place the head of your bed flat to help with coughing."
C. "Restrict fluids to help decrease the amount of sputum."
D. "Splint your chest wall with a pillow for comfort."

QUESTION NUMBER 02.26
Question is about - asthma, acute respiratory distress
Category of the Question - Physiological Integrity, Physiological Adaptation

A 19-year-old patient comes to the ED with acute asthma. His respiratory rate is 44 breaths/minute, and he appears to be in acute respiratory distress. Which of the following actions should you take first?

    A. Take a full medical history.
    B. Give a bronchodilator by nebulizer.
    C. Apply a cardiac monitor to the patient.
    D. Provide emotional support for the patient.

QUESTION NUMBER 02.27
Question is about - smoke inhalation, hypoxia
Category of the Question - Physiological Integrity, Physiological Adaptation

A firefighter who was involved in extinguishing a house fire is being treated for smoke inhalation. He developed severe hypoxia 48 hours after the incident, requiring intubation and mechanical ventilation. Which of the following conditions has he most likely developed?

    A. Atelectasis   C. Bronchitis
    B. Pneumonia   D. Acute respiratory distress syndrome (ARDS)

QUESTION NUMBER 02.28
Question is about - pneumothorax
Category of the Question - Physiological Integrity, Reduction of Risk Potential

Which of the following measures best determines that a patient who had a pneumothorax no longer needs a chest tube?

    A. You see a lot of drainage from the chest tube.
    B. Arterial blood gas (ABG) levels are normal.
    C. The chest X-ray continues to show the lung is 35% deflated.
    D. The water-seal chamber doesn't fluctuate when no suction is applied.

QUESTION NUMBER 02.29
Question is about - subdural hematoma
Category of the Question - Physiological Integrity, Physiological Adaptation

Which of the following nursing interventions should you use to prevent foot drop and contractures in a patient recovering from a subdural hematoma?

    A. High-top sneakers   C. Physical therapy consultation
    B. Low-dose heparin therapy   D. Sequential compressive device

QUESTION NUMBER 02.30
Question is about - increased intracranial pressure
Category of the Question - Physiological Integrity, Physiological Adaptation

Which of the following signs of increased intracranial pressure (ICP) would appear first after head trauma?

A. Bradycardia

B. Large amounts of very dilute urine

C. Restlessness and confusion

D. Widened pulse pressure

QUESTION NUMBER 02.31

Question is about - phenytoin

Category of the Question - Physiological Integrity, Physiological Adaptation

When giving intravenous (I.V.) phenytoin, which of the following methods should you use?

A. Use an in-line filter.

B. Withhold other anticonvulsants.

C. Mix the drug with saline solution only.

D. Flush the I.V. catheter with dextrose solution.

QUESTION NUMBER 02.32

Question is about - hip repair

Category of the Question - Physiological Integrity, Physiological Adaptation

After surgical repair of a hip, which of the following positions is best for the patient's legs and hips?

A. Abduction

B. Adduction

C. Prone

D. Subluxated

QUESTION NUMBER 02.33

Question is about - acute pancreatitis

Category of the Question - Physiological Integrity, Physiological Adaptation

Which of the following factors should be the primary focus of nursing management in a patient with acute pancreatitis?

A. Nutrition management

B. Fluid and electrolyte balance

C. Management of hypoglycemia

D. Pain control

QUESTION NUMBER 02.34

Question is about - liver biopsy

Category of the Question - Physiological Integrity, Reduction of Risk Potential

After a liver biopsy, place the patient in which of the following positions?

A. Left side-lying, with the bed flat

B. Right side-lying, with the bed flat

C. Left side-lying, with the bed in semi-Fowler's position

D. Right side-lying, with the bed in semi-Fowler's position

QUESTION NUMBER 02.35

Question is about - hypothyroidism

Category of the Question - Physiological Integrity, Reduction of Risk Potential

Which of the following potentially serious complications could occur with therapy for hypothyroidism?

A. Acute hemolytic reaction

B. Angina or cardiac arrhythmia

C. Retinopathy

D. Thrombocytopenia

Correct Answer B. Angina or cardiac arrhythmia

Precipitation of angina or cardiac arrhythmia is a potentially serious complication of hypothyroidism treatment.

Option A: Acute hemolytic reaction is a complication of blood transfusions.

Option C: Retinopathy typically is a complication of diabetes mellitus.

Option D: Thrombocytopenia doesn't result from treating hypothyroidism.

QUESTION NUMBER 02.36
Question is about - diabetes insipidus
Category of the Question - Physiological Integrity, Physiological Adaptation

Adequate fluid replacement and vasopressin replacement are objectives of therapy for which of the following disease processes?

A. Diabetes mellitus

B. Diabetes insipidus

C. Diabetic ketoacidosis

D. Syndrome of inappropriate antidiuretic hormone secretion (SIADH)

QUESTION NUMBER 02.37
Question is about - type 1 diabetes mellitus
Category of the Question - Physiological Integrity, Physiological Adaptation

Patients with Type 1 diabetes mellitus may require which of the following changes to their daily routine during periods of infection?

A. No changes

B. Less insulin

C. More insulin

D. Oral diabetic agents

QUESTION NUMBER 02.38
Question Tag:decreased hematocrit
Category of the Question - Physiological Integrity, Reduction of Risk Potential

On a follow-up visit after having a vaginal hysterectomy, a 32-year-old patient has a decreased hematocrit level. Which of the following complications does this suggest?

A. Hematoma

B. Hypovolemia

C. Infection

D. Pulmonary embolus (PE)

QUESTION NUMBER 02.39
Question is about - partial-thickness burn
Category of the Question - Physiological Integrity, Pharmacological and Parenteral Therapies

A patient has partial-thickness burns to both legs and portions of his trunk. Which of the following I.V. fluids are given first?

A. Albumin
B. D5W
C. Lactated Ringer's solution
D. 0.9% sodium chloride solution with 2 mEq of potassium per 100 ml

QUESTION NUMBER 02.40
Question is about - wound culture
Category of the Question - Health Promotion and Maintenance

Which of the following techniques is correct for obtaining a wound culture specimen from a surgical site?

A. Thoroughly irrigate the wound before collecting the specimen.
B. Use a sterile swab and wipe the crusty area around the outside of the wound.
C. Gently roll a sterile swab from the center of the wound outward to collect drainage.
D. Use a sterile swab to collect drainage from the dressing.

QUESTION NUMBER 02.41
Question is about - furosemide, congestive heart failure
Category of the Question - Physiological Integrity, Pharmacological and Parenteral Therapies

A nurse is administering IV furosemide to a patient admitted with congestive heart failure. After the infusion, which of the following symptoms is not expected?

A. Increased urinary output
B. Decreased edema
C. Decreased pain
D. Decreased blood pressure

QUESTION NUMBER 02.42
Question is about - coronary artery disease
Category of the Question - Health Promotion and Maintenance

There are a number of risk factors associated with coronary artery disease. Which of the following is a modifiable risk factor?

A. Gender
B. Age
C. Obesity
D. Heredity

QUESTION NUMBER 02.43
Question is about - myocardial infarction, tissue plasminogen activator
Category of the Question - Physiological Integrity, Physiological Adaptation

Tissue plasminogen activator (t-PA) is considered for the treatment of a patient who arrives in the emergency department following the onset of symptoms of myocardial infarction. Which of the following is a contraindication for treatment with t-PA?

A. Worsening chest pain that began earlier in the evening
B. History of cerebral hemorrhage
C. History of prior myocardial infarction
D. Hypertension

QUESTION NUMBER 02.44
Question is about - myocardial infarction
Category of the Question - Health Promotion and Maintenance

Following myocardial infarction, a hospitalized patient is encouraged to practice frequent leg exercises and ambulate in the hallway as directed by his physician. Which of the following choices reflects the purpose of exercise for this patient?

A. Increases fitness and prevents future heart attacks
B. Prevents bedsores

C. Prevents DVT (deep vein thrombosis)
D. Prevent constipations

QUESTION NUMBER 02.45
Question is about - cardiogenic shock
Category of the Question - Physiological Integrity, Physiological Adaptation

A patient arrives in the emergency department with symptoms of myocardial infarction, progressing to cardiogenic shock. Which of the following symptoms should the nurse expect the patient to exhibit with cardiogenic shock?

A. Hypertension
B. Bradycardia

C. Bounding pulse
D. Confusion

QUESTION NUMBER 02.46
Question is about - congestive heart failure
Category of the Question - Physiological Integrity, Physiological Adaptation

A patient with a history of congestive heart failure arrives at the clinic complaining of dyspnea. Which of the following actions is the first the nurse should perform?

A. Ask the patient to lie down on the exam table.
B. Draw blood for chemistry panel and arterial blood gas (ABG).
C. Send the patient for a chest x-ray.
D. Check blood pressure.

QUESTION NUMBER 02.47
Question is about - nitroglycerin, angina
Category of the Question - Physiological Integrity, Pharmacological and Parenteral Therapies

A clinic patient has recently been prescribed nitroglycerin for treatment of angina. He calls the nurse complaining of frequent headaches. Which of the following responses to the patient is correct?

A. "Stop taking the nitroglycerin and see if the headaches improve."
B. "Go to the emergency department to be checked because nitroglycerin can cause bleeding in the brain."
C. "Headaches are a frequent side effect of nitroglycerine because it causes vasodilation."
D. "The headaches are unlikely to be related to the nitroglycerin, so you should see your doctor for further investigation."

QUESTION NUMBER 02.48
Question is about - colon cancer, chemotherapy
Category of the Question - Physiological Integrity, Reduction of Risk Potential

A patient received surgery and chemotherapy for colon cancer, completing therapy three (3) months previously, and she is now in remission. At a follow-up appointment, she complains of fatigue following activity and difficulty with concentration at her weekly bridge games. Which of the following explanations would account for her symptoms?

A. The symptoms may be the result of anemia caused by chemotherapy.
B. The patient may be immunosuppressed.
C. The patient may be depressed.
D. The patient may be dehydrated.

QUESTION NUMBER 02.49
Question is about - hemoglobin
Category of the Question - Basic Care and Comfort

A clinic patient has a hemoglobin concentration of 10.8 g/dL and reports sticking to a strict vegetarian diet. Which of the following nutritional advice is appropriate?

A. The diet is providing adequate sources of iron and requires no changes.
B. The patient should add meat to her diet; a vegetarian diet is not advised.
C. The patient should use iron cookware to prepare foods, such as dark-green, leafy vegetables and legumes, which are high in iron.
D. A cup of coffee or tea should be added to every meal

QUESTION NUMBER 02.50
Question is about - anemia
Category of the Question - Physiological Integrity, Physiological Adaptation

A hospitalized patient is receiving packed red blood cells (PRBCs) for treatment of severe anemia. Which of the following is the most accurate statement?

A. Transfusion reaction is most likely immediately after the infusion is completed.
B. PRBCs are best infused slowly through a 20g. IV catheter.
C. PRBCs should be flushed with a 5% dextrose solution.
D. A nurse should remain in the room during the first 15 minutes of infusion.

QUESTION NUMBER 02.51
Question is about - Epoetin
Category of the Question - Physiological Integrity, Reduction of Risk Potential

A patient who has received chemotherapy for cancer treatment is given an injection of Epoetin. Which of the following should reflect the findings in a complete blood count (CBC) drawn several days later?

A. An increase in neutrophil count
B. An increase in hematocrit
C. An increase in platelet count
D. An increase in serum iron

QUESTION NUMBER 02.52
Question is about - polycythemia vera
Category of the Question - Physiological Integrity, Physiological Adaptation

A patient is admitted to the hospital with suspected polycythemia vera. Which of the following symptoms is consistent with the diagnosis? Select all Select all that apply.

A. Weight loss
B. Increased clotting time
C. Hypertension
D. Headaches
E. Polyphagia
F. Pruritus

QUESTION NUMBER 02.53
Question is about - platelet count
Category of the Question - Physiological Integrity, Reduction of Risk Potential

A nurse is caring for a patient with a platelet count of 20,000/microliter. Which of the following is an important intervention?

A. Observe for evidence of spontaneous bleeding.
B. Limit visitors to family only.
C. Give aspirin in case of headaches.
D. Impose immune precautions.

QUESTION NUMBER 02.54
Question is about - corticosteroid
Category of the Question - Physiological Integrity, Pharmacological and Parenteral Therapies

A nurse in the emergency department assesses a patient who has been taking long-term corticosteroids to treat renal disease. Which of the following is a typical side effect of corticosteroid treatment? Select all that apply.

A. Hypertension
B. Cushingoid features
C. Hyponatremia
D. Low serum albumin
E. Mood swings

QUESTION NUMBER 02.55
Question is about - neutropenia
Category of the Question - Physiological Integrity, Physiological Adaptation

A nurse is caring for patients in the oncology unit. Which of the following is the most important nursing action when caring for a neutropenic patient?

A. Change the disposable mask immediately after use.
B. Change gloves immediately after use.
C. Minimize patient contact.
D. Minimize conversation with the patient.

QUESTION NUMBER 02.56
Question is about - leukemia
Category of the Question - Health Promotion and Maintenance

A patient is undergoing the induction stage of treatment for leukemia. The nurse teaches family members about infectious precautions. Which of the following statements by family members indicates that the family needs more education?

A. We will bring in books and magazines for entertainment.

B. We will bring in personal care items for comfort.

C. We will bring in fresh flowers to brighten the room.

D. We will bring in family pictures and get well cards.

QUESTION NUMBER 02.57

Question is about - acute lymphoblastic leukemia

Category of the Question - Health Promotion and Maintenance

A nurse is caring for a patient with acute lymphoblastic leukemia (ALL). Which of the following is the most likely age range of the patient?

A. 3-10 years

B. 25-35 years

C. 45-55 years

D. over 60 years

QUESTION NUMBER 02.58

Question is about - Hodgkin's disease

Category of the Question - Physiological Integrity, Physiological Adaptation

A patient is admitted to the oncology unit for diagnosis of suspected Hodgkin's disease. Which of the following symptoms is typical of Hodgkin's disease?

A. Painful cervical lymph nodes

B. Night sweats and fatigue

C. Nausea and vomiting

D. Weight gain

QUESTION NUMBER 02.59

Question is about - Hodgkin's disease

Category of the Question - Physiological Integrity, Physiological Adaptation

The Hodgkin's disease patient described in the question above undergoes a lymph node biopsy for definitive diagnosis. If the diagnosis of Hodgkin's disease were correct, which of the following cells would the pathologist expect to find?

A. Lymphoblastic cells

B. Reed-Sternberg cells

C. Gaucher's cells

D. Rieder's cells

QUESTION NUMBER 02.60

Question is about - bone marrow aspiration

Category of the Question - Physiological Integrity, Physiological Adaptation

A patient is about to undergo bone marrow aspiration and biopsy and expresses fear and anxiety about the procedure. Which of the following is the most effective nursing response?

A. Warn the patient to stay very still because the smallest movement will increase her pain.

B. Encourage the family to stay in the room for the procedure.

C. Stay with the patient and focus on slow, deep breathing for relaxation.

D. Delay the procedure to allow the patient to deal with her feelings.

QUESTION NUMBER 02.61
Question is about - sickle cell anemia
Category of the Question - Physiological Integrity, Reduction of Risk Potential

A 43-year-old African American male is admitted with sickle cell anemia. The nurse plans to assess circulation in the lower extremities every 2 hours. Which of the following outcome criteria would the nurse use?

    A. Body temperature of 99°F or less
    B. Toes moved in active range of motion
    C. Sensation reported when soles of feet are touched
    D. Capillary refill of < 3 seconds

QUESTION NUMBER 02.62
Question is about - sickle cell crisis
Category of the Question - Physiological Integrity, Physiological Adaptation

A 30-year-old male from Haiti is brought to the emergency department in sickle cell crisis. What is the best position for this client?

    A. Side-lying with knees flexed
    B. Knee-chest
    C. High Fowler's with knees flexed
    D. Semi-Fowler's with legs extended on the bed

QUESTION NUMBER 02.63
Question is about - sickle cell crisis
Category of the Question - Physiological Integrity, Physiological Adaptation

A 25-year-old male is admitted in sickle cell crisis. Which of the following interventions would be of the highest priority for this client?

    A. Taking hourly blood pressures with mechanical cuff
    B. Encouraging fluid intake of at least 200mL per hour
    C. Position in high Fowler's with knee gatch raised
    D. Administering Tylenol as ordered

QUESTION NUMBER 02.64
Question is about - sickle cell crisis
Category of the Question - Physiological Integrity, Basic Care and Comfort

Which of the following foods would the nurse encourage the client in sickle cell crisis to eat?

    A. Peaches
    B. Cottage cheese
    C. Popsicle
    D. Lima beans

QUESTION NUMBER 02.65
Question is about - sickle cell crisis
Category of the Question - Physiological Integrity, Physiological Adaptation

A newly admitted client has a sickle cell crisis. The nurse is planning care based on the assessment of the client. The client is complaining of severe pain in his feet and hands. The pulse oximetry is 92. Which of the following interventions would be implemented first? Assume that there are orders for each intervention.

A. Adjust the room temperature

B. Give a bolus of IV fluids

C. Start O2

D. Administer meperidine (Demerol) 75 mg IV push

QUESTION NUMBER 02.66

Question is about - iron-deficiency anemia

Category of the Question - Physiological Integrity, Basic Care and Comfort

The nurse is instructing a client with iron-deficiency anemia. Which of the following meal plans would the nurse expect the client to select?

A. Roast beef, gelatin salad, green beans, and peach pie

B. Chicken salad sandwich, coleslaw, French fries, ice cream

C. Egg salad on wheat bread, carrot sticks, lettuce salad, raisin pie

D. Pork chop, creamed potatoes, corn, and coconut cake

QUESTION NUMBER 02.67

Question is about - sickle cell anemia

Category of the Question - Health Promotion and Maintenance

Clients with sickle cell anemia are taught to avoid activities that cause hypoxia and hypoxemia. Which of the following activities would the nurse recommend?

A. A family vacation in the Rocky Mountains

B. Chaperoning the local boys club on a snow-skiing trip

C. Traveling by airplane for business trips

D. A bus trip to the Museum of Natural History

QUESTION NUMBER 02.68

Question is about - vitamin B12 deficiency

Category of the Question - Physiological Integrity, Physiological Adaptation

The nurse is conducting an admission assessment of a client with vitamin B12 deficiency. Which of the following would the nurse include in the physical assessment?

A. Palpate the spleen

B. Take the blood pressure

C. Examine the feet for petechiae

D. Examine the tongue

QUESTION NUMBER 02.69

Question is about - vitamin B12 deficiency

Category of the Question - Health Promotion and Maintenance

An African American female comes to the outpatient clinic. The physician suspects vitamin B12 deficiency anemia. Because jaundice is often a clinical manifestation of this type of anemia, what body part would be the best indicator?

A. Conjunctiva of the eye

B. Soles of the feet

C. Roof of the mouth

D. Shins

QUESTION NUMBER 02.70

Question is about - anemia

Category of the Question - Physiological Integrity, Physiological Adaptation

The nurse is conducting a physical assessment on a client with anemia. Which of the following clinical manifestations would be most indicative of the anemia?

A. BP 146/88

B. Respirations 28 shallow

C. Weight gain of 10 pounds in 6 months

D. Pink complexion

QUESTION NUMBER 02.71

Question is about - polycythemia vera

Category of the Question - Health Promotion and Maintenance

The nurse is teaching the client with polycythemia vera about prevention of complications of the disease. Which of the following statements by the client indicates a need for further teaching?

A. "I will drink 500mL of fluid or less each day."

B. "I will wear a support hose when I am up."

C. "I will use an electric razor for shaving."

D. "I will eat foods low in iron."

QUESTION NUMBER 02.72

Question is about - acute leukemia

Category of the Question - Health Promotion and Maintenance

A 33-year-old male is being evaluated for possible acute leukemia. Which of the following would the nurse inquire about as a part of the assessment?

A. The client collects stamps as a hobby.

B. The client recently lost his job as a postal worker.

C. The client had radiation for treatment of Hodgkin's disease as a teenager.

D. The client's brother had leukemia as a child.

QUESTION NUMBER 02.73

Question is about - acute leukemia

Category of the Question - Health Promotion and Maintenance

An African American client is admitted with acute leukemia. The nurse is assessing for signs and symptoms of bleeding. Where is the best site for examining the presence of petechiae?

A. The abdomen

B. The thorax

C. The earlobes

D. The soles of the feet

QUESTION NUMBER 02.74
Question is about - acute leukemia
Category of the Question - Health Promotion and Maintenance

A client with acute leukemia is admitted to the oncology unit. Which of the following would be most important for the nurse to inquire?

A. "Have you noticed a change in sleeping habits recently?"
B. "Have you had a respiratory infection in the last 6 months?"
C. "Have you lost weight recently?"
D. "Have you noticed changes in your alertness?"

QUESTION NUMBER 02.75
Question is about - acute leukemia
Category of the Question - Physiological Integrity, Reduction of Risk Potential

Which of the following would be the priority nursing diagnosis for the adult client with acute leukemia?

A. Oral mucous membrane, altered related to chemotherapy
B. Risk for injury related to thrombocytopenia
C. Fatigue related to the disease process
D. Interrupted family processes related to life-threatening illness of a family member

Practice Question Set-3

QUESTION NUMBER 03.01
Which individual is at greatest risk for developing hypertension?

A. 45-year-old African-American attorney
B. 60-year-old Asian-American shop owner
C. 40-year-old Caucasian nurse
D. 55-year-old Hispanic teacher

QUESTION NUMBER 03.02
Question is about - acetaminophen
Category of the Question - Physiological Integrity, Pharmacological and Parenteral Therapies

A 15-year-old female who ingested 15 tablets of maximum strength acetaminophen 45 minutes ago is rushed to the emergency department. Which of these orders should the nurse do first?

A. Gastric lavage
B. Administer acetylcysteine (Mucomyst) orally
C. Start an IV Dextrose 5% with 0.33% normal saline to keep the vein open
D. Have the patient drink activated charcoal mixed with water

QUESTION NUMBER 03.03
Question is about - cardiac catheterization
Category of the Question - Safe and Effective Care Environment, Management of Care

Which complication of cardiac catheterization should the nurse monitor for in the initial 24 hours after the procedure?

A. Angina at rest

B. Thrombus formation

C. Dizziness

D. Falling blood pressure

QUESTION NUMBER 03.04

Question is about - renal calculi, flank pain

Category of the Question - Physiological Integrity, Basic Care and Comfort

A client is admitted to the emergency room with renal calculi and is complaining of moderate to severe flank pain and nausea. The client's temperature is 100.8 degrees Fahrenheit. The priority nursing goal for this client is:

A. Maintain fluid and electrolyte balance

B. Control nausea

C. Manage pain

D. Prevent urinary tract infection

QUESTION NUMBER 03.05

Question is about - growth, school age

Category of the Question - Health Promotion and Maintenance

What would the nurse expect to see while assessing the growth of children during their school age years?

A. Decreasing amounts of body fat and muscle mass

B. Little change in body appearance from year to year

C. Progressive height increase of 4 inches each year

D. Yearly weight gain of about 5.5 pounds per year

QUESTION NUMBER 03.06

Question is about - blood pressure

Category of the Question - Health Promotion and Maintenance

At a community health fair, the blood pressure of a 62-year-old client is 160/96 mmHg. The client states "My blood pressure is usually much lower." The nurse should tell the client to:

A. Go get a blood pressure check within the next 15 minutes

B. Check blood pressure again in two (2) months

C. See the healthcare provider immediately

D. Visit the health care provider within one (1) week for a BP check

QUESTION NUMBER 03.07

Question is about - prioritization

Category of the Question - Safe and Effective Care Environment, Safety and Infection Control

The hospital has sounded the call for a disaster drill on the evening shift. Which of these clients would the nurse put first on the list to be discharged in order to make a room available for a new admission?

A. A middle-aged client with a history of being ventilator dependent for over seven (7) years and admitted with bacterial pneumonia five days ago.

B. A young adult with diabetes mellitus Type 2 for over ten (10) years and admitted with antibiotic-induced diarrhea 24 hours ago.

C. An elderly client with a history of hypertension, hypercholesterolemia, and lupus, and was admitted with Stevens-Johnson syndrome that morning.

D. An adolescent with a positive HIV test and admitted for acute cellulitis of the lower leg 48 hours ago.

QUESTION NUMBER 03.08
Question is about - hypothyroidism, levothyroxine
Category of the Question - Physiological Integrity, Pharmacological and Parenteral Therapies

A 25-year-old male client has been newly diagnosed with hypothyroidism and will take levothyroxine (Synthroid) 50 mcg/day by mouth. As part of the teaching plan, the nurse emphasizes that this medication:

A. Should be taken in the morning
B. May decrease the client's energy level

C. Must be stored in a dark container
D. Will decrease the client's heart rate

QUESTION NUMBER 03.09
Question is about - epiglottis
Category of the Question - Physiological Integrity, Physiological Adaptation

A 3-year-old child was brought to the pediatric clinic after the sudden onset of findings that include irritability, thick muffled voice, croaking on inspiration, hot to touch, sit leaning forward, tongue protruding, drooling and suprasternal retractions. What should the nurse do first?

A. Prepare the child for X-ray of upper airways
B. Examine the child's throat

C. Collect a sputum specimen
D. Notify the healthcare provider of the child's status

QUESTION NUMBER 03.10
Question is about - diabetes, school-age
Category of the Question - Physiological Integrity, Physiological Adaptation

In children suspected to have a diagnosis of diabetes, which one of the following complaints would be most likely to prompt parents to take their school-age child for evaluation?

A. Polyphagia
B. Dehydration

C. Bedwetting
D. Weight loss

QUESTION NUMBER 03.11
Question is about - pelvic inflammatory disease
Category of the Question - Physiological Integrity, Physiological Adaptation

A client comes to the clinic for treatment of recurrent pelvic inflammatory disease. The nurse recognizes that this condition most frequently follows which type of infection?

A. Trichomoniasis
B. Chlamydia

C. Staphylococcus
D. Streptococcus

QUESTION NUMBER 03.12
Question is about - prioritization
Category of the Question - Safe and Effective Care Environment, Management of Care

A registered nurse who usually works in a spinal rehabilitation unit is floated to the emergency department. Which of these clients should the charge nurse assign to this RN?

A. A middle-aged client who says "I took too many diet pills" and "my heart feels like it is racing out of my chest."
B. A young adult who says "I hear songs from heaven. I need money for beer. I quit drinking two (2) days ago for my family. Why are my arms and legs jerking?"
C. An adolescent who has been on pain medications terminal cancer with an initial assessment finding pupils and a relaxed respiratory rate of 11,
D. An elderly client who reports having taken a "large crack hit" 10 minutes prior to walking into the emergency room.

Option D: The client in this option may experience a decrease in sensorium later on due to head trauma.

QUESTION NUMBER 03.13
Question is about - coronary artery disease, nutrition
Category of the Question - Health Promotion and Maintenance

When teaching a client with coronary artery disease about nutrition, the nurse should emphasize:

A. Eating three (3) balanced meals a day
B. Adding complex carbohydrates
C. Avoiding very heavy meals
D. Limiting sodium to 7 gms per day

QUESTION NUMBER 03.14
Question is about - morphine, pain management
Category of the Question - Physiological Integrity, Pharmacological and Parenteral Therapies

Which of these findings indicate that a pump to deliver a basal rate of 10 ml per hour plus PRN for pain breakthrough for morphine drip is not working?

A. The client complains of discomfort at the IV insertion site
B. The client states "I just can't get relief from my pain."
C. The level of drug is 100 ml at 8 AM and is 80 ml at noon
D. The level of the drug is 100 ml at 8 AM and is 50 ml at noon

QUESTION NUMBER 03.15
Question is about - health promotion, chiropractic treatment
Category of the Question - Health Promotion and Maintenance

The nurse is speaking at a community meeting about personal responsibility for health promotion. A participant asks about chiropractic treatment for illnesses. What should be the focus of the nurse's response?

A. Electrical energy fields
B. Spinal column manipulation
C. Mind-body balance
D. Exercise of joints

QUESTION NUMBER 03.16
Question is about - neurological assessment, CVA
Category of the Question - Physiological Integrity, Physiological Adaptation

The nurse is performing a neurological assessment on a client post right cerebrovascular accident. Which finding, if observed by the nurse, would warrant immediate attention?

    A. Decrease in level of consciousness
    B. Loss of bladder control
    C. Altered sensation to stimuli
    D. Emotional lability

QUESTION NUMBER 03.17
Question is about - cystic fibrosis
Category of the Question - Physiological Integrity, Physiological Adaptation

A child who has recently been diagnosed with cystic fibrosis is in a pediatric clinic where a nurse is performing an assessment. Which later finding of this disease would the nurse not expect to see at this time?

    A. Positive sweat test
    B. Bulky greasy stools
    C. Moist, productive cough
    D. Meconium ileus

QUESTION NUMBER 03.18
Question is about - wound care
Category of the Question - Physiological Integrity, Physical Adaptation

The home health nurse visits a male client to provide wound care and finds the client lethargic and confused. His wife states he fell down the stairs two (2) hours ago. The nurse should

    A. Place a call to the client's health care provider for instructions
    B. Send him to the emergency room for evaluation
    C. Reassure the client's wife that the symptoms are transient
    D. Instruct the client's wife to call the doctor if his symptoms become worse

QUESTION NUMBER 03.19
Question is about - KUB radiograph
Category of the Question - Physiological Integrity, Reduction of Risk potential

Which of the following should the nurse implement to prepare a client for a KUB (Kidney, Ureter, Bladder) radiography test?

    A. Client must be NPO before the examination
    B. Enema to be administered prior to the examination
    C. Medicate client with furosemide 20 mg IV 30 minutes prior to the examination
    D. No special orders are necessary for this examination

QUESTION NUMBER 03.20
Question is about - myocardial infarction
Category of the Question - Health Promotion and Maintenance

The nurse is giving discharge teaching to a client seven (7) days post myocardial infarction. He asks the nurse why he must wait six (6) weeks before having sexual intercourse. What is the best response by the nurse to this question?

    A. "You need to regain your strength before attempting such exertion."
    B. "When you can climb 2 flights of stairs without problems, it is generally safe."
    C. "Have a glass of wine to relax you, then you can try to have sex."
    D. "If you can maintain an active walking program, you will have less risk."

QUESTION NUMBER 03.21
Question is about - triaging
Category of the Question - Safe and Effective Care Environment, Management of Care

A triage nurse has these four (4) clients arrive in the emergency department within 15 minutes. Which client should the triage nurse send back to be seen first?

    A. A 2-month-old infant with a history of rolling off the bed and has bulging fontanelle with crying
    B. A teenager who got a singed beard while camping
    C. An elderly client with complaints of frequent liquid brown colored stools
    D. A middle-aged client with intermittent pain behind the right scapula

QUESTION NUMBER 03.22
Question is about - toddler, developmental changes
Category of the Question - Health Promotion and Maintenance

While planning care for a toddler, the nurse teaches the parents about the expected developmental changes for this age. Which statement by the mother shows that she understands the child's developmental needs?

    A. "I want to protect my child from any falls."
    B. "I will set limits on exploring the house."
    C. "I understand the need to use those new skills."
    D. "I intend to keep control over our child."

QUESTION NUMBER 03.23
Question is about - enteral feeding, nasogastric feeding
Category of the Question - Physiological Integrity, Basic Care and Comfort

The nurse is preparing to administer an enteral feeding to a client via a nasogastric feeding tube. The most important action of the nurse is:

    A. Verify correct placement of the tube
    B. Check that the feeding solution matches the dietary order
    C. Aspirate abdominal contents to determine the amount of last feeding remaining in stomach
    D. Ensure that feeding solution is at room temperature

QUESTION NUMBER 03.24
Question is about - potassium, hyperkalemia
Category of the Question - Physiological Integrity, Pharmacological and Parenteral Therapies

The nurse is caring for a client with a serum potassium level of 3.5 mEq/L. The client is placed on a cardiac monitor and receives 40 mEq potassium chloride in 1000 ml of 5% dextrose in water IV. Which of the following EKG patterns indicates to the nurse that the infusions should be discontinued?

A. Narrowed QRS complex
B. Shortened "PR" interval

C. Tall peaked "T" waves
D. Prominent "U" waves

QUESTION NUMBER 03.25
Question is about - rhabdomyosarcoma
Category of the Question - Physiological Integrity, Physiological Adaptation

A nurse prepares to care for a 4-year-old newly admitted for rhabdomyosarcoma. The nurse should alert the staff to pay more attention to the function of which area of the body?

A. All striated muscles
B. The cerebellum

C. The kidneys
D. The leg bones

QUESTION NUMBER 03.26
Question is about - Chinese medicine
Category of the Question - Health Promotion and Maintenance

The nurse anticipates that for a family who practices Chinese medicine the priority goal would be to:

A. Achieve harmony
B. Maintain a balance of energy

C. Respect life
D. Restore yin and yang

QUESTION NUMBER 03.27
Question is about - cardiomyopathy
Category of the Question - Physiological Integrity, Physiological Adaptation

During an assessment of a client with cardiomyopathy, the nurse finds that the systolic blood pressure has decreased from 145 to 110 mm Hg and the heart rate has risen from 72 to 96 beats per minute and the client complains of periodic dizzy spells. The nurse instructs the client to:

A. Increase fluids that are high in protein
B. Restrict fluids
C. Force fluids and reassess blood pressure
D. Limit fluids to non-caffeine beverages

QUESTION NUMBER 03.28
Question is about - pulmonary artery catheter, Swan-Ganz catheter
Category of the Question - Physiological Integrity, Reduction of Risk Potential

The nurse prepares the client for insertion of a pulmonary artery catheter (Swan-Ganz catheter). The nurse teaches the client that the catheter will be inserted to provide information about:

A. Stroke volume
B. Cardiac output
C. Venous pressure
D. Left ventricular functioning

QUESTION NUMBER 03.29
Question is about - chest compressions
Category of the Question - Physiological Integrity, Physiological Adaptation

A nurse enters a client's room to discover that the client has no pulse or respirations. After calling for help, the first action the nurse should take is:

A. Start a peripheral IV
B. Initiate high-quality chest compressions
C. Establish an airway
D. Obtain the crash cart

QUESTION NUMBER 03.30
Question is about - digoxin, metoprolol
Category of the Question - Physiological Integrity, Pharmacological and Parenteral Therapy

A client is receiving digoxin (Lanoxin) 0.25 mg daily. The health care provider has written a new order to give metoprolol (Lopressor) 25 mg B.I.D. In assessing the client prior to administering the medications, which of the following should the nurse report immediately to the health care provider?

A. Blood pressure 94/60 mm Hg
B. Heart rate 76 bpm
C. Urine output 50 ml/hour
D. Respiratory rate 16 bpm

QUESTION NUMBER 03.31
Question is about - infant, assessment
Category of the Question - Health Promotion and Maintenance

While assessing a one-month-old infant, which of the findings warrants further investigation by the nurse? Select all that apply.

A. Abdominal respirations
B. Irregular breathing rate
C. Inspiratory grunt
D. Increased heart rate with crying
E. Nasal flaring
F. Cyanosis
G. Asymmetric chest movement

Correct Answers: C, E, F, & G

Option C. Grunting occurs when an infant attempts to maintain an adequate functional residual capacity in the face of poorly compliant lungs by partial glottic closure. As the infant prolongs the expiratory phase against this partially closed glottis, there is a prolonged and increased residual volume that maintains the airway opening and also an audible expiratory sound.

Option E: Nasal flaring occurs when the nostrils widen while breathing and is a sign of troubled breathing or respiratory distress.

Option F: Cyanosis refers to the bluish discoloration to the skin and indicates a decrease in oxygen attached to the red blood cells in the bloodstream.

Option G: Asymmetric chest movement occurs when the abnormal side of the lungs expands less and lags behind the normal side. This indicates respiratory distress.

Option A: Abdominal respiration is normal among infants and young children. Since their intercostal muscles are not yet fully developed, they use their abdominal muscles much more to pull the diaphragm down for breathing.

Option B: Newborns can have irregular breathing patterns ranging from 30 to 60 breaths per minute with short periods of apnea (15 seconds).

Option D: An increase in heart rate is normal for an infant during activity (including crying). Fluctuations in heart rate follow the changes in the newborn's behavioral state – crying, movement, or wakefulness corresponds to an increase in heart rate.

QUESTION NUMBER 03.32
Question is about - postmature fetus, maternal nursing
Category of the Question - Health Promotion and Maintenance

The nurse practicing in a maternity setting recognizes that the postmature fetus is at risk due to:

A. Excessive fetal weight
B. Low blood sugar levels
C. Depletion of subcutaneous fat
D. Progressive placental insufficiency

QUESTION NUMBER 03.33
Question is about - total hip replacement
Category of the Question - Physiological Integrity, Reduction of Risk Potential

The nurse is caring for a client who had a total hip replacement seven (7) days ago. Which statement by the client requires the nurse's immediate attention?

A. I have bad muscle spasms in my lower leg of the affected extremity.
B. "I just can't 'catch my breath' over the past few minutes and I think I am in grave danger."
C. "I have to use the bedpan to pass my water at least every 1 to 2 hours."
D. "It seems that the pain medication is not working as well today."

QUESTION NUMBER 03.34
Question is about - furosemide, side effect
Category of the Question - Physiological Integrity, Pharmacological and Parenteral Therapies

A 33-year-old male client with heart failure has been taking furosemide for the past week. Which of the following assessment cues below may indicate the client is experiencing a negative side effect from the medication?

A. Weight gain of 5 pounds
B. Edema of the ankles

C. Gastric irritability
D. Decreased appetite

QUESTION NUMBER 03.35
Question is about - obstetrics, miscarriage
Category of the Question - Health Promotion and Maintenance

A 32-year-old pregnant woman comes to the clinic for her prenatal visit. The nurse gathers data about her obstetric history, which includes 3-year-old twins at home and a miscarriage 10 years ago at 12 weeks gestation. How would the nurse accurately document this information? Fill in the blanks.

Gravida {3} para {1}

QUESTION NUMBER 03.36
Question is about - venous stasis ulcer
Category of the Question - Physiological Integrity, Basic care and Comfort

The nurse is caring for a 27-year-old female client with venous stasis ulcer. Which nursing intervention would be most effective in promoting healing?

A. Apply dressing using sterile technique
B. Improve the client's nutrition status

C. Initiate limb compression therapy
D. Begin proteolytic debridement

QUESTION NUMBER 03.37
Question is about - meperidine hydrochloride, atropine sulfate, promethazine hydrochloride
Category of the Question - Physiological Integrity, Pharmacological and Parenteral Therapy

A nurse is to administer meperidine hydrochloride (Demerol) 100 mg, atropine sulfate (Atropisol) 0.4 mg, and promethazine hydrochloride (Phenergan) 50 mg IM to a preoperative client. List the order in which the nurse must carry out the following actions prior to the administration of preoperative medications.

1. Have the client empty bladder
2. Instruct the client to remain in bed
3. Raise the side rails on the bed
4. Place the call bell within reach

Correct order is shown above.

1. Have the client empty the bladder. The first step in the process is to have the client void prior to administering the pre-operative medication. If the client does not have a catheter, it is important to empty the bladder before

receiving preoperative medications to prevent bladder injury (especially in pelvic surgeries). Else, a straight catheter or an indwelling catheter may be ordered to ensure the bladder is empty.

2. Instruct the client to remain in bed. Preoperative medications can cause drowsiness and lightheadedness which may put the client at risk for injury.
3. Raise the side rails on the bed. Raising the side rails on the bed helps prevent accidental falls and injury when the client decides to get out of the bed without assistance.
4. Place the call bell within reach. Call bells should always be within the reach of a client.

QUESTION NUMBER 03.38
Question is about - nursing management and leadership, reward-feedback system
Category of the Question - Health Promotion and Maintenance

Which of these statements best describes the characteristics of an effective reward-feedback system?

A. Specific feedback is given as close to the event as possible
B. Staff is given feedback in equal amounts over time
C. Positive statements are to precede a negative statement
D. Performance goals should be higher than what is attainable

QUESTION NUMBER 03.39
Question is about - multiple sclerosis
Category of the Question - Health Promotion and Maintenance

The nurse is providing information to a client with multiple sclerosis on performing exercises and physical activities. The nurse determines the client needs additional teaching if the client makes which statements? Select all that apply.

A. "I can lift weights and do resistance training."
B. "I should exercise to the point of exhaustion."
C. "I can include aerobic exercises in my routine."
D. "Proper stretching should be done before starting my routine."
E. "I should exercise continuously without rest."

Correct answers: B & E.

Option B: Patients with multiple sclerosis should not exercise to the point of fatigue as strenuous physical exercise raises body temperature and may aggravate symptoms.

Option E: Continuous exercise with no rest periods is contraindicated for patients with multiple sclerosis who want to exercise. The patient should be advised to take short rest periods, preferably lying down. Again, extreme fatigue may contribute to the exacerbation of symptoms.

Option A: Exercises should include activities that would strengthen weak muscles because diminishing muscle strength is often a primary concern in multiple sclerosis. These activities include lifting weights and resistance exercises.

Option C: Aerobic exercises help promote muscle efficiency, increase flexibility, improves mood, and helps eliminate stress.

Option D: Muscle stretching should be included prior to exercise as this helps minimize muscle spasticity and contractures which is common in later stages of multiple sclerosis.

QUESTION NUMBER 03.40
Question is about - home care, Alzheimer's disease
Category of the Question - Safe and Effective Care Environment, Safety and Infection Control

During the evaluation of the quality of home care for a client with Alzheimer's disease, the priority for the nurse is to reinforce which statement by a family member?

A. "At least two (2) full meals a day are eaten."
B. "We go to a group discussion every week at our community center."
C. "We have safety bars installed in the bathroom and have 24-hour alarms on the doors."
D. "The medication is not a problem to have it taken three (3) times a day."

QUESTION NUMBER 03.41
Question is about - medications, pregnancy
Category of the Question - Physiological Integrity, Pharmacological and Parenteral Therapy

A nurse is reviewing a patient's medication during shift change. Which of the following medications would be contraindicated if the patient were pregnant? Select all that apply.

A. Warfarin (Coumadin)
B. Finasteride (Propecia, Proscar)
C. Celecoxib (Celebrex)
D. Clonidine (Catapres)
E. Transdermal nicotine (Habitrol)
F. Clofazimine(Lamprene)

QUESTION NUMBER 03.42
Question is about - history, photosensitivity
Category of the Question - Physiological Integrity, Pharmacological and Parenteral Therapy

A nurse is reviewing a patient's past medical history (PMH). The history indicates the patient has photosensitive reactions to medications. Which of the following drugs is associated with photosensitive reactions? Select all that apply.

A. Ciprofloxacin (Cipro)
B. Sulfonamide
C. Norfloxacin (Noroxin)
D. Sulfamethoxazole and Trimethoprim (Bactrim)
E. Isotretinoin (Accutane)
F. Nitro-Dur patch

QUESTION NUMBER 03.43
Question is about - discolored urine
Category of the Question - Physiological Integrity, Pharmacological and Parenteral Therapy

A patient tells you that her urine is starting to look discolored. If you believe this change is due to medication, which of the following of the patient's medication does not cause urine discoloration?

A. Sulfasalazine
B. Levodopa
C. Phenolphthalein
D. Aspirin

QUESTION NUMBER 03.44
Question is about - refrigerated drugs
Category of the Question - Physiological Integrity, Pharmacological and Parenteral Therapy

You are responsible for reviewing the nursing unit's refrigerator. Which of the following drugs, if found inside the fridge, should be removed?

A. Nadolol (Corgard)
B. Opened (in-use) Humulin N injection

C. Urokinase (Kinlytic)
D. Epoetin alfa IV (Epogen)

QUESTION NUMBER 03.45

Question is about - pregnancy, autoimmune disease, immunoglobulin
Category of the Question - Physiological Integrity, Pharmacological and Parenteral Therapy

A 34-year-old female has recently been diagnosed with an autoimmune disease. She has also recently discovered that she is pregnant. Which of the following is the only immunoglobulin that will provide protection to the fetus in the womb?

A. IgA
B. IgD

C. IgE
D. IgG

QUESTION NUMBER 03.46

Question is about - needlestick, AIDS
Category of the Question - Safe and Effective Care Environment, Safety and Infection Control

A second-year nursing student has just suffered a needlestick while working with a patient that is positive for AIDS. Which of the following is the most significant action that the nursing student should take?

A. Immediately see a social worker
B. Start prophylactic AZT treatment
C. Start prophylactic Pentamidine treatment
D. Seek counseling

QUESTION NUMBER 03.47

Question is about - insulin-dependent, diabetes
Category of the Question - Physiological Integrity, Physiological Adaptation

A thirty-five-year-old male has been an insulin-dependent diabetic for five years and now is unable to urinate. Which of the following would you most likely suspect?

A. Atherosclerosis
B. Diabetic nephropathy

C. Autonomic neuropathy
D. Somatic neuropathy

QUESTION NUMBER 03.48

Question is about - BMI, induced vomiting, constipation
Category of the Question - Physiological Integrity, Physiological Adaptation

You are taking the history of a 14-year-old girl who has a (BMI) of 18. The girl reports inability to eat, induced vomiting and severe constipation. Which of the following would you most likely suspect?

A. Multiple sclerosis
B. Anorexia nervosa

C. Bulimia nervosa
D. Systemic sclerosis

QUESTION NUMBER 03.49
Question is about - myeloma, confusion
Category of the Question - Physiological Integrity, Physiological Adaptation

A 24-year-old female is admitted to the ER for confusion. This patient has a history of a myeloma diagnosis, constipation, intense abdominal pain, and polyuria. Based on the presenting signs and symptoms, which of the following would you most likely suspect?

A. Diverticulosis

B. Hypercalcemia

C. Hypocalcemia

D. Irritable bowel syndrome

QUESTION NUMBER 03.50
Question is about - Rhogam
Category of the Question - Physiological Integrity, Pharmacological and Parenteral Therapy

Rhogam is most often used to treat_____ mothers that have a _____ infant.

A. RH positive, RH positive

B. RH positive, RH negative

C. RH negative, RH positive

D. RH negative, RH negative

QUESTION NUMBER 03.51
Question is about - phenylketonuria
Category of the Question - Health Promotion and Maintenance

A new mother has some questions about phenylketonuria (PKU). Which of the following statements made by a nurse is not correct regarding PKU?

A. A Guthrie test can check the necessary lab values.

B. The urine has a high concentration of phenylpyruvic acid

C. Mental deficits are often present with PKU

D. The effects of PKU are reversible

QUESTION NUMBER 03.52
Question is about - overdose, aspirin
Category of the Question - Physiological Integrity, Pharmacological and Parenteral Therapy

A patient has taken an overdose of aspirin. Which of the following should a nurse must closely monitor during acute management of this patient?

A. Onset of pulmonary edema

B. Metabolic alkalosis

C. Respiratory alkalosis

D. Parkinson's disease type symptoms

QUESTION NUMBER 03.53
Question is about - blind, deaf
Category of the Question - Safe and Effective Care Environment, Safety and Infection Control

A 50-year-old blind and deaf patient has been admitted to your floor. As the charge nurse, your primary responsibility for this patient is?

A. Let others know about the patient's deficits.
B. Communicate with your supervisor your patient safety concerns.
C. Continuously update the patient on the social environment.
D. Provide a secure environment for the patient.

QUESTION NUMBER 03.54
Question is about - COPD, PVD
Category of the Question - Physiological Integrity, Pharmacological and Parenteral Therapy

A patient is getting discharged from a skilled nursing facility (SNF). The patient has a history of severe COPD and PVD. The patient is primarily concerned about his ability to breathe easily. Which of the following would be the best instruction for this patient?

A. Deep breathing techniques to increase oxygen levels.
B. Cough regularly and deeply to clear airway passages.
C. Cough following bronchodilator utilization.
D. Decrease CO2 levels by increased oxygen take output during meals.

QUESTION NUMBER 03.55
Question is about - congenital heart defect
Category of the Question - Physiological Integrity, Physiological Adaptation

A nurse is caring for an infant that has recently been diagnosed with a congenital heart defect. Which of the following clinical signs would most likely be present?

A. Slow pulse rate
B. Weight gain
C. Decreased systolic pressure
D. Irregular WBC lab values

QUESTION NUMBER 03.56
Question is about - Down's syndrome
Category of the Question - Physiological Integrity, Physiological Adaptation

A mother has recently been informed that her child has Down's syndrome. You will be assigned to care for the child at shift change. Which of the following characteristics is not associated with Down's syndrome?

A. Simian crease
B. Brachycephaly

C. Oily skin
D. Hypotonicity

QUESTION NUMBER 03.57
Question is about - myocardial infarction, tissue plasminogen activator, alteplase
Category of the Question - Physiological Integrity, Pharmacological and Parenteral Therapy

A client with myocardial infarction is receiving tissue plasminogen activator, alteplase (Activase, tPA). While on the therapy, the nurse plans to prioritize which of the following?

A. Observe for neurological changes
B. Monitor for any signs of renal failure

C. Check the food diary
D. Observe for signs of bleeding

QUESTION NUMBER 03.58
Question is about - folic acid
Category of the Question - Physiologic Integrity, Basic Care and Comfort

A patient asks a nurse, "My doctor recommended I increase my intake of folic acid. What type of foods contain the highest concentration of folic acids?"

A. Green vegetables and liver
B. Yellow vegetables and red meat

C. Carrots
D. Milk

QUESTION NUMBER 03.59
Question is about - meningitis
Category of the Question - Physiological Integrity, Physiological Adaptation

A nurse is putting together a presentation on meningitis. Which of the following microorganisms has not been linked to meningitis in humans?

A. S. pneumoniae
B. H. influenzae

C. N. meningitidis
D. Cl. difficile

QUESTION NUMBER 03.60
Question is about - hemoglobin, RBC
Category of the Question - Physiologic Integrity, Physiological Adaptation

A nurse is administering blood to a patient who has a low hemoglobin count. The patient asks how long do red blood cells live in my body? The correct response is:

A. The life span of RBC is 45 days
B. The life span of RBC is 60 days

C. The life span of RBC is 90 days
D. The life span of RBC is 120 days

QUESTION NUMBER 03.61
Question is about - spinal stenosis, discharge
Category of the Question - Health Promotion and Maintenance

A 65-year-old man has been admitted to the hospital for spinal stenosis surgery. When should the discharge training and planning begin for this patient?

A. Following surgery
B. Upon admission
C. Within 48 hours of discharge
D. Preoperative discussion

QUESTION NUMBER 03.62
Question is about - psychosocial development, Erik Erikson, school-age
Category of the Question - Psychosocial Integrity

A 5-year-old child and has been recently admitted to the hospital. According to Erik Erikson's psychosocial development stages, the child is in which stage?

A. Trust vs. mistrust
B. Initiative vs. guilt
C. Autonomy vs. shame and doubt
D. Intimacy vs. isolation

QUESTION NUMBER 03.63
Question is about - psychosocial development, Erik Erikson, toddler
Category of the Question - Psychosocial Integrity

A toddler is 26 months old and has been recently admitted to the hospital. According to Erikson, which of the following stages is the toddler in?

A. Trust vs. mistrust
B. Initiative vs. guilt

C. Autonomy vs. shame and doubt
D. Intimacy vs. isolation

QUESTION NUMBER 03.64
Question is about - psychosocial development, Erik Erikson, young adult
Category of the Question - Psychosocial Integrity

A young adult is 20 years old and has been recently admitted to the hospital. According to Erikson, which of the following stages is the adult in?

A. Trust vs. mistrust
B. Initiative vs. guilt

C. Autonomy vs. shame
D. Intimacy vs. isolation

QUESTION NUMBER 03.65
Question is about - vital signs
Category of the Question - Physiological Integrity, Reduction of Risk Potential

A nurse is making rounds taking vital signs. Which of the following vital signs is abnormal?

A. 11-year-old male: 90 BPM, 22 RPM, 100/70 mmHg
B. 13-year-old female: 105 BPM, 22 RPM, 105/50 mmHg
C. 5-year-old male: 102 BPM, 24 RPM, 90/65 mmHg
D. 6-year-old female: 100 BPM, 26 RPM, 90/70 mmHg

QUESTION NUMBER 03.66
Question is about - depression, anxiety disorder, history
Category of the Question - Physiological Integrity, Pharmacological and Parenteral Therapy

When you are taking a patient's history, she tells you she has been depressed and is dealing with an anxiety disorder. Which of the following medications would the patient most likely be taking?

A. Amitriptyline (Elavil)

C. Pergolide mesylate (Permax)

B. Calcitonin

D. Verapamil (Calan)

QUESTION NUMBER 03.67

Question is about - erythromycin

Category of the Question - Physiological Integrity, Pharmacological and Parenteral Therapy

Which of the following conditions would a nurse not administer erythromycin?

A. Campylobacteriosis infection

C. Pneumonia

B. Legionnaires disease

D. Multiple Sclerosis

QUESTION NUMBER 03.68

Question is about - hyperkalemia

Category of the Question - Physiological Integrity, Physiological Adaptation

A patient's chart indicates a history of hyperkalemia. Which of the following would you not expect to see with this patient if this condition were acute?

A. Decreased HR

C. Muscle weakness of the extremities

B. Paresthesias

D. Migraines

QUESTION NUMBER 03.69

Question is about - ketoacidosis

Category of the Question - Physiological Integrity, Physiological Adaptation

A patient's chart indicates a history of ketoacidosis. Which of the following would you not expect to see with this patient if this condition were acute?

A. Vomiting

C. Weight gain

B. Extreme Thirst

D. Acetone breath smell

QUESTION NUMBER 03.70

Question is about - meningitis

Category of the Question - Physiological Integrity, Physiological Adaptation

A patient's chart indicates a history of meningitis. Which of the following would you NOT expect to see with this patient if this condition were acute?

A. Increased appetite

C. Fever

B. Vomiting

D. Poor tolerance of light

QUESTION NUMBER 03.71

Question is about - conjunctivitis

Category of the Question - Physiological Integrity, Physiological Adaptation

A nurse is reviewing a patient's chart and notices that the patient suffers from conjunctivitis. Which of the following microorganisms is related to this condition?

A. Yersinia pestis

B. Helicobacter pylori

C. Vibrio cholerae

D. Haemophilus aegyptius

QUESTION NUMBER 03.72
Question is about - Lyme disease
Category of the Question - Physiological Adaptation

A nurse is reviewing a patient's chart and notices that the patient suffers from Lyme disease. Which of the following microorganisms is related to this condition?

A. Borrelia burgdorferi

B. Streptococcus pyogenes

C. Bacillus anthracis

D. Enterococcus faecalis

QUESTION NUMBER 03.73
Question is about - confusion, falls, hemiparesis
Category of the Question - Physiological Integrity, Reduction of Risk Potential

A fragile 87-year-old female has recently been admitted to the hospital with increased confusion and falls over the last two (2) weeks. She is also noted to have a mild left hemiparesis. Which of the following tests is most likely to be performed?

A. CBC (Complete blood count)

B. ECG (electrocardiogram)

C. Thyroid function tests

D. CT scan

QUESTION NUMBER 03.74
Question is about - mobility, weight gain
Category of the Question - Physiological Integrity, Reduction of Risk Potential

An 85-year-old male has been losing mobility and gaining weight over the last two (2) months. The patient also has the heater running in his house 24 hours a day, even on warm days. Which of the following tests is most likely to be performed?

A. CBC (complete blood count)

B. ECG (electrocardiogram)

C. Thyroid function tests

D. CT scan

QUESTION NUMBER 03.75
Question is about - fever, rash
Category of the Question - Physiological Integrity, Reduction of Risk Potential

A 20-year-old female attending college is found unconscious in her dorm room. She has a fever and a noticeable rash. She has just been admitted to the hospital. Which of the following tests is most likely to be performed first?

A. Blood sugar check

B. CT scan

C. Blood cultures

D. Arterial blood gases

Practice Question Set-4

QUESTION NUMBER 04.01
Question is about - Hodgkin's lymphoma
Category of the Question - Physiological Integrity

A 21-year-old male with Hodgkin's lymphoma is a senior at the local university. He is engaged to be married and is to begin a new job upon graduation. Which of the following diagnoses would be a priority for this client?

A. Sexual dysfunction related to radiation therapy
B. Anticipatory grieving related to terminal illness
C. Tissue integrity related to prolonged bed rest
D. Fatigue related to chemotherapy

QUESTION NUMBER 04.02
Question is about - thrombocytopenic purpura
Category of the Question - Physiological Integrity

A client has autoimmune thrombocytopenic purpura. To determine the client's response to treatment, the nurse would monitor:

A. Platelet count
B. White blood cell count
C. Potassium levels
D. Partial prothrombin time (PTT)

QUESTION NUMBER 04.03
Question is about - thrombocytopenic purpura
Category of the Question - Physiological Integrity

The home health nurse is visiting a client with autoimmune thrombocytopenic purpura (ATP). The client's platelet count currently is 80, it will be most important to teach the client and family about:

A. Bleeding precautions
B. Prevention of falls
C. Oxygen therapy
D. Conservation of energy

QUESTION NUMBER 04.04
Question is about - transsphenoidal hypophysectomy
Category of the Question - Physiological Integrity

A client with a pituitary tumor has had transsphenoidal hypophysectomy. Which of the following interventions would be appropriate for this client?

A. Place the client in Trendelenburg position for postural drainage
B. Encourage coughing and deep breathing every 2 hours
C. Elevate the head of the bed 30°
D. Encourage the Valsalva maneuver for bowel movements

QUESTION NUMBER 04.05
Question is about - diabetes
Category of the Question - Physiological Integrity

The client with a history of diabetes insipidus is admitted with polyuria, polydipsia, and mental confusion. The priority intervention for this client is:

A. Measure the urinary output
B. Check the vital signs

C. Encourage increased fluid intake
D. Weigh the client

QUESTION NUMBER 04.06
Question is about - hemophilia
Category of the Question - Physiological Integrity

A client with hemophilia has a nosebleed. Which nursing action is most appropriate to control the bleeding?
A. Place the client in a sitting position with the head hyperextended
B. Pack the nares tightly with gauze to apply pressure to the source of bleeding
C. Pinch the soft lower part of the nose for a minimum of 5 minutes
D. Apply ice packs to the forehead and back of the neck

QUESTION NUMBER 04.07
Question is about - unilateral adrenalectomy
Category of the Question - Physiological Integrity

A client has had a unilateral adrenalectomy to remove a tumor. To prevent complications, the most important measurement in the immediate postoperative period for the nurse to take is:

A. Blood pressure
B. Temperature

C. Output
D. Specific gravity

QUESTION NUMBER 04.08
Question is about - Addison's disease, glucocorticoids
Category of the Question - Physiological Integrity

A client with Addison's disease has been admitted with a history of nausea and vomiting for the past 3 days. The client is receiving IV glucocorticoids (Solu-Medrol). Which of the following interventions would the nurse implement?

A. Daily weights
B. Intake/output measurements

C. Sodium and potassium levels monitored
D. Glucometer readings as ordered

QUESTION NUMBER 04.09
Question is about - total thyroidectomy
Category of the Question - Physiological Integrity

A client had a total thyroidectomy yesterday. The client is complaining of tingling around the mouth and in the fingers and toes. What would the nurse's next action be?

A. Obtain a crash cart
B. Check the calcium level
C. Assess the dressing for drainage
D. Assess the blood pressure for hypertension

QUESTION NUMBER 04.10
Question is about - hypothyroidism
Category of the Question - Physiological Integrity

A 32-year-old mother of three is brought to the clinic. Her pulse is 52, there is a weight gain of 30 pounds in 4 months, and the client is wearing two sweaters. The client is diagnosed with hypothyroidism. Which of the following nursing diagnoses is of highest priority?

A. Impaired physical mobility related to decreased endurance
B. Hypothermia r/t decreased metabolic rate
C. Disturbed thought processes r/t interstitial edema
D. Decreased cardiac output r/t bradycardia

QUESTION NUMBER 04.11
Question is about - arteriogram
Category of the Question - Physiological Integrity

The client is having an arteriogram. During the procedure, the client tells the nurse, "I'm feeling really hot." Which response would be best?

A. "You are having an allergic reaction. I will get an order for Benadryl."
B. "That feeling of warmth is normal when the dye is injected."
C. "That feeling of warmth indicates that the clots in the coronary vessels are dissolving."
D. "I will tell your doctor and let him explain to you the reason for the hot feeling that you are experiencing."

QUESTION NUMBER 04.12
Question is about - healthcare workers
Category of the Question - Physiological Integrity

The nurse is observing several healthcare workers providing care. Which action by the healthcare worker indicates a need for further teaching?

A. The nursing assistant wears gloves while giving the client a bath.
B. The nurse wears goggles while drawing blood from the client.
C. The doctor washes his hands before examining the client.
D. The nurse wears gloves to take the client's vital signs.

QUESTION NUMBER 04.13
Question is about - electroconvulsive therapy, depression
Category of the Question - Physiological Integrity

The client is having electroconvulsive therapy for treatment of severe depression. Which of the following indicates that the client's ECT has been effective?

A. The client loses consciousness.
B. The client vomits.

C. The client's ECG indicates tachycardia.
D. The client has a grand mal seizure.

QUESTION NUMBER 04.14
Question is about - enterobiasis
Category of the Question - Physiologic Integrity

The 5-year-old is being tested for enterobiasis (pinworms). To collect a specimen for assessment of pinworms, the nurse should teach the mother to:

    A. Examine the perianal area with a flashlight 2 or 3 hours after the child is asleep
    B. Scrape the skin with a piece of cardboard and bring it to the clinic
    C. Obtain a stool specimen in the afternoon
    D. Bring a hair sample to the clinic for evaluation

QUESTION NUMBER 04.15
Question is about - enterobiasis
Category of the Question - Physiological Integrity

The nurse is teaching the mother regarding treatment for enterobiasis. Which instruction should be given regarding the medication?

    A. Treatment is not recommended for children less than 10 years of age.
    B. The entire family should be treated.
    C. Medication therapy will continue for 1 year.
    D. Intravenous antibiotic therapy will be ordered.

QUESTION NUMBER 04.16
Question is about - pregnancy
Category of the Question - Safe and Effective Care Environment

The registered nurse is making assignments for the day. Which client should be assigned to the pregnant nurse?

    A. The client receiving linear accelerator radiation therapy for lung cancer
    B. The client with a radium implant for cervical cancer
    C. The client who has just been administered soluble brachytherapy for thyroid cancer
    D. The client who returned from placement of iridium seeds for prostate cancer

QUESTION NUMBER 04.17
Question is about - room assignments
Category of the Question - Safe and Effective Care Environment

The nurse is planning room assignments for the day. Which client should be assigned to a private room if only one is available?

    A. The client with Cushing's disease
    B. The client with diabetes
    C. The client with acromegaly
    D. The client with myxedema

QUESTION NUMBER 04.18
Question is about - Digitalis
Category of the Question - Safe and Effective Care Environment

The nurse caring for a client in the neonatal intensive care unit administers adult-strength Digitalis to the 3-pound infant. As a result of her actions, the baby suffers permanent heart and brain damage. The nurse can be charged with:

A. Negligence

C. Assault

B. Tort

D. Malpractice

QUESTION NUMBER 04.19

Question is about - licensed practical nurse

Category of the Question - Safe and Effective Care Environment

Which assignment should not be performed by the licensed practical nurse?

A. Inserting a Foley catheter

C. Obtaining a sputum specimen

B. Discontinuing a nasogastric tube

D. Starting a blood transfusion

QUESTION NUMBER 04.20

Question is about - surgery

Category of the Question - Physiological Integrity

The client returns to the unit from surgery with a blood pressure of 90/50, pulse 132, and respirations 30. Which action by the nurse should receive priority?

A. Continuing to monitor the vital signs

C. Asking the client how he feels

B. Contacting the physician

D. Asking the LPN to continue the post-op care

QUESTION NUMBER 04.21

Question is about - preeclampsia

Category of the Question - Safe and Effective Care Environment

Which nurse should be assigned to care for the postpartum client with preeclampsia?

A. The RN with 2 weeks of experience in postpartum

B. The RN with 3 years of experience in labor and delivery

C. The RN with 10 years of experience in surgery

D. The RN with 1 year of experience in the neonatal intensive care unit

QUESTION NUMBER 04.22

Question is about - Board of Nursing

Category of the Question - Safe and Effective Care Environment

Which information should be reported to the state Board of Nursing?

A. The facility fails to provide literature in both Spanish and English.

B. The narcotic count has been incorrect on the unit for the past 3 days.

C. The client fails to receive an itemized account of his bills and services received during his hospital stay.

D. The nursing assistant assigned to the client with hepatitis fails to feed the client and give the bath.

QUESTION NUMBER 04.23
Question is about - medication administration
Category of the Question - Safe and Effective Care Environment

The nurse is suspected of charting medication administration that he did not give. After talking to the nurse, the charge nurse should:

A. Call the Board of Nursing
B. File a formal reprimand

C. Terminate the nurse
D. Charge the nurse with a tort

QUESTION NUMBER 04.24
Question is about - home health care
Category of the Question - Safe and Effective Care Environment

The home health nurse is planning for the day's visits. Which client should be seen first?

A. The 78-year-old who had a gastrectomy 3 weeks ago and has a PEG tube
B. The 5-month-old discharged 1 week ago with pneumonia who is being treated with amoxicillin liquid suspension
C. The 50-year-old with MRSA being treated with Vancomycin via a PICC line
D. The 30-year-old with an exacerbation of multiple sclerosis being treated with cortisone via a centrally placed venous catheter

QUESTION NUMBER 04.25
Question is about - emergency department
Category of the Question - Safe and Effective Care Environment

The emergency room is flooded with clients injured in a tornado. Which clients can be assigned to share a room in the emergency department during the disaster?

A. A schizophrenic client having visual and auditory hallucinations and the client with ulcerative colitis
B. The client who is 6 months pregnant with abdominal pain and the client with facial lacerations and a broken arm
C. A child whose pupils are fixed and dilated and his parents, and a client with a frontal head injury
D. The client who arrives with a large puncture wound to the abdomen and the client with chest pain

QUESTION NUMBER 04.26
Question is about - conjunctivitis
Category of the Question - Physiological Integrity

The nurse is caring for a 6-year-old client admitted with a diagnosis of conjunctivitis. Before administering eye drops, the nurse should recognize that it is essential to consider which of the following?

A. The eye should be cleansed with warm water, removing any exudate, before instilling the eyedrops.
B. The child should be allowed to instill his own eye drops.
C. The mother should be allowed to instill the eyedrops.
D. If the eye is clear from any redness or edema, the eye drops should be held.

QUESTION NUMBER 04.27
Question is about - meal planning
Category of the Question - Health Promotion and Maintenance

The nurse is discussing meal planning with the mother of a 2-year-old toddler. Which of the following statements, if made by the mother, would require a need for further instruction?

A. "It is okay to give my child white grape juice for breakfast."
B. "My child can have a grilled cheese sandwich for lunch."
C. "We are going on a camping trip this weekend, and I have bought hot dogs to grill for his lunch."
D. "For a snack, my child can have ice cream."

QUESTION NUMBER 04.28
Question is about - toddler
Category of the Question - Physiological Integrity

A 2-year-old toddler is admitted to the hospital. Which of the following nursing interventions would you expect?

A. Ask the parent/guardian to leave the room when assessments are being performed.
B. Ask the parent/guardian to take the child's favorite blanket home because anything from the outside should not be brought into the hospital.
C. Ask the parent/guardian to room-in with the child.
D. If the child is screaming, tell him this is inappropriate behavior.

QUESTION NUMBER 04.29
Question is about - hearing aid
Category of the Question - Health Promotion and Maintenance

Which instruction should be given to the client who is fitted for a behind-the-ear hearing aid?

A. Remove the mold and clean every week.
B. Store the hearing aid in a warm place.
C. Clean the lint from the hearing aid with a toothpick.
D. Change the batteries weekly.

QUESTION NUMBER 04.30
Question is about - tonsillectomy
Category of the Question - Physiological Integrity

A priority nursing diagnosis for a child being admitted from surgery following a tonsillectomy is:

A. Body image disturbance
B. Impaired verbal communication
C. Risk for aspiration
D. Pain

QUESTION NUMBER 04.31
Question is about - bacterial pneumonia
Category of the Question - Physiological Integrity

A client with bacterial pneumonia is admitted to the pediatric unit. What would the nurse expect the admitting assessment to reveal?

    A. High fever
    B. Nonproductive cough
    C. Rhinitis
    D. Vomiting and diarrhea

QUESTION NUMBER 04.32
Question is about - epiglottitis
Category of the Question - Safe and Effective Care Environment

The nurse is caring for a client admitted with epiglottitis. Because of the possibility of complete obstruction of the airway, which of the following should the nurse have available?

    A. Intravenous access supplies
    B. A tracheostomy set

    C. Intravenous fluid administration pump
    D. Supplemental oxygen

QUESTION NUMBER 04.33
Question is about - Grave's disease
Category of the Question - Physiological Integrity

A 25-year-old client with Grave's disease is admitted to the unit. What would the nurse expect the admitting assessment to reveal?

    A. Bradycardia
    B. Decreased appetite

    C. Exophthalmos
    D. Weight gain

QUESTION NUMBER 04.34
Question is about - celiac disease
Category of the Question - Health Promotion and Maintenance

The nurse is providing dietary instructions to the mother of an 8-year-old child diagnosed with celiac disease. Which of the following foods, if selected by the mother, would indicate her understanding of the dietary instructions?

    A. Ham sandwich on whole-wheat toast
    B. Spaghetti and meatballs
    C. Hamburger with ketchup
    D. Cheese omelet

QUESTION NUMBER 04.35
Question is about - chronic bronchitis
Category of the Question - Physiological Integrity

The nurse is caring for an 80-year-old with chronic bronchitis. Upon the morning rounds, the nurse finds an O2 sat of 76%. Which of the following actions should the nurse take first?

A. Notify the physician
B. Recheck the O2 saturation level in 15 minutes
C. Apply oxygen by mask
D. Assess the pulse

QUESTION NUMBER 04.36
Question is about - amniotomy
Category of the Question - Physiological Integrity

A gravida 3 para 0 is admitted to the labor and delivery unit. The doctor performs an amniotomy. Which observation would the nurse be expected to make after the amniotomy?

A. Fetal heart tones 160bpm
B. A moderate amount of straw-colored fluid
C. A small amount of greenish fluid
D. A small segment of the umbilical cord

QUESTION NUMBER 04.37
Question is about - vaginal exam
Category of the Question - Physiological Integrity

The client is admitted to the unit. A vaginal exam reveals that she is 2cm dilated. Which of the following statements would the nurse expect her to make?

A. "We have a name picked out for the baby."
B. "I need to push when I have a contraction."
C. "I can't concentrate if anyone is touching me."
D. "When can I get my epidural?"

QUESTION NUMBER 04.38
Question is about - labor
Category of the Question - Physiological Integrity

The client is having fetal heart rates of 90–110 bpm during the contractions. The first action the nurse should take is:

A. Reposition the monitor
B. Turn the client to her left side
C. Ask the client to ambulate
D. Prepare the client for delivery

QUESTION NUMBER 04.39
Question is about - pitocin, dystocia
Category of the Question - Physiological Integrity

In evaluating the effectiveness of IV Pitocin for a client with secondary dystocia, the nurse should expect:

A. A painless delivery
B. Cervical effacement
C. Infrequent contractions
D. Progressive cervical dilation

QUESTION NUMBER 04.40
Question is about - footling breech presentation
Category of the Question - Physiological Integrity

A vaginal exam reveals a footling breech presentation. The nurse should take which of the following actions at this time?

A. Anticipate the need for a Caesarean section
B. Apply the fetal heart monitor

C. Place the client in Genupectoral position
D. Perform an ultrasound exam

QUESTION NUMBER 04.41
Question is about - vaginal exam
Category of the Question - Physiological Integrity

A vaginal exam reveals that the cervix is 4cm dilated, with intact membranes and a fetal heart tone rate of 160–170 bpm. The nurse decides to apply an external fetal monitor. The rationale for this implementation is:

A. The cervix is closed.
B. The membranes are still intact.
C. The fetal heart tones are within normal limits.
D. The contractions are intense enough for insertion of an internal monitor.

QUESTION NUMBER 04.42
Question is about - labor, primigravida
Category of the Question - Physiological Integrity

The following are all nursing diagnoses appropriate for a gravida 1 para 0 in labor. Which one would be most appropriate for the primigravida as she completes the early phase of labor?

A. Impaired gas exchange related to hyperventilation
B. Alteration in placental perfusion related to maternal position
C. Impaired physical mobility related to fetal-monitoring equipment
D. Potential fluid volume deficit related to decreased fluid intake

QUESTION NUMBER 04.43
Question is about - late decelerations
Category of the Question - Physiological Integrity

As the client reaches 8 cm dilation, the nurse notes late decelerations on the fetal monitor. The FHR baseline is 165–175 bpm with variability of 0–2bpm. What is the most likely explanation of this pattern?

A. The baby is asleep.
B. The umbilical cord is compressed.

C. There is a vagal response.
D. There is uteroplacental insufficiency.

QUESTION NUMBER 04.44
Question is about - variable decelerations
Category of the Question - Physiological Integrity

The nurse notes variable decelerations on the fetal monitor strip. The most appropriate initial action would be to:

A. Notify her doctor
B. Start an IV

C. Reposition the client
D. Readjust the monitor

QUESTION NUMBER 04.45
Question is about - fetal heart rate
Category of the Question - Physiological Integrity

Which of the following is a characteristic of a reassuring fetal heart rate pattern?

A. A fetal heart rate of 170–180 bpm
B. A baseline variability of 25–35 bpm

C. Ominous periodic changes
D. Acceleration of FHR with fetal movements

QUESTION NUMBER 04.46
Question is about - epidural anesthesia
Category of the Question - Physiologic Integrity

The rationale for inserting a French catheter every hour for the client with epidural anesthesia is:

A. The bladder fills more rapidly because of the medication used for the epidural.
B. Her level of consciousness is such that she is in a trancelike state.
C. The sensation of the bladder filling is diminished or lost.
D. She is embarrassed to ask for the bedpan that frequently.

QUESTION NUMBER 04.47
Question is about - conception
Category of the Question - Health Promotion and Maintenance

A client in the family planning clinic asks the nurse about the most likely time for her to conceive. The nurse explains that conception is most likely to occur when:

A. Estrogen levels are low.
B. Luteinizing hormone is high.
C. The endometrial lining is thin.
D. The progesterone level is low.

QUESTION NUMBER 04.48
Question is about - rhythm method
Category of the Question - Health Promotion and Maintenance

A client tells the nurse that she plans to use the rhythm method of birth control. The nurse is aware that the success of the rhythm method depends on the:

A. Age of the client
B. Frequency of intercourse

C. Regularity of the menses
D. Range of the client's temperature

QUESTION NUMBER 04.49
Question is about - diabetes, birth control
Category of the Question - Health Promotion and Maintenance

A client with diabetes asks the nurse for advice regarding methods of birth control. Which method of birth control is most suitable for the client with diabetes?

A. Intrauterine device
B. Oral contraceptives

C. Diaphragm
D. Contraceptive sponge

QUESTION NUMBER 04.50
Question is about - ectopic pregnancy
Category of the Question - Physiological Integrity

The doctor suspects that the client has an ectopic pregnancy. Which symptom is consistent with a diagnosis of ectopic pregnancy?

A. Painless vaginal bleeding
B. Abdominal cramping

C. Throbbing pain in the upper quadrant
D. Sudden, stabbing pain in the lower quadrant

QUESTION NUMBER 04.51
Question is about - nutrition, pregnancy
Category of the Question - Health Promotion and Maintenance

The nurse is teaching a pregnant client about nutritional needs during pregnancy. Which menu selection will best meet the nutritional needs of the pregnant client?

A. Hamburger patty, green beans, French fries, and iced tea
B. Roast beef sandwich, potato chips, baked beans, and cola
C. Baked chicken, fruit cup, potato salad, coleslaw, yogurt, and iced tea
D. Fish sandwich, gelatin with fruit, and coffee

QUESTION NUMBER 04.52
Question is about - hyperemesis gravidarum
Category of the Question - Physiological Integrity

The client with hyperemesis gravidarum is at risk for developing:

A. Respiratory alkalosis without dehydration
B. Metabolic acidosis with dehydration
C. Respiratory acidosis without dehydration
D. Metabolic alkalosis with dehydration

QUESTION NUMBER 04.53
Question is about - pregnancy
Category of the Question - Health Promotion and Maintenance

A client tells the doctor that she is about 20 weeks pregnant. The most definitive sign of pregnancy is:

A. Elevated human chorionic gonadotropin
B. The presence of fetal heart tones
C. Uterine enlargement
D. Breast enlargement and tenderness

QUESTION NUMBER 04.54
Question is about - diabetes, neonate
Category of the Question - Physiologic Integrity

The nurse is caring for a neonate whose mother is diabetic. The nurse will expect the neonate to be:

A. Hypoglycemic, small for gestational age
B. Hyperglycemic, large for gestational age
C. Hypoglycemic, large for gestational age
D. Hyperglycemic, small for gestational age

QUESTION NUMBER 04.55
Question is about - oral contraceptives
Category of the Question - Health Promotion and Maintenance

Which of the following instructions should be included in the nurse's teaching regarding oral contraceptives?

A. Weight gain should be reported to the physician.
B. An alternate method of birth control is needed when taking antibiotics.
C. If the client misses one or more pills, two pills should be taken per day for 1 week.
D. Changes in the menstrual flow should be reported to the physician.

QUESTION NUMBER 04.56
Question is about - breastfeeding
Category of the Question - Health Promotion and Maintenance

The nurse is discussing breastfeeding with a postpartum client. Breastfeeding is contraindicated in the postpartum client with:

A. Diabetes
B. Positive HIV
C. Hypertension
D. Thyroid disease

QUESTION NUMBER 04.57
Question is about - vaginal bleeding
Category of the Question - Physiological Integrity

A client is admitted to the labor and delivery unit complaining of vaginal bleeding with very little discomfort. The nurse's first action should be to:

A. Assess the fetal heart tones
B. Check for cervical dilation
C. Check for firmness of the uterus
D. Obtain a detailed history

QUESTION NUMBER 04.58
Question is about - labor

Category of the Question - Physiological Integrity

A client telephones the emergency room stating that she thinks that she is in labor. The nurse should tell the client that labor has probably begun when:

    A. Her contractions are 2 minutes apart.
    B. She has back pain and a bloody discharge.
    C. She experiences abdominal pain and frequent urination.
    D. Her contractions are 5 minutes apart.

QUESTION NUMBER 04.59
Question is about - fetal development, smoking
Category of the Question - Health Promotion and Maintenance

The nurse is teaching a group of prenatal clients about the effects of cigarette smoke on fetal development. Which characteristic is associated with babies born to mothers who smoked during pregnancy?

    A. Low birth weight
    B. Large for gestational age
    C. Preterm birth, but appropriate size for gestation
    D. Growth retardation in weight and length

QUESTION NUMBER 04.60
Question is about - RhoGam
Category of the Question - Physiological Integrity

The physician has ordered an injection of RhoGam for the postpartum client whose blood type is A negative but whose baby is O positive. To provide postpartum prophylaxis, RhoGam should be administered:

    A. Within 72 hours of delivery
    B. Within 1 week of delivery

    C. Within 2 weeks of delivery
    D. Within 1 month of delivery

QUESTION NUMBER 04.61
Question is about - amniotomy
Category of the Question - Physiological Integrity

After the physician performs an amniotomy, the nurse's first action should be to assess the:

    A. Degree of cervical dilation
    B. Fetal heart tones

    C. Client's vital signs
    D. Client's level of discomfort

QUESTION NUMBER 04.62
Question is about - effacement, labor and delivery
Category of the Question - Physiological Integrity

A client is admitted to the labor and delivery unit. The nurse performs a vaginal exam and determines that the client's cervix is 5 cm dilated with 75% effacement. Based on the nurse's assessment the client is in which phase of labor?

A. Active
B. Latent

C. Transition
D. Early

QUESTION NUMBER 04.63
Question is about - narcotic abstinence syndrome
Category of the Question - health

A newborn with narcotic abstinence syndrome is admitted to the nursery. Nursing care of the newborn should include:

A. Teaching the mother to provide tactile stimulation
B. Wrapping the newborn snugly in a blanket
C. Placing the newborn in the infant seat
D. Initiating an early infant-stimulation program

QUESTION NUMBER 04.64
Question is about - epidural anesthesia
Category of the Question -

A client elects to have epidural anesthesia to relieve the discomfort of labor. Following the initiation of epidural anesthesia, the nurse should give priority to:

A. Checking for cervical dilation
B. Placing the client in a supine position

C. Checking the client's blood pressure
D. Obtaining a fetal heart rate

QUESTION NUMBER 04.65
Question is about - postoperative wound infection
Category of the Question - Safe and Effective Care Environment

The nurse is aware that the best way to prevent postoperative wound infection in the surgical client is to:

A. Administer a prescribed antibiotic
B. Wash her hands for 2 minutes before care
C. Wear a mask when providing care
D. Ask the client to cover her mouth when she coughs

QUESTION NUMBER 04.66
Question is about - fractured hip
Category of the Question - Physiological Integrity

The elderly client is admitted to the emergency room. Which symptom is the client with a fractured hip most likely to exhibit?

A. Pain
B. Misalignment

C. Cool extremity
D. Absence of pedal pulses

QUESTION NUMBER 04.67
Question is about - osteoporosis
Category of the Question - Health Promotion and Maintenance

The nurse knows that a 60-year-old female client's susceptibility to osteoporosis is most likely related to:

A. Lack of exercise

B. Hormonal disturbances

C. Lack of calcium

D. Genetic predisposition

QUESTION NUMBER 04.68
Question is about - Bryant's traction
Category of the Question - Physiological Integrity

A 2-year-old is admitted for repair of a fractured femur and is placed in Bryant's traction. Which finding by the nurse indicates that the traction is working properly?

A. The infant no longer complains of pain.

B. The buttocks are 15° off the bed.

C. The legs are suspended in the traction.

D. The pins are secured within the pulley.

QUESTION NUMBER 04.69
Question is about - Buck's traction
Category of the Question - Physiological Integrity

A client with a fractured hip has been placed in Buck's traction. Which statement is true regarding balanced skeletal traction? Balanced skeletal traction:

A. Utilizes a Steinman pin

B. Requires that both legs be secured

C. Utilizes Kirschner wires

D. Is used primarily to heal the fractured hips

QUESTION NUMBER 04.70
Question is about - open reduction internal fixation
Category of the Question - Safe and Effective Care Environment

The client is admitted for an open reduction internal fixation of a fractured hip. Immediately following surgery, the nurse should give priority to assessing the:

A. Serum collection (Davol) drain

B. Client's pain

C. Nutritional status

D. Immobilizer

QUESTION NUMBER 04.71
Question is about - percutaneous gastrostomy tube
Category of the Question - Health Promotion and Maintenance

Which statement made by the family member caring for the client with a percutaneous gastrostomy tube indicates an understanding of the nurse's teaching?

A. "I must flush the tube with water after feeding and clamp the tube."

B. "I must check placement four times per day."

C. "I will report to the doctor any signs of indigestion."

D. "If my father is unable to swallow, I will discontinue the feeding and call the clinic."

QUESTION NUMBER 04.72
Question is about - total knee replacement
Category of the Question - Physiological Integrity

The nurse is assessing the client with a total knee replacement 2 hours postoperative. Which information requires notification of the doctor?

A. Bleeding on the dressing is 3cm in diameter.

B. The client has a temperature of 100.6°F (38.1°C).

C. The client's hematocrit is 26%.

D. The urinary output has been 60 during the last 2 hours.

QUESTION NUMBER 04.73
Question is about - plumbism
Category of the Question - Health Promotion and Maintenance

The nurse is caring for the client with a 5-year-old diagnosis of plumbism. Which information in the health history is most likely related to the development of plumbism?

A. The client has traveled out of the country in the last 6 months.

B. The client's parents are skilled stained-glass artists.

C. The client lives in a house built in one.

D. The client has several brothers and sisters.

QUESTION NUMBER 04.74
Question is about - total hip replacement
Category of the Question - Safe and Effective Care Environment

A client with a total hip replacement requires special equipment. Which equipment would assist the client with a total hip replacement with activities of daily living?

A. High-seat commode

B. Recliner

C. TENS unit

D. Abduction pillow

QUESTION NUMBER 04.75
Question is about - abdominal surgery
Category of the Question - Physiologic Integrity

An elderly client with an abdominal surgery is admitted to the unit following surgery. In anticipation of complications of anesthesia and narcotic administration, the nurse should:

A. Administer oxygen via nasal cannula

B. Have narcan (naloxone) available

C. Prepare to administer blood products

D. Prepare to do cardio resuscitation

Practice Question Set-5

QUESTION NUMBER 05.01
Question is about - confusion
Category of the Question - Physiological Integrity, Reduction of Risk Potential

A 28-year-old male has been found wandering around in a confusing pattern. The male is sweaty and pale. Which of the following tests is most likely to be performed first?

A. Blood sugar check

B. CT scan

C. Blood cultures

D. Arterial blood gases

QUESTION NUMBER 05.02
Question is about - toilet training
Category of the Question - Health Promotion and Maintenance

A mother is inquiring about her child's ability to potty train. Which of the following factors is the most important aspect of toilet training?

A. The age of the child
B. The child's ability to understand instruction.
C. The overall mental and physical abilities of the child.
D. Frequent attempts with positive reinforcement.

QUESTION NUMBER 05.03
Question is about - poisoning
Category of the Question - Safety and infection Control

A parent calls the pediatric clinic and is frantic about the bottle of cleaning fluid her child drank for 20 minutes. Which of the following is the most important instruction the nurse can give the parent?

A. This too shall pass.
B. Take the child immediately to the ER
C. Contact the Poison Control Center quickly
D. Give the child syrup of ipecac

QUESTION NUMBER 05.04
Question is about - vitamin K
Category of the Question - Physiological Integrity, Pharmacological and Parenteral Therapy

A nurse is administering a shot of Vitamin K to a 30 day-old infant. Which of the following target areas is the most appropriate?

A. Gluteus maximus

B. Gluteus minimus

C. Vastus lateralis

D. Vastus medialis

QUESTION NUMBER 05.05
Question is about - toddler, language
Category of the Question - Safe and Effective Care Environment, Safety and Infection Control

A nurse has just started her rounds delivering medication. A new patient on her rounds is a 4-year-old boy who is non-verbal. This child does not have any identification on. What should the nurse do?

    A. Contact the provider
    B. Ask the child to write their name on paper
    C. Ask a coworker about the identification of the child
    D. Ask the father who is in the room the child's name

QUESTION NUMBER 05.06
Question is about - hyperparathyroidism
Category of the Question - Physiological Integrity, Reduction of Risk Potential

A patient is admitted to the hospital with a diagnosis of primary hyperparathyroidism. A nurse checking the patient's lab results would expect which of the following changes in laboratory findings?

    A. Elevated serum calcium
    B. Low serum parathyroid hormone (PTH)
    C. Elevated serum vitamin D
    D. Low urine calcium

QUESTION NUMBER 05.07
Question is about - Addison's disease
Category of the Question - Health Promotion and Maintenance

A patient with Addison's disease asks a nurse for nutrition and diet advice. Which of the following diet modifications is not recommended?

    A. A diet high in grains
    B. A diet with adequate caloric intake
    C. A high protein diet
    D. A restricted sodium diet

QUESTION NUMBER 05.08
Question is about - diabetes mellitus, cholecystectomy
Category of the Question - Physiological Integrity, Physiological Adaptation

A patient with a history of diabetes mellitus is on the second postoperative day following cholecystectomy. She has complained of nausea and isn't able to eat solid foods. The nurse enters the room to find the patient confused and shaky. Which of the following is the most likely explanation for the patient's symptoms?

    A. Anesthesia reaction   C. Hypoglycemia
    B. Hyperglycemia   D. Diabetic ketoacidosis

QUESTION NUMBER 05.09
Question is about - fiberoptic colonoscopy
Category of the Question - Physiological Integrity, Reduction of Risk Potential

A nurse assigned to the emergency department evaluates a patient who underwent fiberoptic colonoscopy 18 hours previously. The patient reports increasing abdominal pain, fever, and chills. Which of the following conditions poses the most immediate concern?

A. Bowel perforation
B. Viral Gastroenteritis

C. Colon cancer
D. Diverticulitis

QUESTION NUMBER 05.10
Question is about - liver biopsy, coagulation
Category of the Question - Physiological Integrity, Reduction of Risk Potential

A patient is admitted to the same-day surgery unit for a liver biopsy. Which of the following laboratory tests assesses coagulation? Select all that apply.

A. Partial thromboplastin time
B. Prothrombin time
C. Platelet count
D. Hemoglobin

QUESTION NUMBER 05.11
Question is about - hepatitis A
Category of the Question - Safe and Effective Care Environment, Safety and Infection Control

A nurse is assessing a clinic patient with a diagnosis of hepatitis A. Which of the following is the most likely route of transmission?

A. Sexual contact with an infected partner
B. Contaminated food
C. Blood transfusion
D. Illegal drug use

QUESTION NUMBER 05.12
Question is about - leukemia, blood transfusion
Category of the Question - Safe and Effective Care Environment, Safety and Infection Control

A leukemia patient has a relative who wants to donate blood for transfusion. Which of the following donor medical conditions would prevent this?

A. A history of hepatitis C five years previously
B. Cholecystitis requiring cholecystectomy one year previously
C. Asymptomatic diverticulosis
D. Crohn's disease in remission

QUESTION NUMBER 05.13
Question is about - acute gastritis
Category of the Question - Physiological Integrity, Pharmacological and Parenteral Therapy

A physician has diagnosed acute gastritis in a clinic patient. Which of the following medications would be contraindicated for this patient?

A. Naproxen sodium (Naprosyn)
B. Calcium carbonate

C. Clarithromycin (Biaxin)
D. Furosemide (Lasix)

QUESTION NUMBER 05.14
Question is about - cholecystitis
Category of the Question - Health Promotion and Maintenance

The nurse is conducting nutrition counseling for a patient with cholecystitis. Which of the following information is important to communicate?

A. The patient must maintain a low-calorie diet
B. The patient must maintain a high protein/low carbohydrate diet.
C. The patient should limit sweets and sugary drinks.
D. The patient should limit fatty foods.

QUESTION NUMBER 05.15
Question is about - myocardial infarction, pulmonary edema
Category of the Question - Physiological Integrity, Physiological Adaptation

A patient admitted to the hospital with myocardial infarction develops severe pulmonary edema. Which of the following symptoms should the nurse expect the patient to exhibit?

A. Slow, deep respirations
B. Stridor

C. Bradycardia
D. Air hunger

QUESTION NUMBER 05.16
Question is about - cardioverter-defibrillator
Category of the Question - Physiological Integrity, Reduction of Risk Potential

A nurse caring for several patients in the cardiac unit is told that one is scheduled for implantation of an automatic internal cardioverter-defibrillator. Which of the following patients is most likely to have this procedure?

A. A patient admitted for myocardial infarction without cardiac muscle damage.
B. A postoperative coronary bypass patient, recovering on schedule.
C. A patient with a history of ventricular tachycardia and syncopal episodes.
D. A patient with a history of atrial tachycardia and fatigue.

QUESTION NUMBER 05.17
Question is about - MRI, lung cancer
Category of the Question - Physiological Integrity, Reduction of Risk Potential

A patient is scheduled for a magnetic resonance imaging (MRI) scan for suspected lung cancer. Which of the following is a contraindication to the study for this patient?

A. The patient is allergic to shellfish.

B. The patient has a pacemaker.

C. The patient suffers from claustrophobia.

D. The patient takes antipsychotic medication.

QUESTION NUMBER 05.18
Question is about - pulmonary embolism
Category of the Question - Physiological Integrity, Physiological Adaptation

A nurse calls a physician with the concern that a patient has developed a pulmonary embolism. Which of the following symptoms has the nurse most likely observed?

A. The patient is somnolent with decreased response to the family.

B. The patient suddenly complains of chest pain and shortness of breath.

C. The patient has developed a wet cough and the nurse hears crackles on auscultation of the lungs.

D. The patient has a fever, chills, and loss of appetite.

QUESTION NUMBER 05.19
Question is about - abdominal aortic aneurysm
Category of the Question - Physiological Integrity, Reduction of Risk Potential

A patient comes to the emergency department with abdominal pain. Work-up reveals the presence of a rapidly enlarging abdominal aortic aneurysm. Which of the following actions should the nurse expect?

A. The patient will be admitted to the medicine unit for observation and medication.

B. The patient will be admitted to the day surgery unit for sclerotherapy.

C. The patient will be admitted to the surgical unit and resection will be scheduled.

D. The patient will be discharged home to follow-up with his cardiologist in 24 hours.

QUESTION NUMBER 05.20
Question is about - leukemia, chemotherapy, platelet count
Category of the Question - Physiological Integrity, Reduction of Risk Potential

A patient with leukemia is receiving chemotherapy that is known to depress bone marrow. A CBC (complete blood count) reveals a platelet count of 25,000/microliter. Which of the following actions related specifically to the platelet count should be included in the nursing care plan?

A. Monitor for fever every 4 hours.

B. Require visitors to wear respiratory masks and protective clothing.

C. Consider transfusion of packed red blood cells.

D. Check for signs of bleeding, including examination of urine and stool for blood.

QUESTION NUMBER 05.21
Question is about - increased intracranial pressure
Category of the Question - Physiological Integrity, Physiological Adaptation

A nurse in the emergency department is observing a 4-year-old child for signs of increased intracranial pressure after a fall from a bicycle, resulting in head trauma. Which of the following signs or symptoms would be cause for concern?

A. Bulging anterior fontanel
B. Repeated vomiting
C. Signs of sleepiness at 10 PM
D. Inability to read short words from a distance of 18 inches

QUESTION NUMBER 05.22
Question is about - rubeola
Category of the Question - Health Promotion and Maintenance

A nonimmunized child appears at the clinic with a visible rash. Which of the following observations indicates the child may have rubeola (measles)?

A. Small blue-white spots are visible on the oral mucosa.
B. The rash begins on the trunk and spreads outward.
C. There is low-grade fever.
D. The lesions have a "teardrop-on-a-rose-petal" appearance.

QUESTION NUMBER 05.23
Question is about - scarlet fever
Category of the Question - Physiological Adaptation

A child is seen in the emergency department for scarlet fever. Which of the following descriptions of scarlet fever is not correct?

A. Scarlet fever is caused by infection with group A Streptococcus bacteria.
B. "Strawberry tongue" is a characteristic sign.
C. Petechiae occur on the soft palate.
D. The pharynx is red and swollen.

QUESTION NUMBER 05.24
Question is about - allergic reaction, diphenhydramine
Category of the Question - Physiological Integrity, Pharmacological and Parenteral Therapy

A child weighing 30 kg arrives at the clinic with diffuse itching as the result of an allergic reaction to an insect bite. Diphenhydramine (Benadryl) 25 mg 3 times a day is prescribed. The correct pediatric dose is 5 mg/kg/day. Which of the following best describes the prescribed drug dose?

A. It is the correct dose
B. The dose is too low
C. The dose is too high
D. The dose should be increased or decreased, depending on the symptoms

QUESTION NUMBER 05.25
Question is about - undescended testis
Category of the Question - Health Promotion and Maintenance

The mother of a 2-month-old infant brings the child to the clinic for a well-baby check. She is concerned because she feels only one testis in the scrotal sac. Which of the following statements about the undescended testis is the most accurate?

A. Normally, the testes are descended by birth.
B. The infant will likely require surgical intervention.
C. The infant probably has only one testis.
D. Normally, the testes descend by one year of age.

QUESTION NUMBER 05.26
Question is about - Wilms tumor
Category of the Question - Physiological Integrity, Physiological Adaptation

A child is admitted to the hospital with a diagnosis of Wilms tumor, stage II. Which of the following statements most accurately describes this stage?

A. The tumor is less than 3 cm. in size and requires no chemotherapy.
B. The tumor did not extend beyond the kidney and was completely resected.
C. The tumor extended beyond the kidney but was completely resected.
D. The tumor has spread into the abdominal cavity and cannot be resected.

QUESTION NUMBER 05.27
Question is about - acute glomerulonephritis
Category of the Question - Physiological Integrity, Reduction of Risk Potential

A teen patient is admitted to the hospital by his physician who suspects a diagnosis of acute glomerulonephritis. Which of the following findings is consistent with this diagnosis? Select all that apply.

A. Urine specific gravity of 1.040.
B. Urine output of 350 ml in 24 hours.
C. Brown ("tea-colored") urine.
D. Generalized edema.

QUESTION NUMBER 05.28
Question is about - acute glomerulonephritis
Category of the Question - Physiological Integrity, Physiological Adaptation

Which of the following conditions most commonly causes acute glomerulonephritis?

A. A congenital condition leading to renal dysfunction.
B. Prior infection with group A Streptococcus within the past 10-14 days.
C. Viral infection of the glomeruli.
D. Nephrotic syndrome.

QUESTION NUMBER 05.29
Question is about - hydrocele
Category of the Question - Physiological Integrity, Physiological Adaptation

An infant with hydrocele is seen in the clinic for a follow-up visit at 1 month of age. The scrotum is smaller than it was at birth, but fluid is still visible on illumination. Which of the following actions is the physician likely to recommend?

A. Massaging the groin area twice a day until the fluid is gone.
B. Referral to a surgeon for repair.
C. No treatment is necessary; the fluid is reabsorbing normally.
D. Keeping the infant in a flat, supine position until the fluid is gone.

QUESTION NUMBER 05.30
Question is about - peripheral vascular disease
Category of the Question - Physiological Integrity, Physiological Adaptation

A nurse is caring for a patient with peripheral vascular disease (PVD). The patient complains of burning and tingling of the hands and feet and cannot tolerate touch of any kind. Which of the following is the most likely explanation for these symptoms?

A. Inadequate tissue perfusion leading to nerve damage.
B. Fluid overload leading to compression of nerve tissue.
C. Sensation distortion due to psychiatric disturbance.
D. Inflammation of the skin on the hands and feet.

QUESTION NUMBER 05.31
Question is about - atherosclerosis
Category of the Question - Health Promotion

A patient in the cardiac unit is concerned about the risk factors associated with atherosclerosis. Which of the following are hereditary risk factors for developing atherosclerosis?

A. Family history of heart disease
B. Overweight
C. Smoking.
D. Age.

QUESTION NUMBER 05.32
Question is about - peripheral vascular disease, claudication
Category of the Question - Physiological Integrity, Physiological Adaptation

Claudication is a well-known effect of peripheral vascular disease. Which of the following facts about claudication is correct? Select all that apply:

A. It results when oxygen demand is greater than oxygen supply.
B. It is characterized by pain that often occurs during rest.
C. It is a result of tissue hypoxia.
D. It is characterized by cramping and weakness.
E. It always affects the upper extremities.

QUESTION NUMBER 05.33
Question is about - peripheral vascular disease
Category of the Question - Health Promotion and Maintenance

A nurse is providing discharge information to a patient with peripheral vascular disease. Which of the following information should be included in instructions?

A. Walk barefoot whenever possible.
B. Use a heating pad to keep feet warm.
C. Avoid crossing the legs.
D. Use antibacterial ointment to treat skin lesions at risk of infection.

QUESTION NUMBER 05.34
Question is about - vasospastic disorder, Raynaud's disease
Category of the Question - Health Promotion and Maintenance

A patient who has been diagnosed with vasospastic disorder (Raynaud's disease) complains of cold and stiffness in the fingers. Which of the following descriptions is most likely to fit the patient?

A. An adolescent male
B. An elderly woman

C. A young woman
D. An elderly man

QUESTION NUMBER 05.35
Question is about - pregnancy, chest pain
Category of the Question - Health Promotion and Maintenance

A 23-year-old patient in the 27th week of pregnancy has been hospitalized on complete bed rest for 6 days. She experiences sudden shortness of breath, accompanied by chest pain. Which of the following conditions is the most likely cause of her symptoms?

A. Myocardial infarction due to a history of atherosclerosis.
B. Pulmonary embolism due to deep vein thrombosis (DVT).
C. Anxiety attacks due to worries about her baby's health.
D. Congestive heart failure due to fluid overload.

QUESTION NUMBER 05.36
Question is about - thrombolytic therapy, stroke
Category of the Question - Health Promotion and Maintenance

Thrombolytic therapy is frequently used in the treatment of suspected stroke. Which of the following is a significant complication associated with thrombolytic therapy?

A. Air embolus.
B. Cerebral hemorrhage.
C. Expansion of the clot.
D. Resolution of the clot.

QUESTION NUMBER 05.37
Question is about - infant, head position
Category of the Question - Health Promotion and Maintenance

An infant is brought to the clinic by his mother, who has noticed that he holds his head in an unusual position and always faces to one side. Which of the following is the most likely explanation?

 A. Torticollis, with shortening of the sternocleidomastoid muscle.
 B. Craniosynostosis, with premature closure of the cranial sutures.
 C. Plagiocephaly, with flattening of one side of the head.
 D. Hydrocephalus, with increased head size.

QUESTION NUMBER 05.38
Question is about - Addison's disease
Category of the Question - Health Promotion and Maintenance

An adolescent brings a physician's note to school stating that he is not to participate in sports due to a diagnosis of Osgood-Schlatter disease. Which of the following statements about the disease is correct?

 A. The condition was caused by the student's competitive swimming schedule.
 B. The student will most likely require surgical intervention.
 C. The student experiences pain in the inferior aspect of the knee.
 D. The student is trying to avoid participation in physical education.

QUESTION NUMBER 05.39
Question is about - assessment
Category of the Question - Health Promotion and Maintenance

The clinic nurse asks a 13-year-old female to bend forward at the waist with arms hanging freely. Which of the following assessments is the nurse most likely conducting?

 A. Spinal flexibility
 B. Leg length disparity
 C. Hypostatic blood pressure
 D. Scoliosis

QUESTION NUMBER 05.40
Question is about - child abuse
Category of the Question - Psychosocial Integrity

A clinic nurse interviews a parent who is suspected of abusing her child. Which of the following characteristics is the nurse least likely to find in an abusing parent?

 A. Low self-esteem
 B. Unemployment
 C. Self-blame for the injury to the child
 D. Single status

QUESTION NUMBER 05.41
Question is about - juvenile idiopathic arthritis
Category of the Question - Physiological Integrity,

A nurse is assigned to the pediatric rheumatology clinic and is assessing a child who has just been diagnosed with juvenile idiopathic arthritis. Which of the following statements about the disease is most accurate?

    A. The child has a poor chance of recovery without joint deformity.
    B. Most children progress to adult rheumatoid arthritis.
    C. Nonsteroidal anti-inflammatory drugs are the first choice in treatment.
    D. Physical activity should be minimized.

QUESTION NUMBER 05.42
Question is about - osteomyelitis
Category of the Question - Safe and Effective Care Environment, Safety and Infection Control

A child is admitted to the hospital several days after stepping on a sharp object that punctured her athletic shoe and entered the flesh of her foot. The physician is concerned about osteomyelitis and has ordered parenteral antibiotics. Which of the following actions is done immediately before the antibiotic is started?

    A. The admission orders are written.
    B. A blood culture is drawn.
    C. A complete blood count with differential is drawn.
    D. The parents arrive.

QUESTION NUMBER 05.43
Question is about - swelling, leg injury
Category of the Question - Physiological Integrity, Physiological Adaptation

A two-year-old child has sustained an injury to the leg and refuses to walk. The nurse in the emergency department documents swelling of the lower affected leg. Which of the following does the nurse suspect is the cause of the child's symptoms?

    A. Possible fracture of the tibia.
    B. Bruising of the gastrocnemius muscle.
    C. Possible fracture of the radius.
    D. No anatomic injury, the child wants his mother to carry him.

QUESTION NUMBER 05.44
Question is about - cerebral palsy
Category of the Question - Health Promotion and Maintenance

A toddler has recently been diagnosed with cerebral palsy. Which of the following information should the nurse provide to the parents? Select all that apply.

    A. Regular developmental screening is important to avoid secondary developmental delays.
    B. Cerebral palsy is caused by injury to the upper motor neurons and results in motor dysfunction, as well as possible ocular and speech difficulties.
    C. Developmental milestones may be slightly delayed but usually will require no additional intervention.
    D. Parent support groups are helpful for sharing strategies and managing health care issues.
    E. Therapies and surgical interventions can cure cerebral palsy.

QUESTION NUMBER 05.45
Question is about - Duchenne's muscular dystrophy
Category of the Question - Health Promotion and Maintenance

A child has recently been diagnosed with Duchenne muscular dystrophy (DMD). The parents are receiving genetic counseling prior to planning another pregnancy. Which of the following statements includes the most accurate information?

    A. Duchenne's is an X-linked recessive disorder, so daughters have a 50% chance of being carriers and sons a 50% chance of developing the disease.
    B. Duchenne's is an X-linked recessive disorder, so both daughters and sons have a 50% chance of developing the disease.
    C. Each child has a 1 in 4 (25%) chance of developing the disorder.
    D. Sons only have a 1 in 4 (25%) chance of developing the disorder.

QUESTION NUMBER 05.46
Question is about - percutaneous transluminal coronary angioplasty
Category of the Question - Physiological Integrity, Reduction of Risk Potential

A client is scheduled for a percutaneous transluminal coronary angioplasty (PTCA). The nurse knows that a PTCA is the

    A. Surgical repair of a diseased coronary artery.
    B. Placement of an automatic internal cardiac defibrillator.
    C. Procedure that compresses plaque against the wall of the diseased coronary artery to improve blood flow.
    D. Non-invasive radiographic examination of the heart.

QUESTION NUMBER 05.47
Question is about - hypothyroidism
Category of the Question - Physiological Integrity, Physiological Adaptation

A newborn has been diagnosed with hypothyroidism. In discussing the condition and treatment with the family, the nurse should emphasize:

    A. They can expect the child will be mentally retarded.
    B. Administration of thyroid hormone will prevent problems.
    C. This rare problem is always hereditary.
    D. Physical growth/development will be delayed.

QUESTION NUMBER 05.48
Question is about - mental illness
Category of the Question - Psychosocial Integrity

A priority goal of involuntary hospitalization of the severely mentally ill client is

    A. Re-orientation to reality
    B. Elimination of symptoms
    C. Protection from harm to self or others
    D. Return to independent functioning

QUESTION NUMBER 05.49
Question is about - suppression
Category of the Question - Psychosocial Integrity

A 19-year-old client is paralyzed in a car accident. Which statement used by the client would indicate to the nurse that the client was using the mechanism of "suppression"?

A. "I don't remember anything about what happened to me."
B. "I'd rather not talk about it right now."
C. "It's the other entire guy's fault! He was going too fast."
D. "My mother is heartbroken about this."

QUESTION NUMBER 05.50
Question is about - premature rupture of membranes
Category of the Question - Health Promotion and Maintenance

The nurse is caring for a woman 2 hours after a vaginal delivery. Documentation indicates that the membranes were ruptured for 36 hours prior to delivery. What are the priority nursing diagnoses at this time?

A. Altered tissue perfusion
B. Risk for fluid volume deficit
C. High risk for hemorrhage
D. Risk for infection

QUESTION NUMBER 05.51
Question is about - hip spica cast
Category of the Question - Physiological Integrity, Physiological Adaptation

A 3-year-old had a hip spica cast applied 2 hours ago. In order to facilitate drying, the nurse should:

A. Expose the cast to air and turn the child frequently.
B. Use a heat lamp to reduce the drying time.
C. Handle the cast with the abductor bar.
D. Turn the child as little as possible.

QUESTION NUMBER 05.52
Question is about - intravenous pyelogram
Category of the Question - Physiological Integrity, Pharmacological and Parenteral Therapy

A client is scheduled for an Intravenous Pyelogram (IVP). In order to prepare the client for this test, the nurse would:

A. Instruct the client to maintain a regular diet the day prior to the examination.
B. Restrict the client's fluid intake 4 hours prior to the examination.
C. Administer a laxative to the client the evening before the examination.
D. Inform the client that only 1 x-ray of his abdomen is necessary.

QUESTION NUMBER 05.53
Question is about - acute glomerulonephritis
Category of the Question - Physiological Integrity, Physiological Adaptation

Following a diagnosis of acute glomerulonephritis (AGN) in their 6-year-old child, the parent's remark: "just don't know how he caught the disease!" The nurse's response is based on an understanding that:

A. AGN is a streptococcal infection that involves the kidney tubules.
B. The disease is easily transmissible in schools and camps.
C. The illness is usually associated with chronic respiratory infections.
D. It is not "caught" but is a response to a previous B-hemolytic strep infection.

QUESTION NUMBER 05.54
Question is about - diarrhea, vomiting
Category of the Question - Physiological Integrity, Physiological Adaptation

The nurse is caring for a 20 lbs (9 kg) 6 month-old with a 3-day history of diarrhea, occasional vomiting and fever. Peripheral intravenous therapy has been initiated, with 5% dextrose in 0.33% normal saline with 20 mEq of potassium per liter infusing at 35 ml/hr. Which finding should be reported to the healthcare provider immediately?

A. 3 episodes of vomiting in 1 hour.
B. Periodic crying and irritability.
C. Vigorous sucking on a pacifier.
D. No measurable voiding in 4 hours.

QUESTION NUMBER 05.55
Question is about - vaginal delivery
Category of the Question - Physiological Integrity, Physiological Adaptation

While caring for the client during the first hour after delivery, the nurse determines that the uterus is boggy and there is vaginal bleeding. What should be the nurse's first action?

A. Check vital signs.
B. Massage the fundus.
C. Offer a bedpan.
D. Check for perineal lacerations.

QUESTION NUMBER 05.56
Question is about - developmental dysplasia
Category of the Question - Physiological Integrity, Physiological Adaptation

The nurse is assessing an infant with developmental dysplasia of the hip. Which finding would the nurse anticipate?

A. Unequal leg length
B. Limited adduction
C. Diminished femoral pulses
D. Symmetrical gluteal folds

QUESTION NUMBER 05.57
Question is about - Valsalva maneuver, acute myocardial infarction
Category of the Question - Physiological Integrity, Pharmacological and Parenteral Therapy

To prevent a Valsalva maneuver in a client recovering from an acute myocardial infarction, the nurse would:

A. Assist the client to use the bedside commode.
B. Administer stool softeners every day as ordered.
C. Administer antidysrhythmics prn as ordered.
D. Maintain the client on strict bed rest.

QUESTION NUMBER 05.58
Question is about - psychiatric unit
Category of the Question - Safe and Effective Care Environment, Management of Care

On admission to the psychiatric unit, the client is trembling and appears fearful. The nurse's initial response should be to:

A. Give the client orientation materials and review the unit rules and regulations.
B. Introduce him/her and accompany the client to the client's room.
C. Take the client to the day room and introduce her to the other clients.
D. Ask the nursing assistant to get the client's vital signs and complete the admission search.

QUESTION NUMBER 05.59
Question is about - glaucoma
Category of the Question - Physiological Integrity, Physiological Adaptation

During the admission assessment on a client with chronic bilateral glaucoma, which statement by the client would the nurse anticipate since it is associated with this problem?

A. "I have constant blurred vision."
B. "I can't see on my left side."
C. "I have to turn my head to see my room."
D. "I have specks floating in my eyes."

QUESTION NUMBER 05.60
Question is about - asthma
Category of the Question - Physiological Integrity, Physiological Adaptation

A client with asthma has low pitched wheezes present in the final half of exhalation. One hour later the client has high pitched wheezes extending throughout exhalation. This change in assessment indicates to the nurse that the client:

A. Has increased airway obstruction.
B. Has improved airway obstruction.
C. Needs to be suctioned.
D. Exhibits hyperventilation.

QUESTION NUMBER 05.61
Question is about - domestic abuse
Category of the Question - Psychosocial Integrity

Which behavioral characteristic describes the domestic abuser?

A. Alcoholic
B. Overconfident
C. High tolerance for frustrations
D. Low self-esteem

QUESTION NUMBER 05.62
Question is about - long leg cast
Category of the Question - Health Promotion and Maintenance

The nurse is caring for a client with a long leg cast. During discharge teaching about appropriate exercises for the affected extremity, the nurse should recommend:

A. Isometric
B. Range of motion
C. Aerobic
D. Isotonic

QUESTION NUMBER 05.63
Question is about - pregnancy
Category of the Question - Physiological Integrity, Reduction of Risk Potential

A client is in her third month of her first pregnancy. During the interview, she tells the nurse that she has several sex partners and is unsure of the identity of the baby's father. Which of the following nursing interventions is a priority?

A. Counsel the woman to consent to HIV screening.
B. Perform tests for sexually transmitted diseases.
C. Discuss her high risk for cervical cancer.
D. Refer the client to a family planning clinic.

QUESTION NUMBER 05.64
Question is about - toddler
Category of the Question - Psychosocial Integrity

A 16-month-old child has just been admitted to the hospital. As the nurse assigned to this child enters the hospital room for the first time, the toddler runs to the mother, clings to her, and begins to cry. What would be the initial action by the nurse?

A. Arrange to change client care assignments.
B. Explain that this behavior is expected.
C. Discuss the appropriate use of "time-out".
D. Explain that the child needs extra attention.

QUESTION NUMBER 05.65
Question is about - toddler, separation anxiety
Category of the Question - Psychosocial Integrity

While planning care for a 2-year-old hospitalized child, which situation would the nurse expect to most likely affect the behavior?

A. Strange bed and surroundings.
B. Separation from parents.
C. Presence of other toddlers.
D. Unfamiliar toys and games.

QUESTION NUMBER 05.66
Question is about - cognitive development
Category of the Question - Psychosocial Integrity

While explaining an illness to a 10-year-old, what should the nurse keep in mind about cognitive development at this age?

A. They are able to make simple associations of ideas.
B. They are able to think logically in organizing facts.
C. Interpretation of events originates from their own perspective.
D. Conclusions are based on previous experiences.

QUESTION NUMBER 05.67
Question is about - depression
Category of the Question - Psychosocial Integrity

The nurse has just admitted a client with severe depression. From which focus should the nurse identify a priority nursing diagnosis?

A. Nutrition
B. Elimination

C. Activity
D. Safety

QUESTION NUMBER 05.68
Question is about - school-age
Category of the Question - Safe and Effective Care Environment, Safety and Infection Control

Which playroom activities should the nurse organize for a small group of 7-year-old hospitalized children?

A. Sports and games with rules.
B. Finger paints and water play.

C. "Dress-up" clothes and props.
D. Chess and television programs

QUESTION NUMBER 05.69
Question is about - congestive heart failure
Category of the Question - Health Promotion and Maintenance

A client is discharged following hospitalization for congestive heart failure. The nurse teaching the family suggests they encourage the client to rest frequently in which of the following positions?

A. High Fowler's
B. Supine

C. Left lateral
D. Low Fowler's

QUESTION NUMBER 05.70
Question is about - burns
Category of the Question - Physiological Integrity, Physiological Adaptation

The nurse is caring for a 10-year-old on admission to the burn unit. One assessment parameter that will indicate that the child has adequate fluid replacement is:

A. Urinary output of 30 ml per hour
B. No complaints of thirst
C. Increased hematocrit
D. Good skin turgor around burn

QUESTION NUMBER 05.71
Question is about - migraine
Category of the Question - Physiological Integrity, Physiological Adaptation

What is the priority nursing diagnosis for a patient experiencing a migraine headache?

A. Acute pain related to biologic and chemical factors
B. Anxiety related to change in or threat to health status
C. Hopelessness related to deteriorating physiological condition
D. Risk for Side effects related to medical therapy

QUESTION NUMBER 05.72
Question is about - migraine
Category of the Question - Health Promotion and Maintenance

You are creating a teaching plan for a patient with newly diagnosed migraine headaches. Which key items should be included in the teaching plan? Select all that apply.

A. Avoid foods that contain tyramine, such as alcohol and aged cheese.
B. Avoid drugs such as Tagamet, nitroglycerin and Nifedipine.
C. Abortive therapy is aimed at eliminating the pain during the aura.
D. A potential side effect of medications is rebound headache.
E. Complementary therapies such as relaxation may be helpful.
F. Continue taking estrogen as prescribed by your physician.

QUESTION NUMBER 05.73
Question is about - seizure
Category of the Question - Safe and Effective Care Environment, Management of Care

The patient with migraine headaches has a seizure. After the seizure, which action can you delegate to the nursing assistant?

A. Document the seizure
B. Perform neurologic checks

C. Take the patient's vital signs
D. Restrain the patient for protection

QUESTION NUMBER 05.74
Question is about - seizure disorder
Category of the Question - Safe and Effective Care Environment, Management of Care

You are preparing to admit a patient with a seizure disorder. Which of the following actions can you delegate to LPN/LVN?

A. Complete admission assessment.
B. Set up oxygen and suction equipment.
C. Place a padded tongue blade at the bedside.
D. Pad the side rails before the patient arrives.

QUESTION NUMBER 05.75
Question is about - epilepsy
Category of the Question - Health Promotion and Maintenance

A nursing student is teaching a patient and family about epilepsy prior to the patient's discharge. For which statement should you intervene?

    A. "You should avoid consumption of all forms of alcohol."
    B. "Wear your medical alert bracelet at all times."
    C. "Protect your loved one's airway during a seizure."
    D. "It's OK to take over-the-counter medications."

Practice Question Set-6

QUESTION NUMBER 06.01
Question is about - room assignments
Category of the Question - Physiological Integrity, Basic Care and Comfort

Which roommate would be most suitable for the 6-year-old male with a fractured femur in Russell's traction?

    A. 16-year-old female with scoliosis
    B. 12-year-old male with a fractured femur

    C. 10-year-old male with sarcoma
    D. 6-year-old male with osteomyelitis

QUESTION NUMBER 06.02
Question is about - celebrex (Celecoxib)
Category of the Question - Health Promotion and Maintenance

A client with osteoarthritis has a prescription for celebrex (Celecoxib). Which instruction should be included in the discharge teaching?

    A. Take the medication with milk.
    B. Report chest pain.
    C. Remain upright after taking for 30 minutes.
    D. Allow 6 weeks for optimal effects.

QUESTION NUMBER 06.03
Question is about - fracture, cast
Category of the Question - Safe and Effective Care Environment,, Safety and Infection Control

A client with a fractured tibia has a plaster-of-Paris cast applied to immobilize the fracture. Which action by the nurse indicates an understanding of a plaster-of-Paris cast? The nurse:

    A. Handles the cast with the fingertips
    B. Petals the cast
    C. Dries the cast with a hair dryer
    D. Allows 24 hours before bearing weight

QUESTION NUMBER 06.04
Question is about - fiberglass cast
Category of the Question - Physiological Integrity, Basic Care and Comfort

The teenager with a fiberglass cast asks the nurse if it will be okay to allow his friends to autograph his cast. Which response would be best?

A. "It will be alright for your friends to autograph the cast."
B. "Because the cast is made of plaster, autographing can weaken the cast."
C. "If they don't use chalk to autograph, it is okay."
D. "Autographing or writing on the cast in any form will harm the cast."

QUESTION NUMBER 06.05
Question is about - Steinmann pin
Category of the Question - Safe and Effective Care Environment, Management of Care

The nurse is assigned to care for the client with a Steinmann pin. During pin care, she notes that the LPN uses sterile gloves and Q-tips to clean the pin. Which action should the nurse take at this time?

A. Assisting the LPN with opening sterile packages and peroxide.
B. Telling the LPN that clean gloves are allowed.
C. Telling the LPN that the registered nurse should perform pin care.
D. Asking the LPN to clean the weights and pulleys with peroxide.

QUESTION NUMBER 06.06
Question is about - scoliosis, spica cast
Category of the Question - Physiological Integrity, Reduction of Risk Potential

A child with scoliosis has a spica cast applied. Which action specific to the spica cast should be taken?

A. Check the bowel sounds
B. Assess the blood pressure
C. Offer pain medication
D. Check for swelling

QUESTION NUMBER 06.07
Question is about - fracture, traction
Category of the Question - Safe and Effective Care Environment,, Safety and Infection Control

The client with a cervical fracture is placed in traction. Which type of traction will be utilized at the time of discharge?

A. Russell's traction
B. Buck's traction
C. Halo traction
D. Crutchfield tong traction

QUESTION NUMBER 06.08
Question is about - continuous passive motion device
Category of the Question - Physiological Integrity, Physiological Adaptation

A client with a total knee replacement has a CPM (continuous passive motion device) applied during the postoperative period. Which statement made by the nurse indicates an understanding of the CPM machine?

A. "Use of the CPM will permit the client to ambulate during the therapy."
B. "The CPM machine controls should be positioned distal to the site."
C. "If the client complains of pain during the therapy, I will turn off the machine and call the doctor."
D. "Use of the CPM machine will alleviate the need for physical therapy after the client is discharged."

QUESTION NUMBER 06.09
Question is about - walker, fracture
Category of the Question - Safe and Effective Care Environment,, Safety and Infection Control

A client with a fractured hip is being taught correct use of the walker. The nurse is aware that the correct use of the walker is achieved if the:

A. Palms rest lightly on the handles
B. Elbows are flexed 0°
C. Client walks to the front of the walker
D. Client carries the walker

QUESTION NUMBER 06.10
Question is about - prolapsed cord
Category of the Question - Physiological Integrity, Physiological Adaptation

When assessing a laboring client, the nurse finds a prolapsed cord. The nurse should:

A. Attempt to replace the cord
B. Place the client on her left side
C. Elevate the client's hips
D. Cover the cord with a dry, sterile gauze

QUESTION NUMBER 06.11
Question is about - rosuvastatin
Category of the Question - Physiological Integrity, Pharmacological and Parenteral Therapies

The client presents to the clinic with a serum cholesterol of 275 mg/dL and is placed on rosuvastatin (Crestor). Which instruction should be given to the client?

A. Report muscle weakness to the physician.
B. Allow six months for the drug to take effect.
C. Take the medication with fruit juice.
D. Ask the doctor to perform a complete blood count before starting the medication.

QUESTION NUMBER 06.12
Question is about - diazoxide, hypertensive crises
Category of the Question - Physiological Integrity, Pharmacological and Parenteral Therapies

The client is admitted to the hospital with hypertensive crises. Diazoxide (Hyperstat) is ordered. During administration, the nurse should:

A. Utilize an infusion pump
B. Check the blood glucose level

C. Place the client in Trendelenburg position
D. Cover the solution with foil

QUESTION NUMBER 06.13
Question is about - ventral septal defect, Digitalis
Category of the Question - Physiological Integrity, Pharmacological and Parenteral Therapies

The 6-month-old client with a ventral septal defect is receiving Digitalis for regulation of his heart rate. Which finding should be reported to the doctor?

A. Blood pressure of 126/80
B. Blood glucose of 110 mg/dL

C. Heart rate of 60 bpm
D. Respiratory rate of 30 per minute

QUESTION NUMBER 06.14
Question is about - angina, nitroglycerin
Category of the Question - Physiological Integrity, Pharmacological and Parenteral Therapies

The client admitted with angina is given a prescription for nitroglycerin. The client should be instructed to:

A. Replenish his supply every 3 months
B. Take one every 15 minutes if pain occurs

C. Leave the medication in the brown bottle
D. Crush the medication and take with water

QUESTION NUMBER 06.15
Question is about - cholesterol
Category of the Question - Physiological Integrity, Basic Care and Comfort

The client is instructed regarding foods that are low in fat and cholesterol. Which diet selection is lowest in saturated fats?

A. Macaroni and cheese
B. Shrimp with rice

C. Turkey breast
D. Spaghetti

QUESTION NUMBER 06.16
Question is about - congestive heart failure
Category of the Question - Physiological Integrity, Reduction of Risk Potential

The client is admitted with right congestive heart failure. In assessing the client for edema, the nurse should check the:

A. Feet
B. Neck

C. Hands
D. Sacrum

QUESTION NUMBER 06.17
Question is about - central venous pressure
Category of the Question - Physiological Integrity, Reduction of Risk Potential

The nurse is checking the client's central venous pressure. The nurse should place the zero of the manometer at the:

A. Phlebostatic axis

B. PMI

C. Erb's point

D. Tail of Spence

QUESTION NUMBER 06.18
Question is about - hypertension
Category of the Question - Physiological Integrity, Pharmacological and Parenteral Therapies

The physician orders lisinopril (Zestril) and furosemide (Lasix) to be administered concomitantly to the client with hypertension. The nurse should:

A. Question the order

B. Administer the medications

C. Administer separately

D. Contact the pharmacy

QUESTION NUMBER 06.19
Question is about - edema
Category of the Question - Physiological Integrity, Physiological Adaptation

The best method of evaluating the amount of peripheral edema is:

A. Weighing the client daily

B. Measuring the extremity

C. Measuring the intake and output

D. Checking for pitting

QUESTION NUMBER 06.20
Question is about - vaginal cancer, radioactive implant
Category of the Question - Physiological Integrity, Physiological Integrity, Reduction of Risk Potential

A client with vaginal cancer is being treated with a radioactive vaginal implant. The client's husband asks the nurse if he can spend the night with his wife. The nurse should explain that:

A. Overnight stays by family members are against hospital policy.

B. There is no need for him to stay because staffing is adequate.

C. His wife will rest much better knowing that he is at home.

D. Visitation is limited to 30 minutes when the implant is in place.

QUESTION NUMBER 06.21
Question is about - facial stroke
Category of the Question - Physiological Integrity, Basic Care and Comfort

The nurse is caring for a client hospitalized with a facial stroke. Which diet selection would be suited to the client?

  A. Roast beef sandwich, potato chips, pickle spear, iced tea
  B. Split pea soup, mashed potatoes, pudding, milk
  C. Tomato soup, cheese toast, Jello, coffee
  D. Hamburger, baked beans, fruit cup, iced tea

QUESTION NUMBER 06.22
Question is about - diabetes mellitus, insulin
Category of the Question - Physiological Integrity, Pharmacological and Parenteral Therapies

The physician has prescribed Novolog insulin for a client with diabetes mellitus. Which statement indicates that the client knows when the peak action of the insulin occurs?

  A. "I will make sure I eat breakfast within 10 minutes of taking my insulin."
  B. "I will need to carry candy or some form of sugar with me all the time."
  C. "I will eat a snack around three o'clock each afternoon."
  D. "I can save my dessert from supper for a bedtime snack."

QUESTION NUMBER 06.23
Question is about - infant care
Category of the Question - Health Promotion and Maintenance

The nurse is teaching basic infant care to a group of first-time parents. The nurse should explain that a sponge bath is recommended for the first 2 weeks of life because:

  A. New parents need time to learn how to hold the baby.
  B. The umbilical cord needs time to separate.
  C. Newborn skin is easily traumatized by washing.
  D. The chance of chilling the baby outweighs the benefits of bathing.

QUESTION NUMBER 06.24
Question is about - leukemia
Category of the Question - Physiological Integrity, Pharmacological and Parenteral Therapies

A client with leukemia is receiving Trimetrexate. After reviewing the client's chart, the physician orders Wellcovorin (leucovorin calcium). The rationale for administering leucovorin calcium to a client receiving Trimetrexate is to:

  A. Treat iron-deficiency anemia caused by chemotherapeutic agents
  B. Create a synergistic effect that shortens treatment time
  C. Increase the number of circulating neutrophils
  D. Reverse drug toxicity and prevent tissue damage

QUESTION NUMBER 06.25
Question is about - immunization
Category of the Question - Health Promotion and Maintenance

A 4-month-old is brought to the well-baby clinic for immunization. In addition to the DPT and polio vaccines, the baby should receive:

A. HibTITER

B. Mumps vaccine

C. Hepatitis B vaccine

D. MMR

QUESTION NUMBER 06.26

Question is about - gastritis

Category of the Question - Physiological Integrity, Pharmacological and Parenteral Therapies

The physician has prescribed esomeprazole (Nexium) for a client with erosive gastritis. The nurse should administer the medication:

A. 30 minutes before meals

B. With each meal

C. In a single dose at bedtime

D. 30 minutes after meals

QUESTION NUMBER 06.27

Question is about - psychiatric unit

Category of the Question - Psychosocial Integrity

A client in the psychiatric unit is in an uncontrolled rage and is threatening other clients and staff. What is the most appropriate action for the nurse to take?

A. Call security for assistance and prepare to sedate the client.

B. Tell the client to calm down and ask him if he would like to play cards.

C. Tell the client that if he continues his behavior he will be punished.

D. Leave the client alone until he calms down.

QUESTION NUMBER 06.28

Question is about - postpartum

Category of the Question - Health Promotion and Maintenance

When the nurse checks the fundus of a client on the first postpartum day, she notes that the fundus is firm, is at the level of the umbilicus, and is displaced to the right. The next action the nurse should take is to:

A. Check the client for bladder distention

B. Assess the blood pressure for hypotension

C. Determine whether an oxytocic drug was given

D. Check for the expulsion of small clots

QUESTION NUMBER 06.29

Question is about - hemoptysis

Category of the Question - Physiological Integrity, Physiological Adaptation

A client is admitted to the hospital with a temperature of 99.8°F, complaints of blood-tinged hemoptysis, fatigue, and night sweats. The client's symptoms are consistent with a diagnosis of:

A. Pneumonia

B. Reaction to antiviral medication

C. Tuberculosis

D. Superinfection due to low CD4 count

QUESTION NUMBER 06.30
Question is about - migraine
Category of the Question - Physiological Integrity, Pharmacological and Parenteral Therapies

The client is seen in the clinic for treatment of migraine headaches. The drug Imitrex (sumatriptan succinate) is prescribed for the client. Which of the following in the client's history should be reported to the doctor?

A. Diabetes

B. Prinzmetal's angina

C. Cancer

D. Cluster headaches

QUESTION NUMBER 06.31
Question is about - meningitis
Category of the Question - Physiological Integrity, Physiological Adaptation

The client with suspected meningitis is admitted to the unit. The doctor is performing an assessment to determine meningeal irritation and spinal nerve root inflammation. A positive Kernig's sign is charted if the nurse notes:

A. Pain on flexion of the hip and knee
B. Nuchal rigidity on flexion of the neck
C. Pain when the head is turned to the left side
D. Dizziness when changing positions

QUESTION NUMBER 06.32
Question is about - Alzheimer's disease
Category of the Question - Psychosocial Integrity

The client with Alzheimer's disease is being assisted with activities of daily living when the nurse notes that the client uses her toothbrush to brush her hair. The nurse is aware that the client is exhibiting:

A. Agnosia

B. Apraxia

C. Anomia

D. Aphasia

QUESTION NUMBER 06.33
Question is about - dementia
Category of the Question - Psychosocial Integrity

The client with dementia is experiencing confusion late in the afternoon and before bedtime. The nurse is aware that the client is experiencing what is known as:

A. Chronic fatigue syndrome
B. Normal aging
C. Sundowning
D. Delusions

QUESTION NUMBER 06.34
Question is about - confusion
Category of the Question - Psychosocial Integrity

The client with confusion says to the nurse, "I haven't had anything to eat all day long. When are they going to bring breakfast?" The nurse saw the client in the day room eating breakfast with other clients 30 minutes before this conversation. Which response would be best for the nurse to make?

A. "You know you had breakfast 30 minutes ago."
B. "I am so sorry that they didn't get you breakfast. I'll report it to the charge nurse."
C. "I'll get you some juice and toast. Would you like something else?"
D. "You will have to wait a while; lunch will be here in a little while."

QUESTION NUMBER 06.35
Question is about - Alzheimer's disease
Category of the Question - Physiological Integrity, Pharmacological and Parenteral Therapies

The doctor has prescribed Exelon (rivastigmine) for the client with Alzheimer's disease. Which side effect is most often associated with this drug?

A. Urinary incontinence
B. Headaches

C. Confusion
D. Nausea

QUESTION NUMBER 06.36
Question is about - labor
Category of the Question - Physiological Integrity, Reduction of Risk Potential

A client is admitted to the labor and delivery unit in active labor. During examination, the nurse notes a papular lesion on the perineum. Which initial action is most appropriate?

A. Document the finding
B. Report the finding to the doctor

C. Prepare the client for a C-section
D. Continue primary care as prescribed

QUESTION NUMBER 06.37
Question is about - human papillomavirus
Category of the Question - Physiological Integrity, Physiological Adaptation

A client with a diagnosis of HPV is at risk for which of the following?

A. Hodgkin's lymphoma
B. Cervical cancer

C. Multiple myeloma
D. Ovarian cancer

QUESTION NUMBER 06.38
Question is about - lesion, vulva
Category of the Question - Physiological integrity, Physiological Adaptation

During the initial interview, the client reports that she has a lesion on the perineum. Further investigation reveals a small blister on the vulva that is painful to touch. The nurse is aware that the most likely source of the lesion is:

A. Syphilis
B. Herpes

C. Gonorrhea
D. Condylomata

QUESTION NUMBER 06.39
Question is about - treponema pallidum
Category of the Question - Physiological Integrity, Physiological Adaptation

A client visiting a family planning clinic is suspected of having an STI. The best diagnostic test for treponema pallidum is:

A. Venereal Disease Research Lab (VDRL)
B. Rapid plasma reagin (RPR)

C. Fluorescent treponemal antibody (FTA)
D. Thayer-Martin culture (TMC)

QUESTION NUMBER 06.40
Question is about - HELLP syndrome
Category of the Question - Physiological Integrity, Reduction of Risk Potential

A 15-year-old primigravida is admitted with a tentative diagnosis of HELLP syndrome. Which laboratory finding is associated with HELLP syndrome?

A. Elevated blood glucose
B. Elevated platelet count

C. Elevated creatinine clearance
D. Elevated hepatic enzymes

QUESTION NUMBER 06.41
Question is about - preeclampsia
Category of the Question - Physiological Integrity, Reduction of Risk Potential

The nurse is assessing the deep tendon reflexes of a client with preeclampsia. Which method is used to elicit the biceps reflex?

A. The nurse places her thumb on the muscle inset in the antecubital space and taps the thumb briskly with the reflex hammer.
B. The nurse loosely suspends the client's arm in an open hand while tapping the back of the client's elbow.
C. The nurse instructs the client to dangle her legs as the nurse strikes the area below the patella with the blunt side of the reflex hammer.
D. The nurse instructs the client to place her arms loosely at her side as the nurse strikes the muscle insert just above the wrist.

QUESTION NUMBER 06.42
Question is about - diabetes, primigravida
Category of the Question - Safe and Effective Care Environment,, Safety and Infection Control

A primigravida with diabetes is admitted to the labor and delivery unit at 34 weeks gestation. Which doctor's order should the nurse question?

A. Magnesium sulfate 4gm (25%) IV
B. Brethine 10 mcg IV

C. Stadol 1 mg IV push every 4 hours as needed prn for pain
D. Ancef 2gm IVPB every 6 hours

QUESTION NUMBER 06.43
Question is about - amniocentesis
Category of the Question - Physiological Integrity, Reduction of Risk Potential

A diabetic multigravida is scheduled for an amniocentesis at 32 weeks gestation to determine the L/S ratio and phosphatidylglycerol level. The L/S ratio is 1:1 and the presence of phosphatidylglycerol is noted. The nurse's assessment of this data is:

A. The infant is at low risk for congenital anomalies.
B. The infant is at high risk for intrauterine growth retardation.
C. The infant is at high risk for respiratory distress syndrome.
D. The infant is at high risk for birth trauma.

QUESTION NUMBER 06.44
Question is about - diabetes
Category of the Question - Health Promotion and Maintenance

Which observation in the newborn of a diabetic mother would require immediate nursing intervention?

A. Crying
B. Wakefulness

C. Jitteriness
D. Yawning

QUESTION NUMBER 06.45
Question is about - magnesium sulfate
Category of the Question - Physiological Integrity, Pharmacological and Parenteral Therapies

The nurse caring for a client receiving intravenous magnesium sulfate must closely observe for side effects associated with drug therapy. An expected side effect of magnesium sulfate is:

A. Decreased urinary output
B. Hypersomnolence

C. Absence of knee jerk reflex
D. Decreased respiratory rate

QUESTION NUMBER 06.46
Question is about - epidural anesthesia
Category of the Question - Physiological Integrity, Reduction of Risk Potential

The client has elected to have epidural anesthesia to relieve labor pain. If the client experiences hypotension, the nurse would:

A. Place her in Trendelenburg position
B. Decrease the rate of IV infusion
C. Administer oxygen per nasal cannula
D. Increase the rate of the IV infusion

QUESTION NUMBER 06.47
Question is about - cancer of the pancreas
Category of the Question - Physiologic Integrity, Physiological Adaptation

A client has cancer of the pancreas. The nurse should be most concerned about which nursing diagnosis?

A. Alteration in nutrition
B. Alteration in bowel elimination

C. Alteration in skin integrity
D. Ineffective individual coping

QUESTION NUMBER 06.48
Question is about - ascites
Category of the Question - Physiological Integrity, Reduction of Risk Potential

The nurse is caring for a client with ascites. Which is the best method to use for determining early ascites?

A. Inspection of the abdomen for enlargement
B. Bimanual palpation for hepatomegaly
C. Daily measurement of abdominal girth
D. Assessment for a fluid wave

QUESTION NUMBER 06.49
Question is about - vehicle accident
Category of the Question - Physiological Integrity, Physiological Adaptation

The client arrives in the emergency department after a motor vehicle accident. Nursing assessment findings include BP 80/34, pulse rate 120, and respirations 20. Which is the client's most appropriate priority nursing diagnosis?

A. Alteration in cerebral tissue perfusion
B. Fluid volume deficit

C. Ineffective airway clearance
D. Alteration in sensory perception

QUESTION NUMBER 06.50
Question is about - osteogenesis imperfecta
Category of the Question - Safe and Effective Care Environment,, Safety and Infection Control

The home health nurse is visiting an 18-year-old with osteogenesis imperfecta. Which information obtained on the visit would cause the most concern? The client:

A. Likes to play football
B. Drinks several carbonated drinks per day

C. Has two sisters with sickle cell tract
D. Is taking acetaminophen to control pain

QUESTION NUMBER 06.51
Question is about - white blood cell count
Category of the Question - Physiological Integrity, Reduction of Risk Potential

The nurse working the organ transplant unit is caring for a client with a decreased white blood cell count. During evening visitation, a visitor brings a basket of fruit. What action should the nurse take?

A. Allow the client to keep the fruit
B. Place the fruit next to the bed for easy access by the client
C. Offer to wash the fruit for the client
D. Tell the family members to take the fruit home

QUESTION NUMBER 06.52
Question is about - laryngectomy
Category of the Question - Physiological Integrity, Physiological Adaptation

The nurse is caring for the client following a laryngectomy when suddenly the client becomes unresponsive and pale, with a BP of 90/40 systolic. The initial nurse's action should be to:

A. Place the client in Trendelenburg position
B. Increase the infusion of Dextrose in normal saline
C. Administer atropine intravenously
D. Move the emergency cart to the bedside

QUESTION NUMBER 06.53
Question is about - chest tube
Category of the Question - Physiological Integrity, Reduction of Risk Potential

The client admitted 2 days earlier that a lung resection accidentally pulls out the chest tube. Which action by the nurse indicates understanding of the management of chest tubes?

A. Order a chest x-ray
B. Reinsert the tube
C. Cover the insertion site with a Vaseline gauze
D. Call the doctor

QUESTION NUMBER 06.54
Question is about - sodium warfarin
Category of the Question - Physiological Integrity, Reduction of Risk Potential

A client being treated with sodium warfarin has a Protime of 120 seconds. Which intervention would be most important to include in the nursing care plan?

A. Assess for signs of abnormal bleeding
B. Anticipate an increase in the Coumadin dosage
C. Instruct the client regarding the drug therapy
D. Increase the frequency of neurological assessments

QUESTION NUMBER 06.55
Question is about - calcium
Category of the Question - Health Promotion and Maintenance

Which selection would provide the most calcium for the client who is 4 months pregnant?

A. A granola bar
B. A bran muffin
C. A cup of yogurt
D. A glass of fruit juice

QUESTION NUMBER 06.56
Question is about - preeclampsia, magnesium sulfate
Category of the Question - Physiological Integrity, Pharmacological and Parenteral Therapies

The client with preeclampsia is admitted to the unit with an order for magnesium sulfate. Which action by the nurse indicates understanding of the possible side effects of magnesium sulfate?

A. The nurse places a sign over the bed not to check blood pressure in the right arm.
B. The nurse places a padded tongue blade at the bedside.
C. The nurse inserts a Foley catheter.
D. The nurse darkens the room.

QUESTION NUMBER 06.57
Question is about - blood transfusion
Category of the Question - Safe and Effective Care Environment, Management of Care

A 6-year-old client is admitted to the unit with a hemoglobin of 6g/dL. The physician has written an order to transfuse 2 units of whole blood. When discussing the treatment, the child's mother tells the nurse that she does not believe in having blood transfusions and that she will not allow her child to have the treatment. What nursing action is most appropriate?

A. Ask the mother to leave while the blood transfusion is in progress
B. Encourage the mother to reconsider
C. Explain the consequences without treatment
D. Notify the physician of the mother's refusal

QUESTION NUMBER 06.58
Question is about - burns
Category of the Question - Physiological Integrity, Physiological Adaptation

A client is admitted to the unit 2 hours after an explosion causes burns to the face. The nurse would be most concerned with the client developing which of the following?

A. Hypovolemia
B. Laryngeal edema

C. Hypernatremia
D. Hyperkalemia

QUESTION NUMBER 06.59
Question is about - anorexia nervosa
Category of the Question - Health Promotion and Maintenance, Physiological Adaptation

The nurse is evaluating nutritional outcomes for a patient with anorexia nervosa. Which data best indicates that the plan of care is effective?

A. The client selects a balanced diet from the menu.
B. The client's hemoglobin and hematocrit improve.
C. The client's tissue turgor improves.
D. The client gains weight.

QUESTION NUMBER 06.60
Question is about - fracture, cast application
Category of the Question - Physiological Integrity, Physiological Adaptation

The client is admitted following repair of a fractured tibia and cast application. Which nursing assessment should be reported to the doctor?

A. Pain beneath the cast

B. Warm toes

C. Pedal pulses weak and rapid

D. Paresthesia of the toes

QUESTION NUMBER 06.61
Question is about - barbiturates
Category of the Question - Psychosocial Integrity

A client with a history of abusing barbiturates abruptly stops taking the medication. The nurse should give priority to assessing the client for:

A. Depression and suicidal ideation

B. Tachycardia and diarrhea

C. Muscle cramping and abdominal pain

D. Tachycardia and euphoric mood

QUESTION NUMBER 06.62
Question is about - labor, FHT
Category of the Question - Physiological Integrity, Physiological Adaptation

During the assessment of a laboring client, the nurse notes that the FHT are loudest in the upper-right quadrant. The infant is most likely in which position?

A. Right breech presentation

B. Right occiput anterior presentation

C. Left sacral anterior presentation

D. Left occiput transverse presentation

QUESTION NUMBER 06.63
Question is about - asthma
Category of the Question - Physiological Integrity, Physiological Adaptation

The primary physiological alteration in the development of asthma is:

A. Bronchial inflammation and dyspnea

B. Hypersecretion of abnormally viscous mucus

C. Infectious processes causing mucosal edema

D. Spasm of bronchial smooth muscle

QUESTION NUMBER 06.64
Question is about - mania
Category of the Question - Physiological Integrity, Basic Care and Comfort

A client with mania is unable to finish her dinner. To help her maintain sufficient nourishment, the nurse should:

A. Serve high-calorie foods she can carry with her

B. Encourage her appetite by sending out for her favorite foods

C. Serve her small, attractively arranged portions

D. Allow her in the unit kitchen for extra food whenever she pleases

QUESTION NUMBER 06.65
Question is about - Bryant's traction
Category of the Question - Physiological Integrity, Basic Care and CoMFORT

To maintain Bryant's traction, the nurse must make certain that the child's:

A. Hips are resting on the bed, with the legs suspended at a right angle to the bed
B. Hips are slightly elevated above the bed and the legs are suspended at a right angle to the bed
C. Hips are elevated above the level of the body on a pillow and the legs are suspended parallel to the bed
D. Hips and legs are flat on the bed, with the traction positioned at the foot of the bed

QUESTION NUMBER 06.66
Question is about - herpes zoster
Category of the Question - Physiological Integrity, Reduction of Risk Potential

Which action by the nurse indicates understanding of herpes zoster?

A. The nurse covers the lesions with a sterile dressing.
B. The nurse wears gloves when providing care.
C. The nurse administers a prescribed antibiotic.
D. The nurse administers oxygen.

QUESTION NUMBER 06.67
Question is about - Vancomycin
Category of the Question - Physiological Integrity, Reduction of Risk Potential

The client has an order for a trough to be drawn on the client receiving Vancomycin. The nurse is aware that the nurse should contact the lab for them to collect the blood:

A. 15 minutes after the infusion
B. 30 minutes before the infusion

C. 1 hour after the infusion
D. 2 hours after the infusion

QUESTION NUMBER 06.68
Question is about - diaphragm
Category of the Question - Health Promotion and Maintenance

The client using a diaphragm should be instructed to:

A. Refrain from keeping the diaphragm in longer than 4 hours
B. Keep the diaphragm in a cool location
C. Have the diaphragm resized if she gains 5 pounds
D. Have the diaphragm resized if she has any surgery

QUESTION NUMBER 06.69
Question is about - postpartum, breastfeeding
Category of the Question - Health Promotion and Maintenance

The nurse is providing postpartum teaching for a mother planning to breastfeed her infant. Which of the client's statements indicates the need for additional teaching?

A. "I'm wearing a support bra."
B. "I'm expressing milk from my breast."
C. "I'm drinking four glasses of fluid during a 24-hour period."
D. "While I'm in the shower, I'll allow the water to run over my breasts."

QUESTION NUMBER 06.70
Question is about - cranial nerve VII
Category of the Question - Physiological Integrity, Physiological Adaptation

Damage to the VII cranial nerve results in:

A. Facial pain
B. Absence of ability to smell

C. Absence of eye movement
D. Tinnitus

QUESTION NUMBER 06.71
Question is about - urinary tract infection
Category of the Question - Physiological Integrity, Pharmacological and Parenteral Therapies

A client is receiving Pyridium (phenazopyridine hydrochloride) for a urinary tract infection. The client should be taught that the medication may:

A. Cause diarrhea
B. Change the color of her urine

C. Cause mental confusion
D. Cause changes in taste

QUESTION NUMBER 06.72
Question is about - Accutane
Category of the Question - Physiological Integrity, Reduction of Risk Potential

Which of the following tests should be performed before beginning a prescription of Accutane?

A. Check the calcium level
B. Perform a pregnancy test

C. Monitor apical pulse
D. Obtain a creatinine level

QUESTION NUMBER 06.73
Question is about - AIDS, acyclovir
Category of the Question - Physiological Integrity, Pharmacological and Parenteral Therapies

A client with AIDS is taking Zovirax (acyclovir). Which nursing intervention is most critical during the administration of acyclovir?

A. Limit the client's activity
B. Encourage a high-carbohydrate diet
C. Utilize an incentive spirometer to improve respiratory function
D. Encourage fluids

QUESTION NUMBER 06.74
Question is about - MRI
Question Category : Physiological Integrity, Reduction of Risk Potential

A client is admitted for an MRI. The nurse should question the client regarding:

A. Pregnancy
B. A titanium hip replacement

C. Allergies to antibiotics
D. Inability to move his feet

QUESTION NUMBER 06.75
Question is about - Amphotericin B
Category of the Question - Physiological Integrity, Pharmacological and Parenteral Therapies

The nurse is caring for the client receiving Amphotericin B. Which of the following indicates that the client has experienced toxicity to this drug?

A. Changes in vision
B. Nausea

C. Urinary frequency
D. Changes in skin color

Practice Question Set-7

QUESTION NUMBER 07.01
Question is about - Parkinson's disease
Category of the Question - Safe and Effective Care Environment, Management of Care

A patient with Parkinson's disease has a nursing diagnosis of Impaired Physical Mobility related to neuromuscular impairment. You observe a nursing assistant performing all of these actions. For which action must you intervene?

A. The NA assists the patient to ambulate to the bathroom and back to bed.
B. The NA reminds the patient not to look at his feet when he is walking.
C. The NA performs the patient's complete bath and oral care.
D. The NA sets up the patient's tray and encourages the patient to feed himself.

QUESTION NUMBER 07.02
Question is about - low back pain
Category of the Question - Health Promotion and Maintenance

The nurse is preparing to discharge a patient with chronic low back pain. Which statement by the patient indicates that additional teaching is necessary?

A. "I will avoid exercise because the pain gets worse."
B. "I will use heat or ice to help control the pain."

C. "I will not wear high-heeled shoes at home or work."
D. "I will purchase a firm mattress to replace my old one."

QUESTION NUMBER 07.03
Question is about - Spinal cord injury
Category of the Question - Physiological Integrity, Physiological Adaptation

A patient with a spinal cord injury (SCI) complains about a severe throbbing headache that suddenly started a short time ago. Assessment of the patient reveals increased blood pressure (168/94) and decreased heart rate (48/minute), diaphoresis, and flushing of the face and neck. What action should you take first?

    A. Administer the ordered acetaminophen (Tylenol).
    B. Check the Foley tubing for kinks or obstruction.
    C. Adjust the temperature in the patient's room.
    D. Notify the physician about the change in status.

QUESTION NUMBER 07.04
Question is about - Neurologic unit
Category of the Question - Safe and Effective Care Environment, Management of Care

Which patient should you, as charge nurse, assign to a new graduate RN who is orienting to the neurologic unit?

    A. A 28-year-old newly admitted patient with spinal cord injury.
    B. A 67-year-old patient with a stroke 3 days ago and left-sided weakness.
    C. An 85-year-old dementia patient to be transferred to long-term care today.
    D. A 54-year-old patient with Parkinson's who needs assistance with bathing.

QUESTION NUMBER 07.05
Question is about - Spinal cord injury
Category of the Question - Physiological Integrity, Physiological Adaptation

A patient with a spinal cord injury at level C3-4 is being cared for in the ED. What is the priority assessment?

    A. Determine the level at which the patient has intact sensation.
    B. Assess the level at which the patient has retained mobility.
    C. Check blood pressure and pulse for signs of spinal shock.
    D. Monitor respiratory effort and oxygen saturation level.

QUESTION NUMBER 07.06
Question is about - delegation
Category of the Question - Safe and Effective Care Environment, Management of Care

You are pulled from the ED to the neurologic floor. Which action should you delegate to the nursing assistant when providing nursing care for a patient with SCI?

    A. Assess the patient's respiratory status every 4 hours.
    B. Take a patient's vital signs and record them every 4 hours.
    C. Monitor nutritional status including calorie counts.
    D. Have the patient turn, cough, and deep breathe every 3 hours.

QUESTION NUMBER 07.07
Question is about - spinal cord injury
Category of the Question - Basic Care and Comfort

You are helping the patient with an SCI to establish a bladder-retraining program. What strategies may stimulate the patient to void? Select all that apply.

A. Stroke the patient's inner thigh.

B. Pull on the patient's pubic hair.

C. Initiate intermittent straight catheterization.

D. Pour warm water over the perineum.

E. Tap the bladder to stimulate detrusor muscle.

Correct Answers: A, B, D, and E

All of the strategies, except straight catheterization, may stimulate voiding in patients with SCI.

Option C: Intermittent bladder catheterization can be used to empty the patient's bladder, but it will not stimulate voiding.

QUESTION NUMBER 07.08
Question is about - cervical SCI
Category of the Question - Safe and Effective Care Environment, Management of Care

The patient with a cervical SCI has been placed in fixed skeletal traction with a halo fixation device. When caring for this patient the nurse may delegate which action (s) to the LPN/LVN? Select all that apply.

A. Check the patient's skin for pressure from the device.

B. Assess the patient's neurologic status for changes.

C. Observe the halo insertion sites for signs of infection.

D. Clean the halo insertion sites with hydrogen peroxide.

QUESTION NUMBER 07.09
Question is about - SCI
Category of the Question - Physiological Integrity, Physiological Adaptation

You are preparing a nursing care plan for the patient with SCI including the nursing diagnosis Impaired Physical Mobility and Self-Care Deficit. The patient tells you, "I don't know why we're doing all this. My life's over." What additional nursing diagnosis takes priority based on this statement?

A. Risk for Injury related to altered mobility

B. Imbalanced Nutrition, Less Than Body Requirements

C. Impaired Adjustment to Spinal Cord Injury

D. Poor Body Image related to immobilization

QUESTION NUMBER 07.10
Question is about - neurologic care
Category of the Question - Safe and Effective Care Environment, Management of Care

Which patient should be assigned to the traveling nurse, new to neurologic nursing care, who has been in the neurologic unit for 1 week?

A. A 34-year-old patient newly diagnosed with multiple sclerosis (MS).

B. A 68-year-old patient with chronic amyotrophic lateral sclerosis (ALS).

C. A 56-year-old patient with Guillain-Barre syndrome (GBS) in respiratory distress.

D. A 25-year-old patient admitted with CA level spinal cord injury (SCI).

144

QUESTION NUMBER 07.11
Question is about - multiple sclerosis
Category of the Question - Physiological Integrity, Basic Care and Comfort

The patient with multiple sclerosis tells the nursing assistant that after physical therapy she is too tired to take a bath. What is your priority nursing diagnosis at this time?

   A. Fatigue related to disease state
   B. Activity Intolerance due to generalized weakness
   C. Impaired Physical Mobility related to neuromuscular impairment
   D. Self-care Deficit related to fatigue and neuromuscular weakness

QUESTION NUMBER 07.12
Question is about - GBS
Category of the Question - Physiological Integrity, Reduction of Risk Potential

The LPN/LVN, under your supervision, is providing nursing care for a patient with GBS. What observation would you instruct the LPN/LVN to report immediately?

   A. Complaints of numbness and tingling.
   B. Facial weakness and difficulty speaking.
   C. Rapid heart rate of 102 beats per minute.
   D. Shallow respirations and decreased breath sounds.

QUESTION NUMBER 07.13
Question is about - myasthenia gravis
Category of the Question - Physiological Adaptation

The nursing assistant reports to you, the RN, that the patient with myasthenia gravis (MG) has an elevated temperature (102.20 F), heart rate of 120/minute, rise in blood pressure (158/94), and was incontinent of urine and stool. What is your best first action at this time?

   A. Administer an acetaminophen suppository
   B. Notify the physician immediately
   C. Recheck vital signs in 1 hour
   D. Reschedule patient's physical therapy session

QUESTION NUMBER 07.14
Question is about - acute hemorrhagic stroke
Category of the Question - Physiological Integrity, Pharmacological and Parenteral Therapies

You are providing care for a patient with an acute hemorrhage stroke. The patient's husband has been reading a lot about strokes and asks why his wife did not receive alteplase. What is your best response?

   A. "Your wife was not admitted within the time frame that alteplase is usually given."
   B. "This drug is used primarily for patients who experience an acute heart attack."
   C. "Alteplase dissolves clots and may cause more bleeding into your wife's brain."
   D. "Your wife had gallbladder surgery just 6 months ago and this prevents the use of alteplase."

QUESTION NUMBER 07.15
Question is about - right hemisphere stroke
Category of the Question - Safe and Effective Care Environment, Management of Care

You are supervising a senior nursing student who is caring for a patient with a right hemisphere stroke. Which action by the student nurse requires that you intervene?

A. The student instructs the patient to sit up straight, resulting in the patient's puzzled expression.
B. The student moves the patient's tray to the right side of her over-bed tray.
C. The student assists the patient with passive range-of-motion (ROM) exercises.
D. The student combs the left side of the patient's hair when the patient combs only the right side.

QUESTION NUMBER 07.16
Question is about - arteries
Category of the Question - Physiological Integrity, Physiological Adaptation

Which of the following arteries primarily feeds the anterior wall of the heart?

A. Circumflex artery
B. Internal mammary artery

C. Left anterior descending artery
D. Right coronary artery

QUESTION NUMBER 07.17
Question is about - coronary arteries
Category of the Question - Physiological Integrity, Physiological Adaptation

When do coronary arteries primarily receive blood flow?

A. During inspiration
B. During diastole

C. During expiration
D. During systole

QUESTION NUMBER 07.18
Question is about - cause of death
Category of the Question - Health Promotion and Maintenance

Which of the following illnesses is the leading cause of death in the US?

A. Cancer
B. Coronary artery disease

C. Liver failure
D. Renal failure

QUESTION NUMBER 07.19
Question is about - coronary artery disease
Category of the Question - Physiological Integrity, Physiological Adaptation

Which of the following conditions most commonly results in CAD?

A. Atherosclerosis
B. DM

C. MI
D. Renal failure

QUESTION NUMBER 07.20
Question is about - atherosclerosis
Category of the Question - Physiological Integrity, Physiological Adaptation

Atherosclerosis impedes coronary blood flow by which of the following mechanisms?

A. Plaques obstruct the vein
B. Plaques obstruct the artery
C. Blood clots form outside the vessel wall
D. Hardened vessels dilate to allow the blood to flow through

QUESTION NUMBER 07.21
Question is about - coronary artery disease
Category of the Question - Health Promotion and Maintenance

Which of the following risk factors for coronary artery disease cannot be corrected?

A. Cigarette smoking
B. DM
C. Heredity
D. HPN

QUESTION NUMBER 07.22
Question is about - cholesterol, coronary artery disease
Category of the Question - Physiological Integrity, Reduction of Risk Potential

Exceeding which of the following serum cholesterol levels significantly increases the risk of coronary artery disease?

A. 100 mg/dl
B. 150 mg/dl
C. 175 mg/dl
D. 200 mg/dl

QUESTION NUMBER 07.23
Question is about - coronary artery disease
Category of the Question - Physiological Integrity, Physiological Adaptation

Which of the following actions is the first priority care for a client exhibiting signs and symptoms of coronary artery disease?

A. Decrease anxiety
B. Enhance myocardial oxygenation
C. Administer sublingual nitroglycerin
D. Educate the client about his symptoms

QUESTION NUMBER 07.24
Question is about - coronary artery disease
Category of the Question - Physiological Integrity, Physiological Adaptation

Medical treatment of coronary artery disease includes which of the following procedures?

A. Cardiac catheterization
B. Coronary artery bypass surgery
C. Oral medication administration
D. Percutaneous transluminal coronary angioplasty

QUESTION NUMBER 07.25
Question is about - infarction
Category of the Question - Physiological Integrity, Physiological Adaptation

Prolonged occlusion of the right coronary artery produces an infarction in which of the following areas of the heart?

A. Anterior
B. Apical

C. Inferior
D. Lateral

QUESTION NUMBER 07.26
Question is about - myocardial infarction
Category of the Question - Physiological Integrity, Physiological Adaptation

Which of the following is the most common symptom of myocardial infarction?

A. Chest pain
B. Dyspnea

C. Edema
D. Palpitations

QUESTION NUMBER 07.27
Question is about - apical pulse
Category of the Question - Physiological Integrity, Physiological Adaptation

Which of the following landmarks is the correct one for obtaining an apical pulse?

A. Left intercostal space, midaxillary line
B. Left fifth intercostal space, midclavicular line
C. Left second intercostal space, midclavicular line
D. Left seventh intercostal space, midclavicular line

QUESTION NUMBER 07.28
Question is about - pain
Category of the Question - Physiological Integrity, Physiological Adaptation

Which of the following systems is the most likely origin of pain the client describes as knifelike chest pain that increases in intensity with inspiration?

A. Cardiac
B. Gastrointestinal

C. Musculoskeletal
D. Pulmonary

QUESTION NUMBER 07.29
Question is about - heart murmurs
Category of the Question - Physiological Integrity, Physiological Adaptation

A murmur is heard at the second left intercostal space along the left sternal border. Which valve area is this?

A. Aortic
B. Mitral

C. Pulmonic
D. Tricuspid

QUESTION NUMBER 07.30
Question is about - cardiac damage
Category of the Question - Physiological Integrity, Reduction of Risk Potential

Which of the following blood tests is most indicative of cardiac damage?

A. Lactate dehydrogenase
B. Complete blood count

C. Troponin I
D. Creatine kinase

QUESTION NUMBER 07.31
Question is about - morphine, myocardial infarction
Category of the Question - Physiological Integrity, Pharmacological and Parenteral therapies

What is the primary reason for administering morphine to a client with myocardial infarction?

A. To sedate the client
B. To decrease the client's pain
C. To decrease the client's anxiety
D. To decrease oxygen demand on the client's heart

QUESTION NUMBER 07.32
Question is about - myocardial infarction
Category of the Question - Physiological Integrity, Physiological Adaptation

Which of the following conditions is most commonly responsible for myocardial infarction?

A. Aneurysm
B. Heart failure

C. Coronary artery thrombosis
D. Renal failure

QUESTION NUMBER 07.33
Question is about - furosemide
Category of the Question - Physiological Integrity, Pharmacological and Parenteral therapies

What supplemental medication is most frequently ordered in conjunction with furosemide (Lasix)?

A. Chloride
B. Digoxin

C. Potassium
D. Sodium

QUESTION NUMBER 07.34
Question is about - glucose, fatty acids
Category of the Question - Physiological Integrity, Physiological Adaptation

After myocardial infarction, serum glucose levels and free fatty acids are both increased. What type of physiologic changes are these?

A. Electrophysiologic
B. Hematologic

C. Mechanical
D. Metabolic

QUESTION NUMBER 07.35
Question is about - heart sounds
Category of the Question - Physiological Integrity, Physiological Adaptation

Which of the following complications is indicated by a third heart sound (S3)?

A. Ventricular dilation

B. Systemic hypertension

C. Aortic valve malfunction

D. Increased atrial contractions

QUESTION NUMBER 07.36
Question is about - crackles
Category of the Question - Physiological Integrity, Physiological Adaptation

After an anterior wall myocardial infarction, which of the following problems is indicated by auscultation of crackles in the lungs?

A. Left-sided heart failure

B. Pulmonic valve malfunction

C. Right-sided heart failure

D. Tricuspid valve malfunction

QUESTION NUMBER 07.37
Question is about - myocardial damage
Category of the Question - Physiological Integrity, Reduction of Risk Potential

Which of the following diagnostic tools is most commonly used to determine the location of myocardial damage?

A. Cardiac catheterization

B. Cardiac enzymes

C. Echocardiogram

D. Electrocardiogram

QUESTION NUMBER 07.38
Question is about - myocardial infarction
Category of the Question - Physiological Integrity, Physiological Adaptation

What is the first intervention for a client experiencing myocardial infarction?

A. Administer morphine

B. Administer oxygen

C. Administer sublingual nitroglycerin

D. Obtain an electrocardiogram

QUESTION NUMBER 07.39
Question is about - myocardial infarction
Category of the Question - Psychosocial Integrity

What is the most appropriate nursing response to a myocardial infarction client who is fearful of dying?

A. "Tell me about your feelings right now."
B. "When the doctor arrives, everything will be fine."
C. "This is a bad situation, but you'll feel better soon."
D. "Please be assured we're doing everything we can to make you feel better."

QUESTION NUMBER 07.40
Question is about - ischemic myocardium
Category of the Question - Physiological Integrity, Pharmacological and Parenteral therapies

Which of the following classes of medications protects the ischemic myocardium by blocking catecholamines and sympathetic nerve stimulation?

A. Beta-adrenergic blockers
B. Calcium channel blockers

C. Narcotics
D. Nitrates

QUESTION NUMBER 07.41
Question is about - myocardial infarction
Category of the Question - Physiological Integrity, Physiological Adaptation

What is the most common complication of a myocardial infarction?

A. Cardiogenic shock
B. Heart failure

C. Arrhythmias
D. Pericarditis

QUESTION NUMBER 07.42
Question is about - jugular vein distention
Category of the Question - Physiological Integrity, Physiological Adaptation

With which of the following disorders is jugular vein distention most prominent?

A. Abdominal aortic aneurysm
B. Heart failure

C. Myocardial infarction
D. Pneumothorax

QUESTION NUMBER 07.43
Question is about - jugular vein distention
Category of the Question - Physiological Integrity, Physiological Adaptation

What position should the nurse place the head of the bed in to obtain the most accurate reading of jugular vein distention?

A. High-Fowler's
B. Raised 10 degrees

C. Raised 30 degrees
D. Supine position

QUESTION NUMBER 07.44
Question is about - digoxin
Category of the Question - Physiological Integrity, Pharmacological and Parenteral therapies

Which of the following parameters should be checked before administering digoxin?

A. Apical pulse
B. Blood pressure

C. Radial pulse
D. Respiratory rate

QUESTION NUMBER 07.45
Question is about - toxicity
Category of the Question - Physiological Integrity, Pharmacological and Parenteral therapies

Toxicity from which of the following medications may cause a client to see a green halo around lights?

A. Digoxin
B. Furosemide

C. Metoprolol
D. Enalapril

QUESTION NUMBER 07.46
Question is about - heart failure
Category of the Question - Physiological Integrity, Physiological Adaptation

Which of the following symptoms is most commonly associated with left-sided heart failure?

A. Crackles
B. Arrhythmias

C. Hepatic engorgement
D. Hypotension

QUESTION NUMBER 07.47
Question is about - sacral edema
Category of the Question - Physiological Integrity, Physiological Adaptation

In which of the following disorders would the nurse expect to assess sacral edema in bedridden client?

A. DM
B. Pulmonary emboli

C. Renal failure
D. Right-sided heart failure

QUESTION NUMBER 07.48
Question is about - right-sided heart failure
Category of the Question - Physiological Integrity, Physiological Adaptation

Which of the following symptoms might a client with right-sided heart failure exhibit?

A. Adequate urine output
B. Polyuria

C. Oliguria
D. Polydipsia

QUESTION NUMBER 07.49
Question is about - ventricular contractility
Category of the Question - Physiological Integrity, Pharmacological and Parenteral Therapies

Which of the following classes of medications maximizes cardiac performance in clients with heart failure by increasing ventricular contractility?

A. Beta-adrenergic blockers
B. Calcium channel blockers

C. Diuretics
D. Inotropic agents

QUESTION NUMBER 07.50
Question is about - sympathetic nervous system
Category of the Question - Physiological Integrity, Physiological Adaptation

Stimulation of the sympathetic nervous system produces which of the following responses?

A. Bradycardia

B. Tachycardia

C. Hypotension

D. Decreased myocardial contractility

QUESTION NUMBER 07.51
Question is about - heart failure
Category of the Question - Physiological Integrity, Physiological Adaptation

Which of the following conditions is most closely associated with weight gain, nausea, and a decrease in urine output?

A. Angina pectoris

B. Cardiomyopathy

C. Left-sided heart failure

D. Right-sided heart failure

QUESTION NUMBER 07.52
Question is about - abdominal aortic aneurysm
Category of the Question - Physiological Integrity, Physiological Adaptation

What is the most common cause of abdominal aortic aneurysm?

A. Atherosclerosis

B. DM

C. HPN

D. Syphilis

QUESTION NUMBER 07.53
Question is about - abdominal aortic aneurysm
Category of the Question - Physiological Integrity, Physiological Adaptation

In which of the following areas is an abdominal aortic aneurysm most commonly located?

A. Distal to the iliac arteries
B. Distal to the renal arteries
C. Adjacent to the aortic branch
D. Proximal to the renal arteries

QUESTION NUMBER 07.54
Question is about - abdominal mass
Category of the Question - Physiological Integrity, Physiological Adaptation

A pulsating abdominal mass usually indicates which of the following conditions?

A. Abdominal aortic aneurysm

B. Enlarged spleen

C. Gastric distention

D. Gastritis

QUESTION NUMBER 07.55
Question is about - abdominal aortic aneurysm
Category of the Question - Physiological Integrity, Physiological Adaptation

What is the most common symptom in a client with abdominal aortic aneurysm?

A. Abdominal pain

B. Diaphoresis

C. Headache

D. Upper back pain

QUESTION NUMBER 07.56
Question is about - abdominal aortic aneurysm
Category of the Question - Physiological Integrity, Physiological Adaptation

Which of the following symptoms usually signifies rapid expansion and impending rupture of an abdominal aortic aneurysm?

A. Abdominal pain

B. Absent pedal pulses

C. Angina

D. Lower back pain

QUESTION NUMBER 07.57
Question is about - abdominal aortic aneurysm
Category of the Question - Physiological Integrity, Reduction of Risk Potential

What is the definitive test used to diagnose an abdominal aortic aneurysm?

A. Abdominal X-ray

B. Arteriogram

C. CT scan

D. Ultrasound

QUESTION NUMBER 07.58
Question is about - abdominal aneurysm
Category of the Question - Physiological Integrity, Reduction of Risk Potential

Which of the following complications is of greatest concern when caring for a preoperative abdominal aneurysm client?

A. HPN

B. Aneurysm rupture

C. Cardiac arrhythmias

D. Diminished pedal pulses

QUESTION NUMBER 07.59
Question is about - aneurysm
Category of the Question - Physiological Integrity, Physiological Adaptation

Which of the following blood vessel layers may be damaged in a client with an aneurysm?

A. Externa

B. Interna

C. Media

D. Interna and Media

QUESTION NUMBER 07.60
Question is about - abdominal aortic aneurysm
Category of the Question - Health Promotion and Maintenance

When assessing a client for an abdominal aortic aneurysm, which area of the abdomen is most commonly palpated?

A. Right upper quadrant

B. Directly over the umbilicus

C. Middle lower abdomen to the left of the midline

D. Midline lower abdomen to the right of the midline

QUESTION NUMBER 07.61
Question is about - aneurysm
Category of the Question - Health Promotion and Maintenance

Which of the following conditions is linked to more than 50% of clients with abdominal aortic aneurysms?

A. DM

B. HPN

C. PVD

D. Syphilis

QUESTION NUMBER 07.62
Question is about - auscultation
Category of the Question - Health Promotion and Maintenance

Which of the following sounds is distinctly heard on auscultation over the abdominal region of an abdominal aortic aneurysm client?

A. Bruit

B. Crackles

C. Dullness

D. Friction rubs

QUESTION NUMBER 07.63
Question is about - ruptured abdominal aneurysm
Category of the Question - Physiological Integrity, Physiological Adaptation

Which of the following groups of symptoms indicated a ruptured abdominal aneurysm?

A. Lower back pain, increased BP, decreased RBC, increased WBC

B. Severe lower back pain, decreased BP, decreased RBC, increased WBC

C. Severe lower back pain, decreased BP, decreased RBC, decreased WBC

D. Intermittent lower back pain, decreased BP, decreased RBC, increased WBC

QUESTION NUMBER 07.64
Question is about - hematoma
Category of the Question - Physiological Integrity, Reduction of Risk Potential

Which of the following complications of an abdominal aortic repair is indicated by detection of a hematoma in the perineal area?

A. Hernia

B. Stage 1 pressure ulcer

C. Retroperitoneal rupture at the repair site

D. Rapid expansion of the aneurysm

QUESTION NUMBER 07.65

Question is about - aneurysm

Category of the Question - Physiological Integrity, Physiological Adaptation

Which hereditary disease is most closely linked to aneurysm?

A. Cystic fibrosis

B. Lupus erythematosus

C. Marfan's syndrome

D. Myocardial infarction

QUESTION NUMBER 07.66

Question is about - ruptured aneurysm

Category of the Question - Physiological Integrity, Physiological Adaptation

Which of the following treatments is the definitive one for a ruptured aneurysm?

A. Antihypertensive medication administration

B. Aortogram

C. Beta-adrenergic blocker administration

D. Surgical intervention

QUESTION NUMBER 07.67

Question is about - cardiovascular diseases

Category of the Question - Physiological Integrity, Reduction of Risk Potential

Which of the following heart muscle diseases is unrelated to other cardiovascular diseases?

A. Cardiomyopathy

B. Coronary artery disease

C. Myocardial infarction

D. Pericardial Effusion

QUESTION NUMBER 07.68

Question is about - cardiomyopathy

Category of the Question - Physiological Integrity, Physiological Adaptation

Which of the following types of cardiomyopathy can be associated with childbirth?

A. Dilated

B. Hypertrophic

C. Myocarditis

D. Restrictive

QUESTION NUMBER 07.69

Question is about - cardiomyopathy

Category of the Question - Physiological Integrity, Physiological Adaptation

Septal involvement occurs in which type of cardiomyopathy?

A. Congestive

B. Dilated

C. Hypertrophic

D. Restrictive

QUESTION NUMBER 07.70
Question is about - cardiomyopathy
Category of the Question - Physiological Integrity, Physiological Adaptation

Which of the following recurring conditions most commonly occurs in clients with cardiomyopathy?

A. Heart failure

B. DM

C. MI

D. Pericardial effusion

QUESTION NUMBER 07.71
Question is about - heart muscle
Category of the Question - Physiological Integrity, Physiological Adaptation

What is the term used to describe an enlargement of the heart muscle?

A. Cardiomegaly

B. Cardiomyopathy

C. Myocarditis

D. Pericarditis

QUESTION NUMBER 07.72
Question is about - heart failure
Category of the Question - Physiological Integrity, Physiological Adaptation

Dyspnea, cough, expectoration, weakness, and edema are classic signs and symptoms of which of the following conditions?

A. Pericarditis

B. Hypertension

C. Obliterative

D. Restrictive

QUESTION NUMBER 07.73
Question is about - cardiomyopathy
Category of the Question - Physiological Integrity, Physiological Adaptation

Which of the following types of cardiomyopathy does not affect cardiac output?

A. Dilated

B. Hypertrophic

C. Restrictive

D. Obliterative

QUESTION NUMBER 07.74
Question is about - heart sounds
Category of the Question - Physiological Integrity, Physiological Adaptation

Which of the following cardiac conditions does a fourth heart sound (S4) indicate?

A. Dilated aorta
B. Normally functioning heart
C. Decreased myocardial contractility
D. Failure of the ventricle to eject all the blood during systole

QUESTION NUMBER 07.75
Question is about - cardiomyopathy
Category of the Question - Pharmacological and Parenteral Therapies

Which of the following classes of drugs is most widely used in the treatment of cardiomyopathy?

A. Antihypertensive
B. Beta-adrenergic blockers
C. Calcium channel blockers
D. Nitrates

Practice Question Set-8

QUESTION NUMBER 08.01
Question is about - prioritization
Category of the Question - Safe and Effective Care Environment, Management of Care

The nurse should visit which of the following clients first?

A. The client with diabetes with a blood glucose of 95 mg/dL
B. The client with hypertension being maintained on Lisinopril
C. The client with chest pain and a history of angina
D. The client with Raynaud's disease

QUESTION NUMBER 08.02
Question is about - cystic fibrosis
Category of the Question - Physiological Integrity, Pharmacological and Parenteral Therapies

A client with cystic fibrosis is taking pancreatic enzymes. The nurse should administer this medication:

A. Once per day in the morning
B. Three times per day with meals
C. Once per day at bedtime
D. Four times per day

QUESTION NUMBER 08.03
Question is about - cataract
Category of the Question - Physiological Integrity, Physiological Adaptation

Cataracts result in opacity of the crystalline lens. Which of the following best explains the functions of the lens?

A. The lens controls stimulation of the retina.
B. The lens orchestrates eye movement.
C. The lens focuses light rays on the retina.
D. The lens magnifies small objects.

QUESTION NUMBER 08.04
Question is about - glaucoma, miotic eye drops
Category of the Question - Physiological Integrity, Pharmacological and Parenteral Therapies

A client who has glaucoma is to have miotic eye drops instilled in both eyes. The nurse knows that the purpose of the medication is to:

A. Anesthetize the cornea

B. Dilate the pupils

C. Constrict the pupils

D. Paralyze the muscles of accommodation

QUESTION NUMBER 08.05
Question is about - corneal ulcer
Category of the Question - Physiological Integrity, Pharmacological and Parenteral Therapies

A client with a severe corneal ulcer has an order for Gentamicin gtt. q 4 hours and Neomycin 1 gtt q 4 hours. Which of the following schedules should be used when administering the drops?

A. Allow 5 minutes between the two medications.

B. The medications may be used together.

C. The medications should be separated by a cycloplegic drug.

D. The medications should not be used in the same client.

QUESTION NUMBER 08.06
Question is about - color blindness
Category of the Question - Physiological Integrity, Physiological Adaptation

The client with color blindness will most likely have problems distinguishing which of the following colors?

A. Orange

B. Violet

C. Red

D. White

QUESTION NUMBER 08.07
Question is about - pacemaker
Category of the Question - Health Promotion and Maintenance

The client with a pacemaker should be taught to:

A. Report ankle edema

B. Check his blood pressure daily

C. Refrain from using a microwave oven

D. Monitor his pulse rate

QUESTION NUMBER 08.08
Question is about - enuresis
Category of the Question - Health Promotion and Maintenance

The client with enuresis is being taught regarding bladder retraining. The nurse should advise the client to refrain from drinking after:

A. 1900

B. 1200

C. 1000

D. 0700

QUESTION NUMBER 08.09
Question is about - urinary tract infection
Category of the Question - Health Promotion and Maintenance

Which of the following diet instructions should be given to the client with recurring urinary tract infections?

A. Increase intake of meat.
B. Avoid citrus fruits.
C. Perform peri care with hydrogen peroxide.
D. Drink a glass of cranberry juice every day.

QUESTION NUMBER 08.10
Question is about - insulin, diabetes mellitus
Category of the Question - Health Promotion and Maintenance

The physician has prescribed NPH insulin for a client with diabetes mellitus. Which statement indicates that the client knows when the peak action of the insulin occurs?

A. "I will make sure I eat breakfast within 2 hours of taking my insulin."
B. "I will need to carry candy or some form of sugar with me all the time."
C. "I will eat a snack around three o'clock each afternoon."
D. "I can save my dessert from supper for a bedtime snack."

QUESTION NUMBER 08.11
Question is about - chest tube
Category of the Question - Physiological Integrity, Physiological Adaptation

The nurse is caring for a 30-year-old male admitted with a stab wound. While in the emergency room, a chest tube is inserted. Which of the following explains the primary rationale for insertion of chest tubes?

A. The tube will allow for equalization of the lung expansion.
B. Chest tubes serve as a method of draining blood and serous fluid and assist in re-inflating the lungs.
C. Chest tubes relieve pain associated with a collapsed lung.
D. Chest tubes assist with cardiac function by stabilizing lung expansion.

QUESTION NUMBER 08.12
Question is about - breastfeeding
Category of the Question - Health Promotion and Maintenance

A client who delivered this morning tells the nurse that she plans to breastfeed her baby. The nurse is aware that successful breastfeeding is most dependent on the:

A. Mother's educational level
B. Infant's birth weight
C. Size of the mother's breast
D. Mother's desire to breastfeed

QUESTION NUMBER 08.13
Question is about - labor
Category of the Question - Health Promotion and Maintenance

The nurse is monitoring the progress of a client in labor. Which finding should be reported to the physician immediately?

A. The presence of scant bloody discharge

B. Frequent urination

C. The presence of green-tinged amniotic fluid

D. Moderate uterine contractions

QUESTION NUMBER 08.14

Question is about - contractions

Category of the Question - Physiological Adaptation

The nurse is measuring the duration of the client's contractions. Which statement is true regarding the measurement of the duration of contractions?

A. Duration is measured by timing from the beginning of one contraction to the beginning of the next contraction.

B. Duration is measured by timing from the end of one contraction to the beginning of the next contraction.

C. Duration is measured by timing from the beginning of one contraction to the end of the same contraction.

D. Duration is measured by timing from the peak of one contraction to the end of the same contraction.

QUESTION NUMBER 08.15

Question is about - Pitocin, labor

Category of the Question - Physiological Integrity, Pharmacological and Parenteral Therapies

The physician has ordered an intravenous infusion of Pitocin for the induction of labor. When caring for the obstetric client receiving intravenous Pitocin, the nurse should monitor for:

A. Maternal hypoglycemia

B. Fetal bradycardia

C. Maternal hyperreflexia

D. Fetal movement

QUESTION NUMBER 08.16

Question is about - pregnancy, insulin

Category of the Question - Physiological Integrity, Physiological Adaptation

A client with diabetes visits the prenatal clinic at 28 weeks gestation. Which statement is true regarding insulin needs during pregnancy?

A. Insulin requirements moderate as the pregnancy progresses.

B. A decreased need for insulin occurs during the second trimester.

C. Elevations in human chorionic gonadotropin decrease the need for insulin.

D. Fetal development depends on adequate insulin regulation.

QUESTION NUMBER 08.17

Question is about - prenatal

Category of the Question - Health Promotion and Maintenance

A client in the prenatal clinic is assessed to have a blood pressure of 180/96. The nurse should give priority to:

A. Providing a calm environment

B. Obtaining a diet history

C. Administering an analgesic

D. Assessing fetal heart tones

QUESTION NUMBER 08.18
Question is about - primigravida
Category of the Question - Physiological Integrity, Physiological Adaptation

A primigravida, age 42, is 6 weeks pregnant. Based on the client's age, her infant is at risk for:

A. Down syndrome

C. Turner's syndrome

B. Respiratory distress syndrome

D. Pathological jaundice

QUESTION NUMBER 08.19
Question is about - abortion
Category of the Question - Physiological Integrity, Physiological Adaptation

A client with a missed abortion at 29 weeks gestation is admitted to the hospital. The client will most likely be treated with: ADVERTISEMENTS

A. Magnesium sulfate
B. Calcium gluconate
C. Dinoprostone (Prostin E.)
D. Bromocriptine (Parlodel)

QUESTION NUMBER 08.20
Question is about - preeclampsia
Category of the Question - Physiological Integrity, Pharmacological and Parenteral Therapies

A client with preeclampsia has been receiving an infusion containing magnesium sulfate for a blood pressure that is 160/80; deep tendon reflexes are 1 plus, and the urinary output for the past hour is 100mL. The nurse should:

A. Continue the infusion of magnesium sulfate while monitoring the client's blood pressure
B. Stop the infusion of magnesium sulfate and contact the physician
C. Slow the infusion rate and turn the client on her left side
D. Administer calcium gluconate IV push and continue to monitor the blood pressure

QUESTION NUMBER 08.21
Question is about - autosomal recessive disorders
Category of the Question - Physiological Integrity, Physiological Adaptation

Which statement made by the nurse describes the inheritance pattern of autosomal recessive disorders?

A. An affected newborn has unaffected parents.
B. An affected newborn has one affected parent.
C. Affected parents have a one in four chance of passing on the defective gene.
D. Affected parents have unaffected children who are carriers.

QUESTION NUMBER 08.22
Question is about - alpha fetoprotein
Category of the Question - Physiological Integrity, Physiological Adaptation

A pregnant client, age 32, asks the nurse why her doctor has recommended a serum alpha fetoprotein. The nurse should explain that the doctor has recommended the test:

A. Because it is a state law
B. To detect cardiovascular defects

C. Because of her age
D. To detect neurological defects

QUESTION NUMBER 08.23
Question is about - hypothyroidism
Category of the Question - Physiological Integrity, Pharmacological and Parenteral Therapies

A client with hypothyroidism asks the nurse if she will still need to take thyroid medication during the pregnancy. The nurse's response is based on the knowledge that:

A. There is no need to take thyroid medication because the fetus's thyroid produces a thyroid-stimulating hormone.
B. Regulation of thyroid medication is more difficult because the thyroid gland increases in size during pregnancy.
C. It is more difficult to maintain thyroid regulation during pregnancy due to a slowing of metabolism.
D. Fetal growth is arrested if thyroid medication is continued during pregnancy.

QUESTION NUMBER 08.24
Question is about - neonatal assessment
Category of the Question - Health Promotion and Maintenance

The nurse is responsible for performing a neonatal assessment on a full-term infant. At 1 minute, the nurse would expect to find:

A. An apical pulse of 100
B. An absence of tonus

C. Cyanosis of the feet and hands
D. Jaundice of the skin and sclera

QUESTION NUMBER 08.25
Question is about - sickle cell anemia
Category of the Question - Health Promotion and Maintenance

A client with sickle cell anemia is admitted to the labor and delivery unit during the first phase of labor. The nurse should anticipate the client's need for:

A. Supplemental oxygen
B. Fluid restriction

C. Blood transfusion
D. Delivery by Caesarean section

QUESTION NUMBER 08.26
Question is about - diabetes
Category of the Question - Physiologic Integrity, Reduction of Risk Potential

A client with diabetes has an order for ultrasonography. Preparation for an ultrasound includes:

A. Increasing fluid intake
B. Limiting ambulation

C. Administering an enema
D. Withholding food for 8 hours

QUESTION NUMBER 08.27
Question is about - infant
Category of the Question - Health Promotion and Maintenance

An infant who weighs 8 pounds at birth would be expected to weigh how many pounds at 1 year?

A. 14 pounds
B. 16 pounds

C. 18 pounds
D. 24 pounds

QUESTION NUMBER 08.28
Question is about - nonstress test
Category of the Question - Physiological Integrity, Reduction of Risk Potential

A pregnant client with a history of alcohol addiction is scheduled for a nonstress test. The nonstress test:

A. Determines the lung maturity of the fetus
B. Measures the activity of the fetus
C. Shows the effect of contractions on the fetal heart rate
D. Measures the neurological well-being of the fetus

QUESTION NUMBER 08.29
Question is about - hypospadias
Category of the Question - Physiological Integrity, Physiological Adaptation

A full-term male has hypospadias. Which statement describes hypospadias?

A. The urethral opening is absent.
B. The urethra opens on the dorsal side of the penis.

C. The penis is shorter than usual.
D. The urethral meatus opens on the underside of the penis.

QUESTION NUMBER 08.30
Question is about - labor
Category of the Question - Health Promotion and Maintenance

A gravida 3 para 2 is admitted to the labor unit. Vaginal exam reveals that the client's cervix is 8 cm dilated, with complete effacement. The priority nursing diagnosis at this time is:

A. Alteration in coping related to pain
B. Potential for injury related to precipitate delivery

C. Alteration in elimination related to anesthesia
D. Potential for fluid volume deficit related to NPO status

QUESTION NUMBER 08.31
Question is about - varicella
Category of the Question - Physiological Integrity, Physiological Adaptation

The client with varicella will most likely have an order for which category of medication?

A. Antibiotics
B. Antipyretics

C. Antivirals
D. Anticoagulants

QUESTION NUMBER 08.32
Question is about - chest pain
Category of the Question - Safe and Effective Care Environment, Safety and Infection Control

A client is admitted complaining of chest pain. Which of the following drug orders should the nurse question?

A. Nitroglycerin

B. Ampicillin

C. Propranolol

D. Verapamil

QUESTION NUMBER 08.33
Question is about - rheumatoid arthritis
Category of the Question - Health Promotion and Maintenance

Which of the following instructions should be included in the teaching for the client with rheumatoid arthritis?

A. Avoid exercise because it fatigues the joints.
B. Take prescribed anti-inflammatory medications with meals.
C. Alternate hot and cold packs to affected joints.
D. Avoid weight-bearing activity.

QUESTION NUMBER 08.34
Question is about - pancreatitis
Category of the Question - Safe and Effective Care Environment, Safety and Infection Control

A client with acute pancreatitis is experiencing severe abdominal pain. Which of the following orders should be questioned by the nurse?

A. Meperidine 100 mg IM q 4 hours PRN pain
B. Mylanta 30 ccs q 4 hours via NG
C. Cimetidine 300 mg PO q.i.d.
D. Morphine 8 mg IM q 4 hours PRN pain

QUESTION NUMBER 08.35
Question is about - chemical dependence
Category of the Question - Psychosocial Integrity

The client is admitted to the chemical dependence unit with an order for continuous observation. The nurse is aware that the doctor has ordered continuous observation because:

A. Hallucinogenic drugs create both stimulant and depressant effects.
B. Hallucinogenic drugs induce a state of altered perception.
C. Hallucinogenic drugs produce severe respiratory depression.
D. Hallucinogenic drugs induce rapid physical dependence.

QUESTION NUMBER 08.36
Question is about - chest pain
Category of the Question - Physiological Integrity, Physiological Adaptation

A patient arrives at the emergency department complaining of midsternal chest pain. Which of the following nursing actions should take priority?

A. A complete history with emphasis on preceding events.
B. An electrocardiogram.
C. Careful assessment of vital signs.
D. Chest exam with auscultation.

QUESTION NUMBER 08.37
Question is about - pneumonia
Category of the Question - Health Promotion and Maintenance

A patient has been hospitalized with pneumonia and is about to be discharged. A nurse provides discharge instructions to a patient and his family. Which misunderstanding by the family indicates the need for more detailed information?

A. The patient may resume normal home activities as tolerated but should avoid physical exertion and get adequate rest.
B. The patient should resume a normal diet with emphasis on nutritious, healthy foods.
C. The patient may discontinue the prescribed course of oral antibiotics once the symptoms have completely resolved.
D. The patient should continue use of the incentive spirometer to keep airways open and free of secretions.

QUESTION NUMBER 08.38
Question is about - lung cancer
ADVERTISEMENTS
Category of the Question - Safe and Effective Care Environment, Management of Care

A nurse is caring for an elderly Vietnamese patient in the terminal stages of lung cancer. Many family members are in the room around the clock performing unusual rituals and bringing ethnic foods. Which of the following actions should the nurse take?

A. Restrict visiting hours and ask the family to limit visitors to two at a time.
B. Notify visitors with a sign on the door that the patient is limited to clear fluids only with no solid food allowed.
C. If possible, keep the other bed in the room unassigned to provide privacy and comfort to the family.
D. Contact the physician to report the unusual rituals and activities.

QUESTION NUMBER 08.39
Question is about - delegation
Category of the Question - Safe and Effective Care Environment, Management of Care

The charge nurse on the cardiac unit is planning assignments for the day. Which of the following is the most appropriate assignment for the float nurse that has been reassigned from labor and delivery?

A. A one-week postoperative coronary bypass patient, who is being evaluated for placement of a pacemaker prior to discharge.
B. A suspected myocardial infarction patient on telemetry, just admitted from the Emergency Department and scheduled for an angiogram.
C. A patient with unstable angina being closely monitored for pain and medication titration.
D. A postoperative valve replacement patient who was recently admitted to the unit because all surgical beds were filled.

QUESTION NUMBER 08.40
Question is about - type 1 diabetes mellitus
Category of the Question - Health Promotion and Maintenance

A newly diagnosed 8-year-old child with type I diabetes mellitus and his mother are receiving diabetes education prior to discharge. The physician has prescribed Glucagon for emergency use. The mother asks the purpose of this medication. Which of the following statements by the nurse is correct?

A. Glucagon enhances the effect of insulin in case the blood sugar remains high one hour after injection.
B. Glucagon treats hypoglycemia resulting from insulin overdose.
C. Glucagon treats lipoatrophy from insulin injections.
D. Glucagon prolongs the effect of insulin, allowing fewer injections.

QUESTION NUMBER 08.41
Question is about - congestive heart failure
Category of the Question - Physiological Integrity, Pharmacological and Parenteral Therapies

An infant with congestive heart failure is receiving diuretic therapy at home. Which of the following symptoms would indicate that the dosage may need to be increased?

A. Sudden weight gain
B. Decreased blood pressure

C. Slow, shallow breathing
D. Bradycardia

QUESTION NUMBER 08.42
Question is about - dilantin, seizure disorder
Category of the Question - Physiological Integrity, Pharmacological and Parenteral Therapies

A patient taking dilantin (Phenytoin) for a seizure disorder is experiencing breakthrough seizures. A blood sample is taken to determine the serum drug level. Which of the following would indicate a sub-therapeutic level?

A. 15 mcg/mL
B. 4 mcg/mL

C. 10 mcg/dL
D. 5 mcg/dL

QUESTION NUMBER 08.43
Question is about - acetaminophen toxicity
Category of the Question - Physiological Integrity, Physiological Adaptation

A patient arrives at the emergency department complaining of back pain. He reports taking at least 3 acetaminophen tablets every three hours for the past week without relief. Which of the following symptoms suggests acetaminophen toxicity?

A. Tinnitus
B. Diarrhea

C. Hypertension
D. Hepatic damage

QUESTION NUMBER 08.44
Question is about - morphine sulfate
Category of the Question - Pharmacological and Parenteral Therapies

A nurse is caring for a cancer patient receiving subcutaneous morphine sulfate for pain. Which of the following nursing actions is most important in the care of this patient?

A. Monitor urine output

B. Monitor respiratory rate

C. Monitor heart rate

D. Monitor temperature

QUESTION NUMBER 08.45

Question is about - leg pain

Category of the Question - Physiological Integrity, Physiological Adaptation

A patient arrives at the emergency department with severe lower leg pain after a fall in a touch football game. Following routine triage, which of the following is the appropriate next step in assessment and treatment?

A. Apply heat to the painful area.

B. Apply an elastic bandage to the leg.

C. X-ray the leg.

D. Give pain medication.

QUESTION NUMBER 08.46

Question is about - cardioverter-defibrillator

Category of the Question - Physiological Integrity, Physiological Adaptation

A nurse caring for several patients in the cardiac unit is told that one is scheduled for implantation of an automatic internal cardioverter-defibrillator. Which of the following patients is most likely to have this procedure?

A. A patient admitted for myocardial infarction without cardiac muscle damage.

B. A postoperative coronary bypass patient, recovering on schedule.

C. A patient with a history of ventricular tachycardia and syncopal episodes.

D. A patient with a history of atrial tachycardia and fatigue.

QUESTION NUMBER 08.47

Question is about - magnetic resonance imaging

Category of the Question - Physiological Integrity, Reduction of Risk Potential

A patient is scheduled for a magnetic resonance imaging (MRI) scan for suspected lung cancer. Which of the following is a contraindication to the study for this patient?

A. The patient is allergic to shellfish.

B. The patient has a pacemaker.

C. The patient suffers from claustrophobia.

D. The patient takes antipsychotic medication.

QUESTION NUMBER 08.48

Question is about - pulmonary embolism

Category of the Question - Physiological Integrity, Physiological Adaptation

A nurse calls a physician with the concern that a patient has developed a pulmonary embolism. Which of the following symptoms has the nurse most likely observed?

    A. The patient is somnolent with decreased response to the family.
    B. The patient suddenly complains of chest pain and shortness of breath.
    C. The patient has developed a wet cough and the nurse hears crackles on auscultation of the lungs.
    D. The patient has a fever, chills, and loss of appetite.

QUESTION NUMBER 08.49
Question is about - abdominal aortic aneurysm
Category of the Question - Physiological Integrity, Reduction of Risk Potential

A patient comes to the emergency department with abdominal pain. Work-up reveals the presence of a rapidly enlarging abdominal aortic aneurysm. Which of the following actions should the nurse expect?

    A. The patient will be admitted to the medicine unit for observation and medication.
    B. The patient will be admitted to the day surgery unit for sclerotherapy.
    C. The patient will be admitted to the surgical unit and resection will be scheduled.
    D. The patient will be discharged home to follow-up with his cardiologist in 24 hours.

QUESTION NUMBER 08.50
Question is about - chemotherapy
Category of the Question - Physiological Integrity, Reduction of Risk Potential

A patient with leukemia is receiving chemotherapy that is known to depress bone marrow. A CBC (complete blood count) reveals a platelet count of 25,000/microliter. Which of the following actions related specifically to the platelet count should be included on the nursing care plan?

    A. Monitor for fever every 4 hours.
    B. Require visitors to wear respiratory masks and protective clothing.
    C. Consider transfusion of packed red blood cells.
    D. Check for signs of bleeding, including examination of urine and stool for blood.

QUESTION NUMBER 08.51
Question is about - leukemia
Category of the Question - Health Promotion and Maintenance

A patient is undergoing the induction stage of treatment for leukemia. The nurse teaches family members about infectious precautions. Which of the following statements by family members indicates that the family needs more education?

    A. We will bring in books and magazines for entertainment.
    B. We will bring in personal care items for comfort.
    C. We will bring in fresh flowers to brighten the room.
    D. We will bring in family pictures and get well cards.

QUESTION NUMBER 08.52
Question is about - acute lymphoblastic leukemia
Category of the Question - Physiological Integrity, Physiological Adaptation

A nurse is caring for a patient with acute lymphoblastic leukemia (ALL). Which of the following is the most likely age range of the patient?

A. 3-10 years

B. 25-35 years

C. 45-55 years

D. over 60 years

QUESTION NUMBER 08.53
Question is about - Hodgkin's disease
Category of the Question - Physiological Integrity, Physiological Adaptation

A patient is admitted to the oncology unit for diagnosis of suspected Hodgkin's disease. Which of the following symptoms is typical of Hodgkin's disease?

A. Painful cervical lymph nodes
B. Night sweats and fatigue
C. Nausea and vomiting
D. Weight gain

QUESTION NUMBER 08.54
Question is about - Hodgkin's disease
Category of the Question - Physiological Integrity, Physiological Adaptation

The Hodgkin's disease patient described in the question above undergoes a lymph node biopsy for definitive diagnosis. If the diagnosis of Hodgkin's disease were correct, which of the following cells would the pathologist expect to find?

A. Reed-Sternberg cells

B. Lymphoblastic cells

C. Gaucher's cells

D. Rieder's cells

QUESTION NUMBER 08.55
Question is about - bone marrow aspiration and biopsy
Category of the Question - Physiological Integrity, Basic Care and Comfort

A patient is about to undergo bone marrow aspiration and biopsy and expresses fear and anxiety about the procedure. Which of the following is the most effective nursing response?

A. Warn the patient to stay very still because the smallest movement will increase her pain.
B. Encourage the family to stay in the room for the procedure.
C. Stay with the patient and focus on slow, deep breathing for relaxation.
D. Delay the procedure to allow the patient to deal with her feelings.

QUESTION NUMBER 08.56
Question is about - toilet training
Category of the Question - Health Promotion and Maintenance

A mother complains to the clinic nurse that her 2 ½-year-old son is not yet toilet trained. She is particularly concerned that, although he reliably uses the potty seat for bowel movements, he isn't able to hold his urine for long periods. Which of the following statements by the nurse is correct?

A. The child should have been trained by age 2 and may have a psychological problem that is responsible for his "accidents."
B. Bladder control is usually achieved before bowel control, and the child should be required to sit on the potty seat until he passes urine.
C. Bowel control is usually achieved before bladder control, and the average age for completion of toilet training varies widely from 24 to 36 months.
D. The child should be told "no" each time he wets so that he learns the behavior is unacceptable.

QUESTION NUMBER 08.57
Question is about - infant
Category of the Question - Health Promotion and Maintenance

The mother of a 14-month-old child reports to the nurse that her child will not fall asleep at night without a bottle of milk in the crib and often wakes during the night asking for another. Which of the following instructions by the nurse is correct?

A. Allow the child to have the bottle at bedtime, but withhold the one later in the night.
B. Put juice in the bottle instead of milk.
C. Give only a bottle of water at bedtime.
D. Do not allow bottles in the crib.

QUESTION NUMBER 08.58
Question is about - infant
Category of the Question - Health Promotion and Maintenance

Which of the following actions is not appropriate in the care of a 2-month-old infant?

A. Place the infant on her back for naps and bedtime.
B. Allow the infant to cry for 5 minutes before responding if she wakes during the night as she may fall back asleep.
C. Talk to the infant frequently and make eye contact to encourage language development.
D. Wait until at least 4 months to add infant cereals and strained fruits to the diet.

QUESTION NUMBER 08.59
Question is about - constipation
Category of the Question - Health Promotion and Maintenance

An older patient asks a nurse to recommend strategies to prevent constipation. Which of the following suggestions would be helpful? Note: More than one answer may be correct. Select all that apply.

A. Get moderate exercise for at least 30 minutes each day.
B. Drink 6-8 glasses of water each day.
C. Eat a diet high in fiber.
D. Take a mild laxative if you don't have a bowel movement every day.
E. Eat a protein-rich diet.

Correct Answers: A, B, and C

A daily bowel movement is not necessary if the patient is comfortable and the bowels move regularly. Moderate exercise, such as walking, encourages bowel health, as does generous water intake. A diet high in fiber is also helpful. Check on the usual pattern of elimination, including frequency and consistency of stool. It is very crucial to carefully know what is "normal" for each patient. The normal frequency of stool passage ranges from twice daily to once every third or fourth day. Dry and hard feces are common characteristics of constipation.

Option A: Urge patient for some physical activity and exercise. Consider isometric abdominal and glute exercises. Movement promotes peristalsis. Abdominal exercises strengthen abdominal muscles that facilitate defecation.

Option B: Encourage the patient to take in fluid 2000 to 3000 mL/day, if not contraindicated medically. Sufficient fluid is needed to keep the fecal mass soft. But take note of some patients or older patients having cardiovascular limitations requiring less fluid intake.

Option C: Assist the patient to take at least 20 g of dietary fiber (e.g. raw fruits, fresh vegetables, whole grains) per day. Fiber adds bulk to the stool and makes defecation easier because it passes through the intestine essentially unchanged.

Option D: Laxatives should be used as a last resort and should not be taken regularly. Over time, laxatives can desensitize the bowel and worsen constipation. The use of laxatives or enemas is indicated for short-term management of constipation.

Option E: Protein-rich foods could cause constipation. A balanced diet that comprises adequate fiber, fresh fruits, vegetables, and grains. Twenty grams of fiber per day is suggested. A regular period for elimination and an adequate time for defection. Successful bowel training relies on routine. Facilitating regular time prevents the bowel from emptying sporadically.

QUESTION NUMBER 08.60
Question is about - rheumatic fever
Category of the Question - Physiological Integrity, Physiological Adaptation

A child is admitted to the hospital with suspected rheumatic fever. Which of the following observations is not confirming the diagnosis?

    A. A reddened rash visible over the trunk and extremities.
    B. A history of sore throat that was self-limited in the past month.
    C. A negative antistreptolysin O titer.
    D. An unexplained fever.

QUESTION NUMBER 08.61
Question is about - congestive heart failure
Category of the Question - Physiological Integrity, Reduction of Risk Potential

A patient with a history of congestive heart failure arrives at the clinic complaining of dyspnea. Which of the following actions is the first the nurse should perform?

    A. Ask the patient to lie down on the exam table.
    B. Draw blood for chemistry panel and arterial blood gas (ABG).
    C. Send the patient for a chest x-ray.
    D. Check blood pressure.

QUESTION NUMBER 08.62
Question is about - nitroglycerin
Category of the Question - Physiological Integrity, Pharmacological and Parenteral Therapies

A clinic patient has recently been prescribed nitroglycerin for treatment of angina. He calls the nurse complaining of frequent headaches. Which of the following responses to the patient is correct?

    A. "Stop taking the nitroglycerin and see if the headaches improve."
    B. "Go to the emergency department to be checked because nitroglycerin can cause bleeding in the brain."
    C. "Headaches are a frequent side effect of nitroglycerine because it causes vasodilation."
    D. "The headaches are unlikely to be related to the nitroglycerin, so you should see your doctor for further investigation."

QUESTION NUMBER 08.63
Question is about - colon cancer
Category of the Question - Physiological Integrity, Reduction of Risk Potential

A patient received surgery and chemotherapy for colon cancer, completing therapy 3 months previously, and she is now in remission. At a follow-up appointment, she complains of fatigue following activity and difficulty with concentration at her weekly bridge games. Which of the following explanations would account for her symptoms?

    A. The symptoms may be the result of anemia caused   C. The patient may be depressed.
       by chemotherapy.   D. The patient may be dehydrated.
    B. The patient may be immunosuppressed.

QUESTION NUMBER 08.64
Question is about - diet, hemoglobin
Category of the Question - Health Promotion and Maintenance

ADVERTISEMENTS

A clinic patient has a hemoglobin concentration of 10.8 g/dL and reports sticking to a strict vegetarian diet. Which of the following nutritional advice is appropriate?

    A. The diet is providing adequate sources of iron and requires no changes.
    B. The patient should add meat to her diet; a vegetarian diet is not advised.
    C. The patient should use iron cookware to prepare foods, such as dark green, leafy vegetables and legumes, which
       are high in iron.
    D. A cup of coffee or tea should be added to every meal.

QUESTION NUMBER 08.65
Question is about - anemia
Category of the Question - Physiological Integrity, Pharmacological and Parenteral Therapies

A hospitalized patient is receiving packed red blood cells (PRBCs) for treatment of severe anemia. Which of the following is the most accurate statement?

    A. Transfusion reaction is most likely immediately after the infusion is completed.
    B. PRBCs are best infused slowly through a 20g. IV catheter.

C. PRBCs should be flushed with a 5% dextrose solution.

D. A nurse should remain in the room during the first 15 minutes of infusion.

QUESTION NUMBER 08.66
Question is about - triage
Category of the Question - Safe and Effective Care Environment, Management of Care

Emergency department triage is an important nursing function. A nurse working the evening shift is presented with four patients at the same time. Which of the following patients should be assigned the highest priority?

A. A patient with low-grade fever, headache, and myalgias for the past 72 hours.

B. A patient who is unable to bear weight on the left foot, with swelling and bruising following a running accident.

C. A patient with abdominal and chest pain following a large, spicy meal.

D. A child with a one-inch bleeding laceration on the chin but otherwise well after falling while jumping on his bed.

QUESTION NUMBER 08.67
Question is about - calcium
Category of the Question - Physiological Integrity, Reduction of Risk Potential

A patient is admitted to the hospital with a calcium level of 6.0 mg/dL. Which of the following symptoms would you not expect to see in this patient?

A. Numbness in hands and feet

B. Muscle cramping

C. Hypoactive bowel sounds

D. Positive Chvostek's sign

QUESTION NUMBER 08.68
Question is about - nasogastric tube, bowel obstruction
Category of the Question - Physiological Integrity, Reduction of Risk Potential

A nurse cares for a patient who has a nasogastric tube attached to low suction because of a suspected bowel obstruction. Which of the following arterial blood gas results might be expected in this patient?

A. pH 7.52, PCO2 54 mmHg.

B. pH 7.42, PCO2 40 mmHg.

C. pH 7.25, PCO2 25 mmHg.

D. pH 7.38, PCO2 36 mmHg.

QUESTION NUMBER 08.69
Question is about - warfarin
Category of the Question - Physiological Integrity, Reduction of Risk Potential

A patient is admitted to the hospital for routine elective surgery. Included in the list of current medications is warfarin (Coumadin) at a high dose. Concerned about the possible effects of the drug, particularly in a patient scheduled for surgery, the nurse anticipates which of the following actions?

A. Draw a blood sample for prothrombin (PT) and international normalized ratio (INR) level.

B. Administer vitamin K.

C. Draw a blood sample for type and crossmatch and request blood from the blood bank.

D. Cancel the surgery after the patient reports stopping the Coumadin one week previously.

QUESTION NUMBER 08.70
Question is about - laboratory results
Category of the Question - Physiological Integrity, Reduction of Risk Potential

The following lab results are received for a patient. Which of the following results are abnormal? Note: More than one answer may be correct. Select all that apply.

    A. Hemoglobin 10.4 g/dL.
    B. Total cholesterol 340 mg/dL.
    C. Total serum protein 7.0 g/dL.
    D. Glycosylated hemoglobin A1C 5.4%.
    E. WBC count 5.5×10^9/L

QUESTION NUMBER 08.71
Question is about - juvenile idiopathic arthritis
Category of the Question - Physiological Integrity, Physiological Adaptation

A nurse is assigned to the pediatric rheumatology clinic and is assessing a child who has just been diagnosed with juvenile idiopathic arthritis. Which of the following statements about the disease is most accurate?

    A. The child has a poor chance of recovery without joint deformity.
    B. Most children progress to adult rheumatoid arthritis.
    C. Nonsteroidal anti-inflammatory drugs are the first choice in treatment.
    D. Physical activity should be minimized.

QUESTION NUMBER 08.72
Question is about - osteomyelitis
Category of the Question - Physiological Integrity, Physiological Adaptation

A child is admitted to the hospital several days after stepping on a sharp object that punctured her athletic shoe and entered the flesh of her foot. The physician is concerned about osteomyelitis and has ordered parenteral antibiotics. Which of the following actions is done immediately before the antibiotic is started?

    A. The admission orders are written.
    B. A blood culture is drawn.

    C. A complete blood count with differential is drawn.
    D. The parents arrive.

QUESTION NUMBER 08.73
Question is about - leg injury
Category of the Question - Physiological Integrity, Physiological Adaptation

A two-year-old child has sustained an injury to the leg and refuses to walk. The nurse in the emergency department documents swelling of the lower affected leg. Which of the following does the nurse suspect is the cause of the child's symptoms?

    A. Possible fracture ogef the tibia.
    B. Bruising of the gastrocnemius muscle.
    C. Possible fracture of the radius.
    D. No anatomic injury, the child wants his mother to carry him.

QUESTION NUMBER 08.74
Question is about - cerebral palsy
Category of the Question - Health Promotion and Maintenance

A toddler has recently been diagnosed with cerebral palsy. Which of the following information should the nurse provide to the parents? Note: More than one answer may be correct. Select all that apply.

    A. Regular developmental screening is important to avoid secondary developmental delays.
    B. Cerebral palsy is caused by injury to the upper motor neurons and results in motor dysfunction, as well as possible ocular and speech difficulties.
    C. Developmental milestones may be slightly delayed but usually will require no additional intervention.
    D. Parent support groups are helpful for sharing strategies and managing health care issues.
    E. Outdoor activities are prohibited for the child.

QUESTION NUMBER 08.75
Question is about - Duchenne's muscular dystrophy
Category of the Question - Physiological Integrity,Physiological Adaptation

A child has recently been diagnosed with Duchenne's muscular dystrophy. The parents are receiving genetic counseling prior to planning another pregnancy. Which of the following statements includes the most accurate information?

    A. Duchenne's is an X-linked recessive disorder, so daughters have a 50% chance of being carriers and sons a 50% chance of developing the disease.
    B. Duchenne's is an X-linked recessive disorder, so both daughters and sons have a 50% chance of developing the disease.
    C. Each child has a 1 in 4 (25%) chance of developing the disorder.
    D. Sons only have a 1 in 4 (25%) chance of developing the disorder.

Practice Question Set-9

QUESTION NUMBER 09.01
Question is about - delegation
Category of the Question - Safe and Effective Care Environment, Management of Care

Which action (s) should you delegate to the experienced nursing assistant when caring for a patient with a thrombotic stroke with residual left-sided weakness? Select all that apply.

    A. Assist the patient to reposition every 2 hours.
    B. Reapply pneumatic compression boots.
    C. Remind the patient to perform active ROM.
    D. Check extremities for redness and edema.

QUESTION NUMBER 09.02
Question is about - stroke
Category of the Question - Safe and Effective Care Environment, Management of Care

The patient who had a stroke needs to be fed. What instruction should you give to the nursing assistant who will feed the patient?

A. Position the patient sitting up in bed before you feed her.
B. Check the patient's gag and swallowing reflexes.
C. Feed the patient quickly because there are three more waiting.
D. Suction the patient's secretions between bites of food.

QUESTION NUMBER 09.03
Question is about - bacterial meningitis
Category of the Question - Physiological Integrity, Physiological Adaptation

You have just admitted a patient with bacterial meningitis to the medical-surgical unit. The patient complains of a severe headache with photophobia and has a temperature of 102.60 F orally. Which collaborative intervention must be accomplished first?

A. Administer codeine 15 mg orally for the patient's headache.
B. Infuse ceftriaxone (Rocephin) 2000 mg IV to treat the infection.
C. Give acetaminophen (Tylenol) 650 mg orally to reduce the fever.
D. Give furosemide (Lasix) 40 mg IV to decrease intracranial pressure.

QUESTION NUMBER 09.04
Question is about - meningococcal meningitis
Category of the Question - Physiological Integrity, Management of Care

You are mentoring a student nurse in the intensive care unit (ICU) while caring for a patient with meningococcal meningitis. Which action by the student requires that you intervene immediately?

A. The student enters the room without putting on a mask and gown.
B. The student instructs the family that visits are restricted to 10 minutes.
C. The student gives the patient a warm blanket when he says he feels cold.
D. The student checks the patient's pupil response to light every 30 minutes.

QUESTION NUMBER 09.05
Question is about - delegation
Category of the Question - Safe and Effective Care Environment, Management of Care

A 23-year-old patient with a recent history of encephalitis is admitted to the medical unit with new onset generalized tonic-clonic seizures. Which nursing activities included in the patient's care will be best to delegate to an LPN/LVN whom you are supervising? Select all that apply.

A. Document the onset time, nature of seizure activity, and postictal behaviors for all seizures.
B. Administer phenytoin (Dilantin) 200 mg PO daily.
C. Teach the patient about the need for good oral hygiene.
D. Develop a discharge plan, including physician visits and referral to the Epilepsy Foundation.
E. Gather information about the seizure activity

QUESTION NUMBER 09.06
Question is about - seizure disorder
Category of the Question - Physiological Integrity, Physiological Adaptation

While working in the ICU, you are assigned to care for a patient with a seizure disorder. Which of these nursing actions will you implement first if the patient has a seizure?

    A. Place the patient on a non-rebreather mask will the oxygen at 15 L/minute.
    B. Administer lorazepam (Ativan) 1 mg IV.
    C. Turn the patient to the side and protect the airway.
    D. Assess level of consciousness during and immediately after the seizure.

QUESTION NUMBER 09.07
Question is about - phenytoin
Category of the Question - Physiological Integrity, Pharmacological and Parenteral therapies

A patient recently started on phenytoin (Dilantin) to control simple complex seizures is seen in the outpatient clinic. Which information obtained during his chart review and assessment will be of greatest concern?

    A. The gums appear enlarged and inflamed.
    B. The white blood cell count is 2300/mm3.
    C. Patient occasionally forgets to take the phenytoin until after lunch.
    D. Patient wants to renew his driver's license next month.

QUESTION NUMBER 09.08
Question is about - prioritization
Category of the Question - Safe and Effective Care Environment, Management of Care

After receiving a change-of-shift report at 7:00 AM, which of these patients will you assess first?

    A. A 23-year-old with a migraine headache who is complaining of severe nausea associated with retching.
    B. A 45-year-old who is scheduled for a craniotomy in 30 minutes and needs preoperative teaching.
    C. A 59-year-old with Parkinson's disease who will need a swallowing assessment before breakfast.
    D. A 63-year-old with multiple sclerosis who has an oral temperature of 101.80 F and flank pain.

QUESTION NUMBER 09.09
Question is about - delegation
Category of the Question - Safe and Effective Care Environment, Management of Care

All of these nursing activities are included in the care plan for a 78-year-old man with Parkinson's disease who has been referred to your home health agency. Which ones will you delegate to a nursing assistant (NA)? Select all that apply.

    A. Check for orthostatic changes in pulse and blood pressure.
    B. Monitor for improvement in tremor after levodopa (L-dopa) is given.
    C. Remind the patient to allow adequate time for meals.
    D. Monitor for abnormal involuntary jerky movements of extremities.
    E. Assist the patient with prescribed strengthening exercises.

F. Adapt the patient's preferred activities to his level of function.

QUESTION NUMBER 09.10
Question is about - delegation
Category of the Question - Safe and Effective Care Environment, Management of Care

As the manager in a long-term-care (LTC) facility, you are in charge of developing a standard plan of care for residents with Alzheimer's disease. Which of these nursing tasks is best to delegate to the LPN team leaders working in the facility?

A. Check for improvement in resident memory after medication therapy is initiated.
B. Use the Mini-Mental State Examination to assess residents every 6 months.
C. Assist residents to the toilet every 2 hours to decrease the risk for urinary intolerance.
D. Develop individualized activity plans after consulting with residents and family.

QUESTION NUMBER 09.11
Question is about - Alzheimer's disease
Category of the Question - Physiological Integrity, Basic Care and Comfort

A patient who has been admitted to the medical unit with new-onset angina also has a diagnosis of Alzheimer's disease. Her husband tells you that he rarely gets a good night's sleep because he needs to be sure she does not wander during the night. He insists on checking each of the medications you give her to be sure they are the same as the ones she takes at home. Based on this information, which nursing diagnosis is most appropriate for this patient?

A. Decreased Cardiac Output related to poor myocardial contractility
B. Caregiver Role Strain related to continuous need for providing care
C. Ineffective Therapeutic Regimen Management related to poor patient memory
D. Risk for Falls related to patient wandering behavior during the night

QUESTION NUMBER 09.12
Question is about - glioblastoma
Category of the Question - Physiological Integrity, Pharmacological and Parenteral therapies

You are caring for a patient with a recurrent glioblastoma who is receiving dexamethasone (Decadron) 4 mg IV every 6 hours to relieve symptoms of right arm weakness and headache. Which assessment information concerns you the most?

A. The patient does not recognize family members.
B. The blood glucose level is 234 mg/dL.
C. The patient complains of a continued headache.
D. The daily weight has increased by 1 kg.

QUESTION NUMBER 09.13
Question is about - lethargy
Category of the Question - Safe and Effective Care Environment, Management of Care

A 70-year-old alcoholic patient with acute lethargy, confusion, and incontinence is admitted to the hospital ED. His wife tells you that he fell down the stairs about a month ago, but "he didn't have a scratch afterward." She feels that he has become gradually less active and sleepier over the last 10 days or so. Which of the following collaborative interventions will you implement first?

A. Place on the hospital alcohol withdrawal protocol.
B. Transfer to radiology for a CT scan.
C. Insert a retention catheter to straight drainage.
D. Give phenytoin (Dilantin) 100 mg PO.

QUESTION NUMBER 09.14
Question is about - delegation
Category of the Question - Safe and Effective Care Environment, Management of Care

Which of these patients in the neurologic ICU will be best to assign to an RN who has floated from the medical unit?

A. A 26-year-old patient with a basilar skull structure who has clear drainage coming out of the nose.
B. A 42-year-old patient admitted several hours ago with a headache and diagnosed with a ruptured berry aneurysm.
C. A 46-year-old patient who was admitted 48 hours ago with bacterial meningitis and has an antibiotic dose due.
D. A 65-year-old patient with an astrocytoma who has just returned to the unit after having a craniotomy.

QUESTION NUMBER 09.15
Question is about - migraine
Category of the Question - Physiological Integrity, Physiological Adaptation

What is the priority nursing diagnosis for a patient experiencing a migraine headache?

A. Acute pain related to biologic and chemical factors
B. Anxiety related to change in or threat to health status
C. Hopelessness related to deteriorating physiological condition
D. Risk for Side effects related to medical therapy

QUESTION NUMBER 09.16
Question is about - sigmoid colostomy
Category of the Question - Physiological Integrity, Reduction of Risk Potential

Nurse Michelle should know that the drainage is normal four (4) days after a sigmoid colostomy when the stool is:

A. Green liquid
B. Solid formed
C. Loose, bloody
D. Semiformed

QUESTION NUMBER 09.17
Question is about - right-sided brain attack, hemianopsia
Category of the Question - Physiological Integrity, Physiological Adaptation

Where would nurse Kristine place the call light for a male client with a right-sided brain attack and left homonymous hemianopsia?

A. On the client's right side
B. On the client's left side
C. Directly in front of the client
D. Where the client like

QUESTION NUMBER 09.18
Question is about - accident
Category of the Question - Physiological Integrity, Physiological Adaptation

A male client is admitted to the emergency department following an accident. What are the first nursing actions of the nurse?

A. Check respiration, circulation, neurological response
B. Align the spine, check pupils, and check for hemorrhage
C. Check respirations, stabilize the spine and check the circulation
D. Assess level of consciousness and circulation

QUESTION NUMBER 09.19
Question is about - nitroglycerin
Category of the Question - Physiological Integrity, Pharmacological and Parenteral therapies

In evaluating the effect of nitroglycerin, Nurse Arthur should know that it reduces preload and relieves angina by:

A. Increasing contractility and slowing heart rate
B. Increasing AV conduction and heart rate
C. Decreasing contractility and oxygen consumption
D. Decreasing venous return through vasodilation

QUESTION NUMBER 09.20
Question is about - myocardial infarction
Category of the Question - Physiological Integrity, Physiological Adaptation

Nurse Patricia finds a female client who is post-myocardial infarction (MI) slumped on the side rails of the bed and unresponsive to shaking or shouting. Which is the nurse's next action?

A. Call for help and note the time
B. Clear the airway
C. Give two sharp thumps to the precordium, and check the pulse
D. Administer two quick blows

QUESTION NUMBER 09.21
Question is about - gastrointestinal bleeding
Category of the Question - Physiological Integrity, Physiological Adaptation

Nurse Monett is caring for a client recovering from gastrointestinal bleeding. The nurse should:

   A. Plan care so the client can receive 8 hours of uninterrupted sleep each night.
   B. Monitor vital signs every 2 hours.
   C. Make sure that the client takes food and medications at prescribed intervals.
   D. Provide milk every 2 to 3 hours.

QUESTION NUMBER 09.22
Question is about - heparin
Category of the Question - Physiological Integrity, Pharmacological and Parenteral therapies

A male client was on warfarin (Coumadin) before admission and has been receiving heparin I.V. for 2 days. The partial thromboplastin time (PTT) is 68 seconds. What should Nurse Carla do?

   A. Stop the I.V. infusion of heparin and notify the physician.
   B. Continue treatment as ordered.
   C. Expect the warfarin to increase the PTT.
   D. Increase the dosage, because the level is lower than normal.

QUESTION NUMBER 09.23
Question is about - ileostomy, stoma
Category of the Question - Physiological Integrity, Physiological Adaptation

A client underwent an ileostomy, when should the drainage appliance be applied to the stoma?

   A. 24 hours later, when edema has subsided
   B. In the operating room
   C. After the ileostomy begins to function
   D. When the client is able to begin self-care procedures

QUESTION NUMBER 09.24
Question is about - spinal anesthesia
Category of the Question - Physiological Integrity, Reduction of Risk Potential

A client has undergone spinal anesthetic, it will be important that the nurse immediately position the client in:

   A. On the side, to prevent obstruction of the airway by the tongue
   B. Flat on back
   C. On the back, with knees flexed 15 degrees
   D. Flat on the stomach, with the head turned to the side

QUESTION NUMBER 09.25
Question is about - increased intracranial pressure
Category of the Question - Physiological Integrity, Physiological Adaptation

While monitoring a male client several hours after a motor vehicle accident, which assessment data suggest increasing intracranial pressure?

A. Blood pressure has decreased from 160/90 to 110/70.
B. Pulse is increased from 87 to 95, with an occasional skipped beat.
C. The client is oriented when aroused from sleep and goes back to sleep immediately.
D. The client refuses dinner because of anorexia.

QUESTION NUMBER 09.26
Question is about - pneumonia
Category of the Question - Physiological Integrity, Physiological Adaptation

Mrs. Cruz, 80 years old is diagnosed with pneumonia. Which of the following symptoms may appear first?

A. Altered mental status and dehydration

B. Fever and chills

C. Hemoptysis and Dyspnea

D. Pleuritic chest pain and cough

QUESTION NUMBER 09.27
Question is about - tuberculosis
Category of the Question - Physiological Integrity, Physiological Adaptation

A male client has active tuberculosis (TB). Which of the following symptoms will be exhibited?

A. Chest and lower back pain
B. Chills, fever, night sweats, and hemoptysis
C. Fever of more than 104°F (40°C) and nausea
D. Headache and photophobia

QUESTION NUMBER 09.28
Question is about - asthma
Category of the Question - Physiological Integrity, Physiological Adaptation

Mark, a 7-year-old client, is brought to the emergency department. He's tachypneic and afebrile and has a respiratory rate of 36 breaths/minute and has a nonproductive cough. He recently had a cold. From this history; the client may have which of the following conditions?

A. Acute asthma
B. Bronchial pneumonia
C. Chronic obstructive pulmonary disease (COPD)
D. Emphysema

QUESTION NUMBER 09.29
Question is about - morphine
Category of the Question - Physiological Integrity, Pharmacological and Parenteral Therapies

Marichu was given morphine sulfate for pain. She is sleeping and her respiratory rate is 4 breaths/minute. If action isn't taken quickly, she might have which of the following reactions?

A. Asthma attack
B. Respiratory arrest

C. Seizure
D. Wake up on her own

QUESTION NUMBER 09.30
Question is about - elective knee surgery
Category of the Question - Health Promotion and Maintenance

A 77-year-old male client is admitted for elective knee surgery. Physical examination reveals shallow respirations but no sign of respiratory distress. Which of the following is a normal physiologic change related to aging?

A. Increased elastic recoil of the lungs
B. Increased number of functional capillaries in the alveoli
C. Decreased residual volume
D. Decreased vital capacity

QUESTION NUMBER 09.31
Question is about - lidocaine
Category of the Question - Physiological Integrity, Pharmacological and Parenteral Therapies

Nurse John is caring for a male client receiving lidocaine I.V. Which factor is the most relevant to the administration of this medication?

A. Decrease in arterial oxygen saturation (SaO2) when measured with a pulse oximeter.
B. Increase in systemic blood pressure
C. Presence of premature ventricular contractions (PVCs) on a cardiac monitor
D. Increase in intracranial pressure (ICP)

QUESTION NUMBER 09.32
Question is about - anticoagulant
Category of the Question - Physiological Integrity, Pharmacological and Parenteral Therapies

Nurse Ron is caring for a male client taking an anticoagulant. The nurse should teach the client to:

A. Report incidents of diarrhea
B. Avoid foods high in vitamin K

C. Use a straight razor when shaving
D. Take aspirin for pain relief

QUESTION NUMBER 09.33
Question is about - I.V. catheter
Category of the Question - Physiological Integrity, Reduction of Risk Potential

Nurse Lynette is preparing a site for the insertion of an I.V. catheter. The nurse should treat excess hair at the site by:

A. Leaving the hair intact
B. Shaving the area
C. Clipping the hair in the area
D. Removing the hair with a depilatory

QUESTION NUMBER 09.34
Question is about - osteoporosis
Category of the Question - Health Promotion and Maintenance

Nurse Michelle is caring for an elderly female with osteoporosis. When teaching the client, the nurse should include information about which major complication:

A. Bone fracture
B. Loss of estrogen
C. Negative calcium balance
D. Dowager's hump

QUESTION NUMBER 09.35
Question is about - BSE
Category of the Question - Health Promotion and Maintenance

Nurse Len is teaching a group of women to perform BSE. The nurse should explain that the purpose of performing the examination is to discover:

A. Cancerous lumps
B. Areas of thickness or fullness
C. Changes from previous examinations
D. Fibrocystic masses

QUESTION NUMBER 09.36
Question is about - hyperthyroidism
Category of the Question - Physiological Integrity, Basic Care and Comfort

When caring for a female client who is being treated for hyperthyroidism, it is important to:

A. Provide extra blankets and clothing to keep the client warm.
B. Monitor the client for signs of restlessness, sweating, and excessive weight loss during thyroid replacement therapy.
C. Balance the client's periods of activity and rest.
D. Encourage the client to be active to prevent constipation.

QUESTION NUMBER 09.37
Question is about - atherosclerosis
Category of the Question - Health Promotion and Maintenance

Nurse Kris is teaching a client with a history of atherosclerosis. To decrease the risk of atherosclerosis, the nurse should encourage the client to:

A. Avoid focusing on his weight
B. Increase his activity level
C. Follow a regular diet
D. Continue leading a high-stress lifestyle.

QUESTION NUMBER 09.38
Question is about - logroll
Category of the Question - Physiological Integrity, Physiological Adaptation

Nurse Greta is working on a surgical floor. Nurse Greta must logroll a client following a:

A. Laminectomy
B. Thoracotomy

C. Hemorrhoidectomy
D. Cystectomy

QUESTION NUMBER 09.39
Question is about - intraocular lens implant
Category of the Question - Health Promotion and Maintenance

A 55-year old client underwent cataract removal with intraocular lens implant. Nurse Oliver is giving the client discharge instructions. These instructions should include which of the following?

A. Avoid lifting objects weighing more than 5 lb (2.25 kg)
B. Lie on your abdomen when in bed
C. Keep rooms brightly lit
D. Avoiding straining during a bowel movement or bending at the waist

QUESTION NUMBER 09.40
Question is about - testicular exams
Category of the Question - Health Promotion and Maintenance

George should be taught about testicular examinations during:

A. When sexual activity starts
B. After age 69

C. After age 40
D. Before age 20

QUESTION NUMBER 09.41
Question is about - wound dehiscence
Category of the Question - Physiological Integrity, Physiological Adaptation

A male client has undergone a colon resection. While turning him, wound dehiscence with evisceration occurs. Nurse Trish first response is to:

A. Call the physician
B. Place a saline-soaked sterile dressing on the wound
C. Take blood pressure and pulse
D. Pull the dehiscence closed

QUESTION NUMBER 09.42
Question is about - Cheyne-Stokes respirations
Category of the Question - Physiological Integrity, Physiological Adaptation

Nurse Audrey is caring for a client who has suffered a severe cerebrovascular accident. During routine assessment, the nurse notices Cheyne- Stokes respirations. Cheyne-stokes respirations are:

A. Progressively deeper breath followed by shallower breaths with apneic periods.
B. Rapid, deep breathing with abrupt pauses between each breath.
C. Rapid, deep breathing and irregular breathing without pauses.
D. Shallow breathing with an increased respiratory rate.

QUESTION NUMBER 09.43
Question is about - heart failure
Category of the Question - Physiological Integrity, Physiological Adaptation

Nurse Bea is assessing a male client with heart failure. The breath sounds commonly auscultated in clients with heart failure are:

A. Tracheal
B. Fine crackles
C. Coarse crackles
D. Friction rubs

QUESTION NUMBER 09.44
Question is about - acute asthma
Category of the Question - Physiological Integrity, Physiological Adaptation

The nurse is caring for Kenneth experiencing an acute asthma attack. The client stops wheezing and breath sounds aren't audible. The reason for this change is that:

A. The attack is over.
B. The airways are so swollen that no air cannot get through.
C. The swelling has decreased.
D. Crackles have replaced wheezes.

QUESTION NUMBER 09.45
Question is about - seizure
Category of the Question - Safe & Effective Care Environment, Safety and infection Control

Mike with epilepsy is having a seizure. During the active seizure phase, the nurse should:

A. Place the client on his back, remove dangerous objects, and insert a bite block.
B. Place the client on his side, remove dangerous objects, and insert a bite block.
C. Place the client on his back, remove dangerous objects, and hold down his arms.
D. Place the client on his side, remove dangerous objects, and protect his head.

QUESTION NUMBER 09.46
Question is about - chest tube, pneumothorax
Category of the Question - Physiological Integrity,Reduction of Risk Potential

After insertion of a chest tube for a pneumothorax, a client becomes hypotensive with neck vein distention, tracheal shift, absent breath sounds, and diaphoresis. Nurse Amanda suspects a tension pneumothorax has occurred. What cause of tension pneumothorax should the nurse check for?

A. Infection of the lung

B. Kinked or obstructed chest tube

C. Excessive water in the water-seal chamber

D. Excessive chest tube drainage

QUESTION NUMBER 09.47

Question is about - choking

Category of the Question - Safe & Effective Care Environment, Safety and infection Control

Nurse Maureen is talking to a male client, the client begins choking on his lunch. He's coughing forcefully. The nurse should:

A. Stand him up and perform the abdominal thrust maneuver from behind.

B. Lay him down, straddle him, and perform the abdominal thrust maneuver.

C. Leave him to get assistance.

D. Stay with him but not intervene at this time.

QUESTION NUMBER 09.48

Question is about - health history

Category of the Question - Health Promotion and Maintenance

Nurse Ron is taking the health history of an 84-year-old client. Which information will be most useful to the nurse for planning care?

A. General health for the last 10 years

B. Current health promotion activities

C. Family history of diseases

D. Marital status

QUESTION NUMBER 09.49

Question is about - oral care

Category of the Question - Physiological Integrity, Physiological Adaptation

When performing oral care on a comatose client, Nurse Krina should:

A. Apply lemon glycerin to the client's lips at least every 2 hours.

B. Brush the teeth with a client lying supine.

C. Place the client in a side-lying position, with the head of the bed lowered.

D. Clean the client's mouth with hydrogen peroxide.

QUESTION NUMBER 09.50

Question is about - pneumonia

Category of the Question - Physiological Integrity, Physiological Adaptation

A 77-year-old male client is admitted with a diagnosis of dehydration and change in mental status. He's being hydrated with L.V. fluids. When the nurse takes his vital signs, she notes he has a fever of 103°F (39.4°C), a cough producing yellow sputum and pleuritic chest pain. The nurse suspects this client may have which of the following conditions?

A. Adult respiratory distress syndrome (ARDS)

B. Myocardial infarction (MI)

C. Pneumonia

D. Tuberculosis

QUESTION NUMBER 09.51

Question is about - tuberculosis

Category of the Question - Health Promotion and Maintenance

Nurse Oliver is working in an outpatient clinic. He has been alerted that there is an outbreak of tuberculosis (TB). Which of the following clients entering the clinic today is most likely to have TB?

A. A 16-year-old female high school student

B. A 33-year-old daycare worker

C. A 43-year-old homeless man with a history of alcoholism

D. A 54-year-old businessman

QUESTION NUMBER 09.52

Question is about - Mantoux test

Category of the Question - Physiological Integrity, Reduction of Risk Potential

Virgie with a positive Mantoux test result will be sent for a chest X-ray. The nurse is aware that which of the following reasons this is done?

A. To confirm the diagnosis

B. To determine if a repeat skin test is needed

C. To determine the extent of lesions

D. To determine if this is a primary or secondary infection

QUESTION NUMBER 09.53

Question is about - acute asthma

Category of the Question - Physiological Integrity, Physiological Adaptation

Kennedy with acute asthma showing inspiratory and expiratory wheezes and a decreased forced expiratory volume should be treated with which of the following classes of medication right away?

A. Beta-adrenergic blockers

B. Bronchodilators

C. Inhaled steroids

D. Oral steroids

QUESTION NUMBER 09.54

Question is about - bronchitis

Category of the Question - Physiological Integrity, Physiological Adaptation

Mr. Vasquez 56-year-old client with a 40-year history of smoking one to two packs of cigarettes per day has a chronic cough producing thick sputum, peripheral edema, and cyanotic nail beds. Based on this information, he most likely has which of the following conditions?

    A. Adult respiratory distress syndrome (ARDS)
    B. Asthma
    C. Chronic obstructive bronchitis
    D. Emphysema

QUESTION NUMBER 09.55
Question is about - chronic lymphocytic anemia
Category of the Question - Physiological Integrity, Reduction of Risk Potential

Situation: Francis, age 46 is admitted to the hospital with diagnosis of Chronic Lymphocytic Leukemia.

The treatment for patients with leukemia is bone marrow transplantation. Which statement about bone marrow transplantation is not correct?

    A. The patient is under local anesthesia during the procedure.
    B. The aspirated bone marrow is mixed with heparin.
    C. The aspiration site is the posterior or anterior iliac crest.
    D. The recipient receives cyclophosphamide (Cytoxan) for 4 consecutive days before the procedure.

QUESTION NUMBER 09.56
Question is about - disorientation
Category of the Question - Safe and Effective Care Environemnt

After several days of admission, Francis becomes disoriented and complains of frequent headaches. The nurse in-charge first action would be:

    A. Call the physician
    B. Document the patient's status in his charts
    C. Prepare oxygen treatment
    D. Raise the side rails

QUESTION NUMBER 09.57
Question is about - WBC
Category of the Question - Physiological Integrity, Physiological Adaptation

During routine care, Francis asks the nurse, "How can I be anemic if this disease causes increased white blood cell production?" The nurse in-charge best response would be that the increased number of white blood cells (WBC) is:

    A. Crowded red blood cells
    B. Is not responsible for the anemia
    C. Uses nutrients from other cells
    D. Have an abnormally short lifespan of cells

QUESTION NUMBER 09.58
Question is about - leukocytosis
Category of the Question - Physiological Integrity, Reduction of Risk Potential

Diagnostic assessment of Francis would probably not reveal:

A. Predominance of lymphoblasts

B. Leukocytosis

C. Abnormal blast cells in the bone marrow

D. Elevated thrombocyte counts

QUESTION NUMBER 09.59
Question is about - embolectomy
Category of the Question - Physiological Integrity, Reduction of Risk Potential

Robert, a 57-year-old client with acute arterial occlusion of the left leg undergoes an emergency embolectomy. Six hours later, the nurse isn't able to obtain pulses in his left foot using Doppler ultrasound. The nurse immediately notifies the physician and asks her to prepare the client for surgery. As the nurse enters the client's room to prepare him, he states that he won't have any more surgery. Which of the following is the best initial response by the nurse?

A. Explain the risks of not having the surgery

B. Notifying the physician immediately

C. Notifying the nursing supervisor

D. Recording the client's refusal in the nurses' notes

QUESTION NUMBER 09.60
Question is about - prioritization
Category of the Question - Safe and Effective Care Environment, Management of Care

During the endorsement, which of the following clients should the on-duty nurse assess first?

A. The 58-year-old client who was admitted 2 days ago with heart failure, blood pressure of 126/76 mm Hg, and a respiratory rate of 22 breaths/minute.

B. The 89-year-old client with end-stage right-sided heart failure, blood pressure of 78/50 mm Hg, and a "do not resuscitate" order.

C. The 62-year-old client who was admitted 1 day ago with thrombophlebitis and is receiving L.V. heparin.

D. The 75-year-old client who was admitted 1 hour ago with new-onset atrial fibrillation and is receiving L.V. diltiazem (Cardizem).

QUESTION NUMBER 09.61
Question is about - cocaine use
Category of the Question - Physiological Integrity, Pharmacological and Parenteral Therapies

Honey, a 23-year old client complains of substernal chest pain and states that her heart feels like "it's racing out of the chest". She reports no history of cardiac disorders. The nurse attaches her to a cardiac monitor and notes sinus tachycardia with a rate of 136beats/minutes. Breath sounds are clear and the respiratory rate is 26 breaths/minutes. Which of the following drugs should the nurse question the client about using?

A. Barbiturates

B. Opioids

C. Cocaine

D. Benzodiazepines

QUESTION NUMBER 09.62
Question is about - breast lump
Category of the Question - Health Promotion and Maintenance

A 51-year-old female client tells the nurse-in-charge that she has found a painless lump in her right breast during her monthly self-examination. Which assessment finding would strongly suggest that this client's lump is cancerous?

    A. Eversion of the right nipple and mobile mass.
    B. Nonmobile mass with irregular edges.
    C. Mobile mass that is soft and easily delineated.
    D. Nonpalpable right axillary lymph nodes.

QUESTION NUMBER 09.63
Question is about - vaginal cancer
Category of the Question - Physiological Integrity, Physiological Adaptation

A 35-year-old client with vaginal cancer asks the nurse, "What is the usual treatment for this type of cancer?" Which treatment should the nurse name?

    A. Surgery
    B. Chemotherapy
    C. Radiation
    D. Immunotherapy

QUESTION NUMBER 09.64
Question is about - TNM staging
Category of the Question - Physiological Integrity, Reduction of Risk Potential

Cristina undergoes a biopsy of a suspicious lesion. The biopsy report classifies the lesion according to the TNM staging system as follows: TIS, N0, M0. What does this classification mean?

    A. No evidence of primary tumor, no abnormal regional lymph nodes, and no evidence of distant metastasis.
    B. Carcinoma in situ, no abnormal regional lymph nodes, and no evidence of distant metastasis.
    C. Can't assess tumor or regional lymph nodes and no evidence of metastasis.
    D. Carcinoma in situ, no demonstrable metastasis of the regional lymph nodes, and ascending degrees of distant metastasis.

QUESTION NUMBER 09.65
Question is about - laryngectomy, stoma
Category of the Question - Physiological Integrity, Reduction of Risk Potential

Lydia undergoes a laryngectomy to treat laryngeal cancer. When teaching the client how to care for the neck stoma, the nurse should include which instruction?

    A. "Keep the stoma uncovered."
    B. "Keep the stoma dry."
    C. "Have a family member perform stoma care initially until you get used to the procedure."
    D. "Keep the stoma moist."

QUESTION NUMBER 09.66
Question is about - cancer
Category of the Question - Physiological Integrity, Physiological Adaptation

A 37-year-old client with uterine cancer asks the nurse, "Which is the most common type of cancer in women?" The nurse replies that it's breast cancer. Which type of cancer causes the most deaths in women?

    A. Breast cancer
    B. Lung cancer
    C. Brain cancer
    D. Colon and rectal cancer

QUESTION NUMBER 09.67
Question is about - Horner's syndrome, lung cancer
Category of the Question - Physiological Integrity, Physiological Adaptation

Antonio, with lung cancer, develops Horner's syndrome when the tumor invades the ribs and affects the sympathetic nerve ganglia. When assessing for signs and symptoms of this syndrome, the nurse should note:

    A. Miosis, partial eyelid ptosis, and anhidrosis on the affected side of the face.
    B. Chest pain, dyspnea, cough, weight loss, and fever.
    C. Arm and shoulder pain and atrophy of arm and hand muscles, both on the affected side.
    D. Hoarseness and dysphagia.

QUESTION NUMBER 09.68
Question is about - PSA
Category of the Question - Physiological Integrity, Reduction of Risk Potential

Vic asks the nurse what PSA is. The nurse should reply that it stands for:

    A. Prostate-specific antigen, which is used to screen for prostate cancer.
    B. Protein serum antigen, which is used to determine protein levels.
    C. Pneumococcal strep antigen, which is a bacteria that causes pneumonia.
    D. Papanicolaou-specific antigen, which is used to screen for cervical cancer.

QUESTION NUMBER 09.69
Question is about - subarachnoid block
Category of the Question - Physiological Integrity, Reduction of Risk Potential

What is the most important postoperative instruction that nurse Kate must give a client who has just returned from the operating room after receiving a subarachnoid block?

    A. "Avoid drinking liquids until the gag reflex returns."
    B. "Avoid eating milk products for 24 hours."
    C. "Notify a nurse if you experience blood in your urine."
    D. "Remain supine for the time specified by the physician."

QUESTION NUMBER 09.70
Question is about - colorectal cancer
Category of the Question - Physiological Integrity, Reduction of Risk Potential

A male client suspected of having colorectal cancer will require which diagnostic study to confirm the diagnosis?

   A. Stool Hematest
   B. Carcinoembryonic antigen (CEA)
   C. Sigmoidoscopy
   D. Abdominal computed tomography (CT) scan

QUESTION NUMBER 09.71
Question is about - breast cancer
Category of the Question - Physiological Integrity, Physiological Adaptation

During a breast examination, which finding most strongly suggests that the Luz has breast cancer?

   A. Slight asymmetry of the breasts.
   B. A fixed nodular mass with dimpling of the overlying skin.
   C. Bloody discharge from the nipple.
   D. Multiple firm, round, freely movable masses that change with the menstrual cycle.

QUESTION NUMBER 09.72
Question is about - cancer
Category of the Question - Physiological Integrity, Physiological Adaptation

A female client with cancer is being evaluated for possible metastasis. Which of the following is one of the most common metastasis sites for cancer cells?

   A. Liver
   B. Colon
   C. Reproductive tract
   D. White blood cells (WBCs)

QUESTION NUMBER 09.73
Question is about - MRI
Category of the Question - Physiological Integrity,Reduction of Risk Potential

Nurse Mandy is preparing a client for magnetic resonance imaging (MRI) to confirm or rule out a spinal cord lesion. During the MRI scan, which of the following would pose a threat to the client?

   A. The client lies still
   B. The client asks questions
   C. The client hears thumping sounds
   D. The client wears a watch and wedding band

QUESTION NUMBER 09.74
Question is about - osteoporosis
Category of the Question - Health Promotion and Maintenance

Nurse Cecile is teaching a female client about preventing osteoporosis. Which of the following teaching points is correct?

A. Obtaining an X-ray of the bones every 3 years is recommended to detect bone loss.
B. To avoid fractures, the client should avoid strenuous exercise.
C. The recommended daily allowance of calcium may be found in a wide variety of foods
D. Obtaining the recommended daily allowance of calcium requires taking a calcium supplement.

QUESTION NUMBER 09.75
Question is about - arthroscopy
Category of the Question - Physiological Integrity, Reduction of Risk Potential

Before Jacob undergoes arthroscopy, the nurse reviews the assessment findings for contraindications for this procedure. Which finding is a contraindication?

A. Joint pain
B. Joint deformity

C. Joint flexion of less than 50%
D. Joint stiffness

Practice Question Set-10

QUESTION NUMBER 10.01
Question is about - mitral regurgitation
Category of the Question - Physiological Integrity, Physiological Adaptation

Among the following signs and symptoms, which would most likely be present in a client with mitral regurgitation?

A. Altered level of consciousness
B. Exertional Dyspnea
C. Increase creatine phosphokinase concentration
D. Chest pain

QUESTION NUMBER 10.02
Question is about - urinary frequency
Category of the Question - Physiological Integrity, Physiological Adaptation

Kris with a history of chronic infection of the urinary system complains of urinary frequency and burning sensation. To figure out whether the current problem is of renal origin, the nurse should assess whether the client has discomfort or pain in the:

A. Urinary meatus
B. Pain in the labium
C. Suprapubic area
D. Right or left costovertebral angle

QUESTION NUMBER 10.03
Question is about - renal function
Category of the Question - Physiological Integrity, Physiological Adaptation

Nurse Perry is evaluating the renal function of a male client. After documenting urine volume and characteristics, Nurse Perry assesses which signs as the best indicator of renal function.

A. Blood pressure
B. Consciousness
C. Distension of the bladder
D. Pulse rate

QUESTION NUMBER 10.04
Question is about - seizure
Category of the Question - Physiological Integrity, Physiological Adaptation

John suddenly experiences a seizure, and Nurse Gina notices that John exhibits uncontrollable jerking movements. Nurse Gina documents that John experienced which type of seizure?

A. Tonic seizure
B. Absence seizure

C. Myoclonic seizure
D. Clonic seizure

QUESTION NUMBER 10.05
Question is about - smoking cessation, Buerger's disease
Category of the Question - Health Promotion and Maintenance

Smoking cessation is a critical strategy for the client with Buerger's disease, Nurse Jasmin anticipates that the male client will go home with a prescription for which medication?

A. Paracetamol
B. Ibuprofen

C. Nitroglycerin
D. Nicotine (Nicotrol)

QUESTION NUMBER 10.06
Question is about - Raynaud's disease
Category of the Question - Physiological Integrity, Physiological Adaptation

Nurse Lilly has been assigned to a client with Raynaud's disease. Nurse Lilly realizes that the etiology of the disease is unknown but it is characterized by:

A. Episodic vasospastic disorder of capillaries
B. Episodic vasospastic disorder of small veins
C. Episodic vasospastic disorder of the aorta
D. Episodic vasospastic disorder of the small arteries

QUESTION NUMBER 10.07
Question is about - diabetes
Category of the Question - Health Promotion and Maintenance

Nurse Jamie should explain to a male client with diabetes that self-monitoring of blood glucose is preferred to urine glucose testing because:

A. More accurate

B. Can be done by the client

C. It is easy to perform

D. It is not influenced by drugs

QUESTION NUMBER 10.08

Question is about - diuretic therapy

Category of the Question - Physiological Integrity, Physiological Adaptation

Jessie weighed 210 pounds on admission to the hospital. After 2 days of diuretic therapy, Jessie weighs 205.5 pounds. The nurse could estimate the amount of fluid Jessie has lost:

A. 0.3 L

B. 1.5 L

C. 2.0 L

D. 3.5 L

QUESTION NUMBER 10.09

Question is about - albumin

Category of the Question - Physiological Integrity, Physiological Adaptation

Nurse Donna is aware that the shift of body fluids associated with Intravenous administration of albumin occurs in the process of:

A. Osmosis

B. Diffusion

C. Active transport

D. Filtration

QUESTION NUMBER 10.10

Question is about - crutch walking

Category of the Question - Physiological Integrity, Reduction of Risk Potential

Myrna, a 52-year-old client with a fractured left tibia, has a long leg cast and she is using crutches to ambulate. Nurse Joy assesses for which sign and symptom that indicates complication associated with crutch walking?

A. Left leg discomfort

B. Weak biceps brachii

C. Triceps muscle spasm

D. Forearm weakness

QUESTION NUMBER 10.11

Question is about - neutropenia

Category of the Question - Health Promotion and Maintenance

Which of the following statements should the nurse teach the neutropenic client and his family to avoid?

A. Performing oral hygiene after every meal

B. Using suppositories or enemas

C. Performing perineal hygiene after each bowel movement

D. Using a filter mask

QUESTION NUMBER 10.12
Question is about - perforated peptic ulcer
Category of the Question - Physiological Integrity, Physiological Adaptation

A female client is experiencing a painful and rigid abdomen and is diagnosed with perforated peptic ulcer. A surgery has been scheduled and a nasogastric tube is inserted. The nurse should place the client before surgery in

A. Sims position

B. Supine position

C. Semi-fowlers position

D. Dorsal recumbent position

QUESTION NUMBER 10.13
Question is about - ventilating exchange
Category of the Question - Physiological Integrity, Physiological Adaptation

Which nursing intervention ensures adequate ventilating exchange after surgery?

A. Remove the airway only when the client is fully conscious

B. Assess for hypoventilation by auscultating the lungs

C. Position client laterally with the neck extended

D. Maintain humidified oxygen via nasal cannula

QUESTION NUMBER 10.14
Question is about - chest tube
Category of the Question - Physiological Integrity, Reduction of Risk Potential

George, who has undergone thoracic surgery has a chest tube connected to a water-seal drainage system attached to suction. Presence of excessive bubbling is identified in the water-seal chamber, the nurse should:

A. "Strip" the chest tube catheter

B. Check the system for air leaks

C. Recognize the system is functioning correctly

D. Decrease the amount of suction pressure

QUESTION NUMBER 10.15
Question is about - hypertension
Category of the Question - Health Promotion and Maintenance

A client who has been diagnosed with hypertension is being taught to restrict intake of sodium. The nurse would know that the teachings are effective if the client states that:

A. I can eat celery sticks and carrots

B. I can eat broiled scallops

C. I can eat shredded wheat cereal

D. I can eat spaghetti on rye bread

QUESTION NUMBER 10.16
Question is about - cirrhosis
Category of the Question - Physiological Integrity, Physiological Adaptation

A male client with a history of cirrhosis and alcoholism is admitted with severe dyspnea resulting from ascites. The nurse should be aware that the ascites is most likely the result of increased:

A. Pressure in the portal vein

B. Production of serum albumin

C. Secretion of bile salts

D. Interstitial osmotic pressure

QUESTION NUMBER 10.17
Question is about - Hodgkin's disease
Category of the Question - PSafe and Effective Care Environment, Management of Care

A newly admitted client diagnosed with Hodgkin's disease undergoes an excisional cervical lymph node biopsy under local anesthesia. What does the nurse assess first after the procedure?

A. Vital signs
B. Incision site
C. Airway
D. Level of consciousness

QUESTION NUMBER 10.18
Question is about - hypovolemic shock
Category of the Question - Physiological Integrity, Physiological Adaptation

A client has 15% blood loss. Which of the following nursing assessment findings indicates hypovolemic shock?

A. Systolic blood pressure less than 90 mm Hg
B. Pupils unequally dilated
C. Respiratory rate of 4 breath/min
D. Pulse rate less than 60 bpm

QUESTION NUMBER 10.19
Question is about - rhinoplasty
Category of the Question - Physiological Integrity, Reduction of Risk Potential

ADVERTISEMENTS

Nurse Lucy is planning to give preoperative teaching to a client who will be undergoing rhinoplasty. Which of the following should be included?

A. Results of the surgery will be immediately noticeable postoperatively
B. Normal saline nose drops will need to be administered preoperatively
C. After surgery, nasal packing will be in place 8 to 10 days
D. Aspirin-containing medications should not be taken 14 days before surgery

QUESTION NUMBER 10.20
Question is about - diabetic ketoacidosis
Category of the Question - Physiological Integrity, Physiological Adaptation

Paul is admitted to the hospital due to metabolic acidosis caused by Diabetic ketoacidosis (DKA). The nurse prepares which of the following medications as an initial treatment for this problem?

A. Regular insulin
B. Potassium
C. Sodium bicarbonate
D. Calcium gluconate

QUESTION NUMBER 10.21
Question is about - beta-carotene
Category of the Question - Health Promotion and Maintenance

Dr. Marquez tells a client that an increased intake of foods that are rich in Vitamin E and beta-carotene are important for healthier skin. The nurse teaches the client that excellent food sources of both of these substances are:

A. Fish and fruit jam
B. Oranges and grapefruit

C. Carrots and potatoes
D. Spinach and mangoes

QUESTION NUMBER 10.22
Question is about - gastroesophageal reflux
Category of the Question - Health Promotion and Maintenance

A client has Gastroesophageal Reflux Disease (GERD). The nurse should teach the client that after every meal, the client should:

A. Rest in sitting position
B. Take a short walk

C. Drink plenty of water
D. Lie down at least 30 minutes

QUESTION NUMBER 10.23
Question is about - gastroscopy
Category of the Question - PPhysiological Integrity, Reduction of Risk Potential

After gastroscopy, an adaptation that indicates major complication would be:

A. Nausea and vomiting
B. Abdominal distention
C. Increased GI motility
D. Difficulty in swallowing

QUESTION NUMBER 10.24
Question is about - cholecystectomy
Category of the Question - Health Promotion and Maintenance

A client who has undergone a cholecystectomy asks the nurse whether there are any dietary restrictions that must be followed. Nurse Hilary would recognize that the dietary teaching was well understood when the client tells a family member that:

A. "Most people need to eat a high protein diet for 12 months after surgery"
B. "I should not eat those foods that upset me before the surgery"
C. "I should avoid fatty foods as long as I live"
D. "Most people can tolerate regular diet after this type of surgery"

QUESTION NUMBER 10.25
Question is about - hepatitis A
Category of the Question - Physiological Integrity, Physiological Adaptation

Nurse Rachel teaches a client who has been recently diagnosed with hepatitis A about untoward signs and symptoms related to Hepatitis that may develop. The one that should be reported immediately to the physician is:

A. Restlessness

B. Yellow urine

C. Nausea

D. Clay-colored stools

QUESTION NUMBER 10.26

Question is about - antituberculosis

Category of the Question - Physiological Integrity, Pharmacological and Parenteral Therapies

Which of the following antituberculosis drugs can damage the 8th cranial nerve?

A. Isoniazid (INH)

B. Para Aminosalicylic acid (PAS)

C. Ethambutol hydrochloride (Myambutol)

D. Streptomycin

QUESTION NUMBER 10.27

Question is about - peptic ulcer disease

Category of the Question - Physiological Integrity, Physiological Adaptation

The client asks Nurse Annie the causes of peptic ulcer. Nurse Annie responds that recent research indicates that peptic ulcers are the result of which of the following:

A. Genetic defect in gastric mucosa

B. Stress

C. Diet high in fat

D. Helicobacter pylori infection

QUESTION NUMBER 10.28

Question is about - gastrectomy

Category of the Question - Physiological Integrity, Physiological Adaptation

Ryan has undergone subtotal gastrectomy. The nurse should expect that nasogastric tube drainage will be what color for about 12 to 24 hours after surgery?

A. Bile green

B. Bright red

C. Cloudy white

D. Dark brown

QUESTION NUMBER 10.29

Question is about - eye surgery

Category of the Question - Physiological Integrity, Physiological Adaptation

Nurse Joan is assigned to come for a client who has just undergone eye surgery. Nurse Joan plans to teach the client activities that are permitted during the postoperative period. Which of the following is best recommended for the client?

A. Watching circus

B. Bending over

C. Watching TV

D. Lifting objects

QUESTION NUMBER 10.30
Question is about - leg injury
Category of the Question - Physiological Integrity, Physiological Adaptation

A client suffered from a lower leg injury and seeks treatment in the emergency room. There is a prominent deformity to the lower aspect of the leg, and the injured leg appears shorter than the other leg. The affected leg is painful, swollen and beginning to become ecchymotic. The nurse interprets that the client is experiencing:

A. Fracture
B. Strain
C. Sprain
D. Contusion

QUESTION NUMBER 10.31
Question is about - otic solution
Category of the Question - Physiological Integrity, Pharmacological and Parenteral Therapies

Nurse Jenny is instilling an otic solution into an adult male client's left ear. Nurse Jenny avoids doing which of the following as part of the procedure

A. Pulling the auricle backward and upward.
B. Warming the solution to room temperature.
C. Pacing the tip of the dropper on the edge of the ear canal.
D. Placing the client in a side lying position.

QUESTION NUMBER 10.32
Question is about - ileostomy
Category of the Question - Physiological Integrity, Reduction of Risk Potential

Nurse Bea should instruct the male client with an ileostomy to report immediately which of the following symptoms?

A. Absence of drainage from the ileostomy for 6 or more hours
B. Passage of liquid stool in the stoma
C. Occasional presence of undigested food
D. A temperature of 37.6 °C

QUESTION NUMBER 10.33
Question is about - appendicitis
Category of the Question - Physiological Integrity, Physiological Adaptation

Jerry has been diagnosed with appendicitis. He develops a fever, hypotension, and tachycardia. The nurse suspects which of the following complications?

A. Intestinal obstruction
B. Peritonitis
C. Bowel ischemia
D. Deficient fluid volume

QUESTION NUMBER 10.34
Question is about - pancreatitis
Category of the Question - Physiological Integrity, Physiological Adaptation

Which of the following complications should the nurse carefully monitor a client with acute pancreatitis?

A. Myocardial Infarction

B. Cirrhosis

C. Peptic ulcer

D. Pneumonia

QUESTION NUMBER 10.35
Question is about - viral hepatitis
Category of the Question - Physiological Integrity, Physiological Adaptation

Which of the following symptoms during the icteric phase of viral hepatitis should the nurse expect the client to inhibit?

A. Watery stool

B. Yellow sclera

C. Tarry stool

D. Shortness of breath

QUESTION NUMBER 10.36
Question is about - craniotomy
Category of the Question - Physiological Integrity, Physiological Adaptation

Marco, who was diagnosed with a brain tumor, was scheduled for craniotomy. In preventing the development of cerebral edema after surgery, the nurse should expect the use of:

A. Diuretics

B. Antihypertensive

C. Steroids

D. Anticonvulsants

QUESTION NUMBER 10.37
Question is about - blood transfusion
Category of the Question - Physiological Integrity, Pharmacological and Parenteral Therapies

Halfway through the administration of blood, the female client complains of lumbar pain. After stopping the infusion Nurse Hazel should:

A. Increase the flow of normal saline

B. Assess the pain further

C. Notify the blood bank

D. Obtain vital signs

QUESTION NUMBER 10.38
Question is about - HIV infection
Category of the Question - Physiological Integrity, Physiological Adaptation

Nurse Maureen knows that the positive diagnosis of HIV infection is made based on which of the following:

A. A history of high-risk sexual behaviors.

B. Positive ELISA and western blot tests

C. Identification of an associated opportunistic infection

D. Evidence of extreme weight loss and high fever

QUESTION NUMBER 10.39
Question is about - chronic renal failure
Category of the Question - Health Promotion and Maintenance

Nurse Maureen is aware that a client who has been diagnosed with chronic renal failure recognizes an adequate amount of high-biological-value protein when the food the client selected from the menu was:

A. Raw carrots
B. Apple juice

C. Whole wheat bread
D. Cottage cheese

QUESTION NUMBER 10.40
Question is about - uremic syndrome
Category of the Question - Physiological Integrity, Physiological Adaptation

Kenneth, who was diagnosed with uremic syndrome has the potential to develop complications. Which among the following complications should the nurse anticipates:

A. Flapping hand tremors
B. An elevated hematocrit level

C. Hypotension
D. Hypokalemia

QUESTION NUMBER 10.41
Question is about - benign prostatic hyperplasia
Category of the Question - Physiological Integrity, Physiological Adaptation

A client is admitted to the hospital with benign prostatic hyperplasia, the nurse most relevant assessment would be:

A. Flank pain radiating in the groin
B. Distention of the lower abdomen

C. Perineal edema
D. Urethral discharge

QUESTION NUMBER 10.42
Question is about - penile implant
Category of the Question - Physiological Integrity, Reduction of Risk Potential

A client has undergone a penile implant. After 24 hrs of surgery, the client's scrotum was edematous and painful. The nurse should:

A. Assist the client with sitz bath
B. Apply warm soaks in the scrotum

C. Elevate the scrotum using a soft support
D. Prepare for a possible incision and drainage

QUESTION NUMBER 10.43
Question is about - chest pain
Category of the Question - Physiological Integrity, Physiological Adaptation

Nurse Hazel receives emergency laboratory results for a client with chest pain and immediately informs the physician. An increased myoglobin level suggests which of the following?

A. Liver disease
B. Myocardial damage

C. Hypertension
D. Cancer

QUESTION NUMBER 10.44
Question is about - mitral stenosis
Category of the Question - Physiological Integrity, Physiological Adaptation

Nurse Maureen would expect a client with mitral stenosis would demonstrate symptoms associated with congestion in the:

A. Right atrium

B. Superior vena cava

C. Aorta

D. Pulmonary

QUESTION NUMBER 10.45
Question is about - hypertension
Category of the Question - Physiological Integrity, Reduction of Risk Potential

A client has been diagnosed with hypertension. The nurse priority nursing diagnosis would be:

A. Ineffective health maintenance

B. Impaired skin integrity

C. Deficient fluid volume

D. Pain

QUESTION NUMBER 10.46
Question is about - angina
Category of the Question - Physiological Integrity, Pharmacological and Parenteral Therapies

Nurse Hazel teaches the client with angina about common expected side effects of nitroglycerin including:

A. High blood pressure

B. Stomach cramps

C. Headache

D. Shortness of breath

QUESTION NUMBER 10.47
Question is about - atherosclerosis, PVD
Category of the Question - Physiological Integrity, Physiological Adaptation

The following are lipid abnormalities. Which of the following is a risk factor for the development of atherosclerosis and PVD?

A. High levels of low-density lipid (LDL) cholesterol

B. High levels of high-density lipid (HDL) cholesterol

C. Low concentration triglycerides

D. Low levels of LDL cholesterol.

QUESTION NUMBER 10.48
Question is about - aortic aneurysm
Category of the Question - Physiological Integrity, Reduction of Risk Potential

Which of the following represents a significant risk immediately after surgery for repair of aortic aneurysm?

A. Potential wound infection

B. Potential ineffective coping

C. Potential electrolyte imbalance

D. Potential alteration in renal perfusion

QUESTION NUMBER 10.49
Question is about - vitamin B12
Category of the Question - Physiological Integrity, Basic Care and Comfort

Nurse Josie should instruct the client to eat which of the following foods to obtain the best supply of Vitamin B12?

A. Dairy products
B. Vegetables
C. Grains
D. Broccoli

QUESTION NUMBER 10.50
Question is about - aplastic anemia
Category of the Question - Physiological Integrity, Reduction of Risk Potential

Karen has been diagnosed with aplastic anemia. The nurse monitors for changes in which of the following physiologic functions?

A. Bowel function
B. Peripheral sensation
C. Bleeding tendencies
D. Intake and output

QUESTION NUMBER 10.51
Question is about - splenectomy
Category of the Question - Physiological Integrity, Reduction of Risk Potential

Lydia is scheduled for elective splenectomy. Before the client goes to surgery, the nurse in charge final assessment would be:

A. Signed consent
B. Vital signs
C. Name band
D. Empty bladder

QUESTION NUMBER 10.52
Question is about - acute lymphocytic anemia
Category of the Question - Physiological Integrity, Physiological Adaptation

What is the peak age range for acquiring acute lymphocytic leukemia (ALL)?

A. 4 to 12 years
B. 20 to 30 years
C. 40 to 50 years
D. 60 to 70 years

QUESTION NUMBER 10.53
Question is about - acute lymphocytic leukemia
Category of the Question - Physiological Integrity, Physiological Adaptation

Marie with acute lymphocytic leukemia suffers from nausea and headache. These clinical manifestations may indicate all of the following except:

A. Effects of radiation
B. Chemotherapy side effects
C. Meningeal irritation
D. Gastric distension

QUESTION NUMBER 10.54

Question is about - disseminated intravascular coagulation
Category of the Question - Physiological Integrity, Physiological Integrity, Reduction of Risk Potential

A client has been diagnosed with Disseminated Intravascular Coagulation (DIC). Which of the following is contraindicated with the client?

    A. Administering Heparin
    B. Administering Coumadin
    C. Treating the underlying cause
    D. Replacing depleted blood products

QUESTION NUMBER 10.55

Question is about - hypovolemic shock
Category of the Question - Physiological Integrity, Physiological Adaptation

Which of the following findings is the best indication that fluid replacement for the client with hypovolemic shock is adequate?

    A. Urine output greater than 30ml/hr
    B. Respiratory rate of 21 breaths/minute
    C. Diastolic blood pressure greater than 90 mmHg
    D. Systolic blood pressure greater than 110 mmHg

QUESTION NUMBER 10.56

Question is about - laryngeal cancer
Category of the Question - Physiological Integrity, Physiological Adaptation

Which of the following signs and symptoms would Nurse Maureen include in her teaching plan as an early manifestation of laryngeal cancer?

    A. Stomatitis
    B. Airway obstruction
    C. Hoarseness
    D. Dysphagia

QUESTION NUMBER 10.57

Question is about - myasthenia gravis
Category of the Question - Physiological Integrity, Physiological Adaptation

Karina, a client with myasthenia gravis, is to receive immunosuppressive therapy. The nurse understands that this therapy is effective because it:

    A. Promotes the removal of antibodies that impair the transmission of impulses
    B. Stimulates the production of acetylcholine at the neuromuscular junction.
    C. Decreases the production of autoantibodies that attack the acetylcholine receptors.
    D. Inhibits the breakdown of acetylcholine at the neuromuscular junction.

QUESTION NUMBER 10.58
Question is about - Mannitol
Category of the Question - Pharmacological and Parenteral Therapies

A female client is receiving IV Mannitol. An assessment specific to safe administration of the said drug is:

A. Vital signs q4h

B. Weighing daily

C. Urine output hourly

D. Level of consciousness q4h

QUESTION NUMBER 10.59
Question is about - diabetes mellitus
Category of the Question - Health Promotion and Maintenance

Patricia, a 20-year-old college student with diabetes mellitus, requests additional information about the advantages of using a pen-like insulin delivery device. The nurse explains that the advantages of these devices over syringes include:

A. Accurate dose delivery

B. Shorter injection time

C. Lower cost with reusable insulin cartridges

D. Use of a smaller gauge needle.

QUESTION NUMBER 10.60
Question is about - fracture
Category of the Question - Physiological Integrity, Reduction of Risk Potential

A male client's left tibia was fractured in an automobile accident, and a cast is applied. To assess for damage to major blood vessels from the fracture tibia, the nurse in charge should monitor the client for:

A. Swelling of the left thigh

B. Increased skin temperature of the foot

C. Prolonged reperfusion of the toes after blanching

D. Increased blood pressure

QUESTION NUMBER 10.61
Question is about - cast
Category of the Question - Physiological Integrity, Basic Care and Comfort

After a long leg cast is removed, the male client should:

A. Cleanse the leg by scrubbing with a brisk motion

B. Put leg through full range of motion twice daily

C. Report any discomfort or stiffness to the physician

D. Elevate the leg when sitting for long periods of time.

QUESTION NUMBER 10.62
Question is about - tophi
Category of the Question - Physiological Integrity, Reduction of Risk Potential

While performing a physical assessment of a male client with gout of the great toe, Nurse Vivian should assess for additional tophi (urate deposits) on the:

A. Buttocks

B. Ears

C. Face

D. Abdomen

QUESTION NUMBER 10.63
Question is about - crutch walking
Category of the Question - Safe and Effective Care Environment,, Safety and Infection Control

Nurse Katrina would recognize that the demonstration of crutch walking with tripod gait was understood when the client places weight on the:

A. Palms of the hands and axillary regions
B. Palms of the hand
C. Axillary regions
D. Feet, which are set apart

QUESTION NUMBER 10.64
Question is about - rheumatoid arthritis
Category of the Question - Physiological Integrity, Physiological Adaptation

Mang Jose with rheumatoid arthritis states, "The only time I am without pain is when I lie in bed perfectly still". During the convalescent stage, the nurse in charge with Mang Jose should encourage:

ADVERTISEMENTS

A. Active joint flexion and extension
B. Continued immobility until pain subsides
C. Range of motion exercises twice daily
D. Flexion exercises three times daily

QUESTION NUMBER 10.65
Question is about - spinal surgery
Category of the Question - Physiological Integrity, Reduction of Risk Potential

A male client has undergone spinal surgery, the nurse should:
A. Observe the client's bowel movement and voiding patterns
B. Log-roll the client to prone position
C. Assess the client's feet for sensation and circulation
D. Encourage client to drink plenty of fluids

QUESTION NUMBER 10.66
Question is about - acute renal failure
Category of the Question - Physiological Integrity, Physiological Adaptation

Marina with acute renal failure moves into the diuretic phase after one week of therapy. During this phase the client must be assessed for signs of developing:

A. Hypovolemia
B. Renal failure
C. Metabolic acidosis
D. Hyperkalemia

QUESTION NUMBER 10.67
Question Tag:
Category of the Question - Physiological Integrity, Reduction of Risk Potential

Nurse Judith obtains a specimen of clear nasal drainage from a client with a head injury. Which of the following tests differentiates mucus from cerebrospinal fluid (CSF)?

A. Protein
B. Specific gravity

C. Glucose
D. Microorganism

QUESTION NUMBER 10.68
Question is about - seizure
Category of the Question - Physiological Integrity, Physiological Adaptation

A 22-year-old client suffered from his first tonic-clonic seizure. Upon awakening, the client asks the nurse, "What caused me to have a seizure? Which of the following would the nurse include in the primary cause of tonic-clonic seizures in adults more than 20 years?

A. Electrolyte imbalance
B. Head trauma
C. Epilepsy
D. Congenital defect

QUESTION NUMBER 10.69
Question is about - thrombotic CVA
Category of the Question - Physiological Integrity, Reduction of Risk Potential

What is the priority nursing assessment in the first 24 hours after admission of the client with thrombotic CVA?

A. Pupil size and pupillary response
B. Cholesterol level
C. Echocardiogram
D. Bowel sounds

QUESTION NUMBER 10.70
Question is about - multiple sclerosis
Category of the Question - Health Promotion and Maintenance

Nurse Linda is preparing a client with multiple sclerosis for discharge from the hospital to home. Which of the following instructions is most appropriate?

A. "Practice using the mechanical aids that you will need when future disabilities arise".
B. "Follow good health habits to change the course of the disease".
C. "Keep active, use stress reduction strategies, and avoid fatigue".
D. "You will need to accept the necessity for a quiet and inactive lifestyle".

QUESTION NUMBER 10.71
Question is about - hypoxia
Category of the Question - Physiological Integrity, Physiological Adaptation

The nurse is aware the early indicator of hypoxia in the unconscious client is:

A. Cyanosis

B. Increased respirations

C. Hypertension

D. Restlessness

QUESTION NUMBER 10.72
Question is about - spinal shock
Category of the Question - Physiological Integrity, Physiological Adaptation

A client is experiencing spinal shock. Nurse Myrna should expect the function of the bladder to be which of the following?

A. Normal

B. Atonic

C. Spastic

D. Uncontrolled

QUESTION NUMBER 10.73
Question is about - carcinogen
Category of the Question - Physiological Integrity, Physiological Adaptation

Which of the following stages is the carcinogen irreversible?

A. Progression stage

B. Initiation stage

C. Regression stage

D. Promotion stage

QUESTION NUMBER 10.74
Question is about - pain assessment
Category of the Question - Physiological Integrity, Physiological Adaptation

Among the following components thorough pain assessment, which is the most significant?

A. Effect

B. Cause

C. Causing factors

D. Intensity

QUESTION NUMBER 10.75
Question is about - pruritus
Category of the Question - Physiological Integrity, Physiological Adaptation

A 65 year old female is experiencing a flare-up of pruritus. Which of the client's actions could aggravate the cause of flare-ups?

A. Sleeping in cool and humidified environment

B. Daily baths with fragrant soap

C. Using clothes made from 100% cotton

D. Increasing fluid intake

Practice Question Set-11

QUESTION NUMBER 11.01
Question is about - arthritis
Category of the Question - Physiological Integrity,

Mr. Rodriguez is admitted with severe pain in the knees. Which form of arthritis is characterized by urate deposits and joint pain, usually in the feet and legs, and occurs primarily in men over age 30?

    A. Septic arthritis
    B. Traumatic arthritis
    C. Intermittent arthritis
    D. Gouty arthritis

QUESTION NUMBER 11.02
Question is about - heparin
Category of the Question - Physiological Integrity, Pharmacological and Parenteral Therapies

A heparin infusion at 1,500 units/hour is ordered for a 64-year-old client with stroke in evolution. The infusion contains 25,000 units of heparin in 500 ml of saline solution. How many milliliters per hour should be given?

    A. 15 ml/hour
    B. 30 ml/hour

    C. 45 ml/hour
    D. 50 ml/hour

QUESTION NUMBER 11.03
Question is about - stroke
Category of the Question - Physiological Integrity, Physiological Adaptation

A 76-year-old male client had a thromboembolic right stroke; his left arm is swollen. Which of the following conditions may cause swelling after a stroke?

    A. Elbow contracture secondary to spasticity.
    B. Loss of muscle contraction decreasing venous return.
    C. Deep vein thrombosis (DVT) due to immobility of the ipsilateral side.
    D. Hypoalbuminemia due to protein escaping from an inflamed glomerulus.

QUESTION NUMBER 11.04
Question is about - osteoarthritis
Category of the Question - Physiological Integrity, Physiological Adaptation

Heberden's nodes are a common sign of osteoarthritis. Which of the following statements is correct about this deformity?

    A. It appears only in men.
    B. It appears on the distal interphalangeal joint.
    C. It appears on the proximal interphalangeal joint.
    D. It appears on the dorsolateral aspect of the interphalangeal joint.

QUESTION NUMBER 11.05
Question is about - arthritis
Category of the Question - Physiological Integrity, Physiological Adaptation

Which of the following statements explains the main difference between rheumatoid arthritis and osteoarthritis?

A. Osteoarthritis is gender-specific, rheumatoid arthritis isn't.
B. Osteoarthritis is a localized disease rheumatoid arthritis is systemic.
C. Osteoarthritis is a systemic disease, rheumatoid arthritis is localized.
D. Osteoarthritis has dislocations and subluxations, rheumatoid arthritis doesn't.

QUESTION NUMBER 11.06
Question is about - assistive devices
Category of the Question - Basic Care and Comfort

Mrs. Cruz uses a cane for assistance in walking. Which of the following statements is true about a cane or other assistive devices?

A. A walker is a better choice than a cane.
B. The cane should be used on the affected side.
C. The cane should be used on the unaffected side.
D. A client with osteoarthritis should be encouraged to ambulate without the cane.

QUESTION NUMBER 11.07
Question is about - insulin
Category of the Question - Physiological Integrity, Pharmacological and Parenteral Therapies

A male client with type 1 diabetes is scheduled to receive 30 U of 70/30 insulin. There is no 70/30 insulin available. As a substitution, the nurse may give the client:

A. 9 U regular insulin and 21 U neutral protamine Hagedorn (NPH).
B. 21 U regular insulin and 9 U NPH.
C. 10 U regular insulin and 20 U NPH.
D. 20 U regular insulin and 10 U NPH.

QUESTION NUMBER 11.08
Question is about - gout
Category of the Question - Physiological Integrity, Pharmacological and Parenteral Therapies

Nurse Len should expect to administer which medication to a client with gout?

A. Aspirin
B. Furosemide (Lasix)

C. Colchicines
D. Calcium gluconate (Kalcinate)

QUESTION NUMBER 11.09
Question is about - hyperaldosteronism
Category of the Question - Physiological Integrity, Physiological Adaptation

Mr. Domingo with a history of hypertension is diagnosed with primary hyperaldosteronism. This diagnosis indicates that the client's hypertension is caused by excessive hormone secretion from which of the following glands?

A. Adrenal cortex
B. Pancreas
C. Adrenal medulla
D. Parathyroid

QUESTION NUMBER 11.10
Question is about - ulcer
Category of the Question - Health Promotion and Maintenance

For a diabetic male client with a foot ulcer, the doctor orders bed rest, a wet to- dry dressing change every shift, and blood glucose monitoring before meals and bedtime. Why are wet-to-dry dressings used for this client?

A. They contain exudate and provide a moist wound environment.
B. They protect the wound from mechanical trauma and promote healing.
C. They debride the wound and promote healing by secondary intention.
D. They prevent the entrance of microorganisms and minimize wound discomfort.

QUESTION NUMBER 11.11
Question is about - Addisonian crisis
Category of the Question - Physiological Integrity, Reduction of Risk Potential

Nurse Zeny is caring for a client in an acute Addisonian crisis. Which laboratory data would the nurse expect to find?

A. Hyperkalemia
B. Reduced blood urea nitrogen (BUN)
C. Hypernatremia
D. Hyperglycemia

QUESTION NUMBER 11.12
Question is about - SIADH
Category of the Question - Physiological Integrity, Physiological Adaptation

A client is admitted for treatment of the syndrome of inappropriate antidiuretic hormone (SIADH). Which nursing intervention is appropriate?

A. Infusing I.V. fluids rapidly as ordered.
B. Encouraging increased oral intake.
C. Restricting fluids.
D. Administering glucose-containing I.V. fluids as ordered.

QUESTION NUMBER 11.13
Question is about - diabetes mellitus
Category of the Question - Physiological Integrity, Reduction of Risk Potential

A female client tells nurse Nikki that she has been working hard for the last 3 months to control her type 2 diabetes mellitus with diet and exercise. To determine the effectiveness of the client's efforts, the nurse should check:

A. Urine glucose level.
B. Fasting blood glucose level.
C. Serum fructosamine level.
D. Glycosylated hemoglobin level.

QUESTION NUMBER 11.14
Question is about - insulin
Category of the Question - Physiological Integrity, Pharmacological and Parenteral Therapies

Nurse Trinity administered neutral protamine Hagedorn (NPH) insulin to a diabetic client at 7 a.m. At what time would the nurse expect the client to be most at risk for a hypoglycemic reaction?

A. 10:00 am
B. Noon
C. 4:00 pm
D. 10:00 pm

QUESTION NUMBER 11.15
Question is about - adrenal cortex
Category of the Question - Physiological Integrity, Physiological Adaptation

The adrenal cortex is responsible for producing which substances?

A. Glucocorticoids and androgens
B. Catecholamines and epinephrine
C. Mineralocorticoids and catecholamines
D. Norepinephrine and epinephrine

QUESTION NUMBER 11.16
Question is about - partial thyroidectomy
Category of the Question - Physiological Integrity, Physiological Adaptation

On the third day after a partial thyroidectomy, Proserfina exhibits muscle twitching and hyperirritability of the nervous system. When questioned, the client reports numbness and tingling of the mouth and fingertips. Suspecting a life-threatening electrolyte disturbance, the nurse notifies the surgeon immediately. Which electrolyte disturbance most commonly follows thyroid surgery?

A. Hypocalcemia
B. Hyponatremia
C. Hyperkalemia
D. Hypermagnesemia

QUESTION NUMBER 11.17
Question is about - cancer
Category of the Question - Physiological Integrity, Reduction of Risk Potential

Which laboratory test value is elevated in clients who smoke and can't be used as a general indicator of cancer?

A. Acid phosphatase level
B. Serum calcitonin level
C. Alkaline phosphatase level
D. Carcinoembryonic antigen level

QUESTION NUMBER 11.18
Question is about - iron-deficiency anemia
Category of the Question - Physiological Integrity, Physiological Adaptation

Francis with anemia has been admitted to the medical-surgical unit. Which assessment findings are characteristic of iron-deficiency anemia?

  A. Nights sweats, weight loss, and diarrhea
  B. Dyspnea, tachycardia, and pallor
  C. Nausea, vomiting, and anorexia
  D. Itching, rash, and jaundice

QUESTION NUMBER 11.19
Question is about - HIV, pregnancy
Category of the Question - Health Promotion and Maintenance

In teaching a female client who is HIV-positive about pregnancy, the nurse would know more teaching is necessary when the client says:

  A. The baby can get the virus from my placenta."
  B. "I'm planning on starting on birth control pills."
  C. "Not everyone who has the virus gives birth to a baby who has the virus."
  D. "I'll need to have a C-section if I become pregnant and have a baby."

QUESTION NUMBER 11.20
Question is about - AIDS
Category of the Question - Health Promotion and Maintenance

When preparing Judy with acquired immunodeficiency syndrome (AIDS) for discharge to the home, the nurse should be sure to include which instruction?

  A. "Put on disposable gloves before bathing."
  B. "Sterilize all plates and utensils in boiling water."
  C. "Avoid sharing such articles as toothbrushes and razors."
  D. "Avoid eating foods from serving dishes shared by other family members."

QUESTION NUMBER 11.21
Question is about - pernicious anemia
Category of the Question - Physiological Integrity, Physiological Adaptation

Nurse Marie is caring for a 32-year-old client admitted with pernicious anemia. Which set of findings should the nurse expect when assessing the client?

  A. Pallor, bradycardia, and reduced pulse pressure
  B. Pallor, tachycardia, and a sore tongue
  C. Sore tongue, dyspnea, and weight gain
  D. Angina, double vision, and anorexia

QUESTION NUMBER 11.22

Question is about - anaphylactic shock

Category of the Question - Management of Care

After receiving a dose of penicillin, a client develops dyspnea and hypotension. Nurse Celestina suspects the client is experiencing anaphylactic shock. What should the nurse do first?

    A. Page an anesthesiologist immediately and prepare to intubate the client.
    B. Administer epinephrine, as prescribed, and prepare to intubate the client if necessary.
    C. Administer the antidote for penicillin, as prescribed, and continue to monitor the client's vital signs.
    D. Insert an indwelling urinary catheter and begin to infuse I.V. fluids as ordered.

QUESTION NUMBER 11.23

Question is about - aspirin

Category of the Question - Physiological Integrity, Physiological Adaptation

Mr. Marquez with rheumatoid arthritis is about to begin aspirin therapy to reduce inflammation. When teaching the client about aspirin, the nurse discusses adverse reactions to prolonged aspirin therapy. These include:

    A. Weight gain.
    B. Fine motor tremors.
    C. Respiratory acidosis.
    D. Bilateral hearing loss.

QUESTION NUMBER 11.24

Question is about - HIV, AIDS

Category of the Question - Health Promotion and Maintenance

A 23-year-old client is diagnosed with human immunodeficiency virus (HIV). After recovering from the initial shock of the diagnosis, the client expresses a desire to learn as much as possible about HIV and acquired immunodeficiency syndrome (AIDS). When teaching the client about the immune system, the nurse states that adaptive immunity is provided by which type of white blood cell?

    A. Neutrophil   C. Monocyte
    B. Basophil   D. Lymphocyte

QUESTION NUMBER 11.25

Question is about - Sjögren's syndrome

Category of the Question - Physiological Integrity, Physiological Adaptation

In an individual with Sjögren's syndrome, nursing care should focus on:

    A. Moisture replacement.
    B. Electrolyte balance.
    C. Nutritional supplementation.
    D. Arrhythmia management.

QUESTION NUMBER 11.26
Question is about - chemotherapy
Category of the Question - Physiological Integrity, Reduction of Risk Potential

During chemotherapy for lymphocytic leukemia, Mathew develops abdominal pain, fever, and "horse barn" smelling diarrhea. It would be most important for the nurse to advise the physician to order:

A. Enzyme-linked immunosuppressant assay (ELISA) test.
B. Electrolyte panel and hemogram.
C. Stool for Clostridium difficile test.
D. Flat plate X-ray of the abdomen.

QUESTION NUMBER 11.27
Question is about - HIV
Category of the Question - Physiological Integrity, Reduction of Risk Potential

A male client seeks medical evaluation for fatigue, night sweats, and a 20-lb weight loss in 6 weeks. To confirm that the client has been infected with the human immunodeficiency virus (HIV), the nurse expects the physician to order:

A. E-rosette immunofluorescence.
B. Quantification of T-lymphocytes.
C. Enzyme-linked immunosorbent assay (ELISA).
D. Western blot test with ELISA.

QUESTION NUMBER 11.28
Question is about - blood count
Category of the Question - Physiological Integrity, Reduction of Risk Potential

A complete blood count is commonly performed before Joe goes into surgery. What does this test seek to identify?

A. Potential hepatic dysfunction indicated by decreased blood urea nitrogen (BUN) and creatinine levels.
B. Low levels of urine constituents normally excreted in the urine.
C. Abnormally low hematocrit (HCT) and hemoglobin (Hb) levels.
D. Electrolyte imbalance that could affect the blood's ability to coagulate properly.

QUESTION NUMBER 11.29
Question is about - disseminated intravascular coagulation
Category of the Question - Physiological Integrity, Reduction of Risk Potential

While monitoring a client for the development of disseminated intravascular coagulation (DIC), the nurse should take note of what assessment parameters?

A. Platelet count, prothrombin time, and partial thromboplastin time
B. Platelet count, blood glucose levels, and white blood cell (WBC) count
C. Thrombin time, calcium levels, and potassium levels
D. Fibrinogen level, WBC, and platelet count

QUESTION NUMBER 11.30
Question is about - allergen, diet
Category of the Question - Basic Care and Comfort

When taking a dietary history from a newly admitted female client, Nurse Len should remember which of the following foods is a common allergen?

A. Bread
B. Carrots

C. Orange
D. Strawberries

QUESTION NUMBER 11.31
Question is about - outpatient, prioritization
Category of the Question - Safe and Effective Care Environment, Management of Care

Nurse John is caring for clients in the outpatient clinic. Which of the following phone calls should the nurse return first?

A. A client with hepatitis A who states, "My arms and legs are itching."
B. A client with a cast on the right leg who states, "I have a funny feeling in my right leg."
C. A client with osteomyelitis of the spine who states, "I am so nauseous that I can't eat."
D. A client with rheumatoid arthritis who states, "I am having trouble sleeping."

QUESTION NUMBER 11.32
Question is about - prioritization
Category of the Question - Safe and Effective Care Environment, Management of Care

Nurse Sarah is caring for clients on the surgical floor and has just received a report from the previous shift. Which of the following clients should the nurse see first?

A. A 35-year-old admitted three hours ago with a gunshot wound; 1.5 cm area of dark drainage noted on the dressing.
B. A 43-year-old who had a mastectomy two days ago; 23 ml of serosanguinous fluid noted in the Jackson-Pratt drain.
C. A 59-year-old with a collapsed lung due to an accident; no drainage noted in the previous eight hours.
D. A 62-year-old who had an abdominal-perineal resection three days ago; client complains of chills.

QUESTION NUMBER 11.33
Question is about - thyroidectomy
Category of the Question - Physiological Integrity, Physiological Adaptation

Nurse Eve is caring for a client who had a thyroidectomy 12 hours ago for treatment of Grave's disease. The nurse would be most concerned if which of the following was observed?

A. Blood pressure 138/82, respirations 16, oral temperature 99 degrees Fahrenheit.
B. The client supports his head and neck when turning his head to the right.
C. The client spontaneously flexes his wrist when the blood pressure is obtained.
D. The client is drowsy and complains of sore throat.

QUESTION NUMBER 11.34
Question is about - pain relief
Category of the Question - Physiological Integrity, Physiological Adaptation

Julius is admitted with complaints of severe pain in the lower right quadrant of the abdomen. To assist with pain relief, the nurse should take which of the following actions?

A. Encourage the client to change positions frequently in bed.
B. Administer Demerol 50 mg IM q 4 hours and PRN.
C. Apply warmth to the abdomen with a heating pad.
D. Use comfort measures and pillows to position the client.

QUESTION NUMBER 11.35
Question is about - peritoneal dialysis
Category of the Question - Physiological Integrity, Physiological Adaptation

Nurse Tina prepares a client for peritoneal dialysis. Which of the following actions should the nurse take first?

A. Assess for a bruit and a thrill.
B. Warm the dialysate solution.
C. Position the client on the left side.
D. Insert a Foley catheter

QUESTION NUMBER 11.36
Question is about - cane
Category of the Question - Health Promotion and Maintenance

Nurse Jannah teaches an elderly client with right-sided weakness how to use a cane. Which of the following behaviors, if demonstrated by the client to the nurse, indicates that the teaching was effective?

A. The client holds the cane with his right hand, moves the cane forward followed by the right leg, and then moves the left leg.
B. The client holds the cane with his right hand, moves the cane forward followed by his left leg, and then moves the right leg.
C. The client holds the cane with his left hand, moves the cane forward followed by the right leg, and then moves the left leg.
D. The client holds the cane with his left hand, moves the cane forward followed by his left leg, and then moves the right leg.

QUESTION NUMBER 11.37
Question is about - confusion
Category of the Question - Physiological Adaptation, Physiological Adaptation

An elderly client is admitted to the nursing home setting. The client is occasionally confused and her gait is often unsteady. Which of the following actions, if taken by the nurse, is most appropriate?

A. Ask the woman's family to provide personal items such as photos or mementos.
B. Select a room with a bed by the door so the woman can look down the hall.
C. Suggest the woman eat her meals in the room with her roommate.
D. Encourage the woman to ambulate in the halls twice a day.

QUESTION NUMBER 11.38
Question is about - walker
Category of the Question - Health Promotion and Maintenance

Nurse Evangeline teaches an elderly client how to use a standard aluminum walker. Which of the following behaviors, if demonstrated by the client, indicates that the nurse's teaching was effective?

A. The client slowly pushes the walker forward 12 inches, then takes small steps forward while leaning on the walker.
B. The client lifts the walker, moves it forward 10 inches, and then takes several small steps forward.
C. The client supports his weight on the walker while advancing it forward, then takes small steps while balancing on the walker.
D. The client slides the walker 18 inches forward, then takes small steps while holding onto the walker for balance.

QUESTION NUMBER 11.39
Question is about - sensory deprivation
Category of the Question - Health Promotion and Maintenance

Nurse Derek is supervising a group of elderly clients in a residential home setting. The nurse knows that the elderly are at greater risk of developing sensory deprivation for what reason?

A. Increased sensitivity to the side effects of medications.
B. Decreased visual, auditory, and gustatory abilities.
C. Isolation from their families and familiar surroundings.
D. Decrease musculoskeletal function and mobility.

QUESTION NUMBER 11.40
Question is about - emphysema
Category of the Question - Physiological Integrity, Physiological Adaptation

A male client with emphysema becomes restless and confused. What step should nurse Jasmine take next?

A. Encourage the client to perform pursed-lip breathing.
B. Check the client's temperature.
C. Assess the client's potassium level.
D. Increase the client's oxygen flow rate.

QUESTION NUMBER 11.41
Question is about - organ rejection
Category of the Question - Physiological Integrity, Reduction of Risk Potential

Randy has undergone a kidney transplant, what assessment would prompt Nurse Katrina to suspect organ rejection?

A. Sudden weight loss
B. Polyuria
C. Hypertension
D. Shock

QUESTION NUMBER 11.42
Question is about - ureteral colic
Category of the Question - Physiological Integrity, Physiological Adaptation

The immediate objective of nursing care for an overweight, mildly hypertensive male client with ureteral colic and hematuria is to decrease:

A. Pain
B. Weight

C. Hematuria
D. Hypertension

QUESTION NUMBER 11.43
Question is about - Lugol's iodine solution
Category of the Question - Physiological Integrity, Pharmacological and Parenteral Therapy

Matilda, with hyperthyroidism, is to receive Lugol's iodine solution before a subtotal thyroidectomy is performed. The nurse is aware that this medication is given to:

A. Decrease the total basal metabolic rate.
B. Maintain the function of the parathyroid glands.
C. Block the formation of thyroxine by the thyroid gland.
D. Decrease the size and vascularity of the thyroid gland.

QUESTION NUMBER 11.44
Question is about - acute hypoglycemia
Category of the Question - Physiological Integrity, Physiological Adaptation

Ricardo was diagnosed with type I diabetes. The nurse is aware that acute hypoglycemia also can develop in the client who is diagnosed with:

A. Liver disease
B. Hypertension
C. Type 2 diabetes
D. Hyperthyroidism

QUESTION NUMBER 11.45
Question is about - carcinoma
Category of the Question - Physiological Integrity, Physiological Adaptation

Tracy is receiving combination chemotherapy for treatment of metastatic carcinoma. Nurse Ruby should monitor the client for the systemic side effect of:

A. Ascites
B. Nystagmus
C. Leukopenia
D. Polycythemia

QUESTION NUMBER 11.46
Question is about - colostomy
Category of the Question - Health Promotion and Maintenance

Norma, with recent colostomy, expresses concern about the inability to control the passage of gas. Nurse Oliver should suggest that the client plan to:

A. Eliminate foods high in cellulose.
B. Decrease fluid intake at mealtimes.
C. Avoid foods that in the past caused flatus.
D. Adhere to a bland diet prior to social events.

QUESTION NUMBER 11.47
Question is about - colostomy
Category of the Question - Health Promotion and Maintenance

Nurse Ron begins to teach a male client how to perform colostomy irrigations. The nurse would evaluate that the instructions were understood when the client states, "I should:

A. Lie on my left side while instilling the irrigating solution."
B. Keep the irrigating container less than 18 inches above the stoma."
C. Instill a minimum of 1200 ml of irrigating solution to stimulate evacuation of the bowel."
D. Insert the irrigating catheter deeper into the stoma if cramping occurs during the procedure."

QUESTION NUMBER 11.48
Question is about - electrolyte imbalance
Category of the Question - Physiological Integrity, Physiological Adaptation

Patrick is in the oliguric phase of acute tubular necrosis and is experiencing fluid and electrolyte imbalances. The client is somewhat confused and complains of nausea and muscle weakness. As part of the prescribed therapy to correct this electrolyte imbalance, the nurse would expect to:

A. Administer Kayexalate
B. Restrict foods high in protein
C. Increase oral intake of cheese and milk.
D. Administer large amounts of normal saline via I.V.

QUESTION NUMBER 11.49
Question is about - burn injury
Category of the Question - Pharmacological and Parenteral Therapies

Mario has a burn injury. After 48 hours, the physician orders for Mario 2 liters of IV fluid to be administered q12 h. The drop factor of the tubing is 10 gtt/ml. The nurse should set the flow to provide:

A. 18 gtt/min
B. 28 gtt/min
C. 32 gtt/min
D. 36 gtt/min

QUESTION NUMBER 11.50
Question is about - burn injury
Category of the Question - Physiological Integrity, Physiological Adaptation

Terence suffered from burn injury. Using the rule of nines, which has the largest percent of burns?

    A. Face and neck
    B. Right upper arm and penis
    C. Right thigh and penis
    D. Upper trunk

QUESTION NUMBER 11.51
Question is about - fall
Category of the Question - Physiological Integrity, Physiological Adaptation

Herbert, a 45-year-old construction engineer, is brought to the hospital unconscious after falling from a 2-story building. When assessing the client, the nurse would be most concerned if the assessment revealed:

    A. Reactive pupils
    B. A depressed fontanel
    C. Bleeding from ears
    D. An elevated temperature

QUESTION NUMBER 11.52
Question is about - pacemaker
Category of the Question - Physiological Integrity, Physiological Adaptation

Nurse Sherry is teaching male client regarding his permanent artificial pacemaker. Which information given by the nurse shows her knowledge deficit about the artificial cardiac pacemaker?

    A. Take the pulse rate once a day, in the morning upon awakening.
    B. May be allowed to use electrical appliances.
    C. Have regular follow up care.
    D. May engage in contact sports.

QUESTION NUMBER 11.53
Question is about - COPD
Category of the Question - Physiological Integrity, Physiological Adaptation

The nurse is aware that the most relevant knowledge about oxygen administration to a male client with COPD is:

    A. Oxygen at 1-2L/min is given to maintain the hypoxic stimulus for breathing.
    B. Hypoxia stimulates the central chemoreceptors in the medulla that makes the client breathe.
    C. Oxygen is administered best using a non-rebreathing mask.
    D. Blood gases are monitored using a pulse oximeter.

QUESTION NUMBER 11.54
Question is about - thoracotomy, pneumonectomy
Category of the Question - Physiological Integrity, Physiological Adaptation

Tonny has undergone a left thoracotomy and a partial pneumonectomy. Chest tubes are inserted, and one-bottle water-seal drainage is instituted in the operating room. In the postanesthesia care unit, Tonny is placed in Fowler's position on either his right side or on his back. The nurse is aware that this position:

A. Reduce incisional pain.
B. Facilitate ventilation of the left lung.
C. Equalize pressure in the pleural space.
D. Increase venous return.

QUESTION NUMBER 11.55
Question is about - bronchoscopy
Category of the Question - Physiological Integrity, Reduction of Risk Potential

Kristine is scheduled for a bronchoscopy. When teaching Kristine what to expect afterward, the nurse's highest priority of information would be:

A. Food and fluids will be withheld for at least 2 hours.
B. Warm saline gargles will be done q 2h.
C. Coughing and deep-breathing exercises will be done q2h.
D. Only ice chips and cold liquids will be allowed initially.

QUESTION NUMBER 11.56
Question is about - acute renal failure
Category of the Question - Physiological Integrity, Physiological Adaptation

Nurse Tristan is caring for a male client with acute renal failure. The nurse should expect hypertonic glucose, insulin infusions, and sodium bicarbonate to be used to treat:

A. Hypernatremia.
B. Hypokalemia.

C. Hyperkalemia.
D. Hypercalcemia.

QUESTION NUMBER 11.57
Question is about - genital warts
Category of the Question - Physiological Integrity, Physiological Adaptation

Ms. X has just been diagnosed with condylomata acuminata (genital warts). What information is appropriate to tell this client?

A. This condition puts her at a higher risk for cervical cancer; therefore, she should have a Papanicolaou (Pap) smear annually.
B. The most common treatment is metronidazole (Flagyl), which should eradicate the problem within 7 to 10 days.
C. The potential for transmission to her sexual partner will be eliminated if condoms are used every time they have sexual intercourse.
D. The human papillomavirus (HPV), which causes condylomata acuminata, can't be transmitted during oral sex.

QUESTION NUMBER 11.58
Question is about - palpation
Category of the Question - Physiological Integrity, Physiological Adaptation

Maritess was recently diagnosed with a genitourinary problem and is being examined in the emergency department. When palpating her kidneys, the nurse should keep which anatomical fact in mind?

A. The left kidney usually is slightly higher than the right one.
B. The kidneys are situated just above the adrenal glands.
C. The average kidney is approximately 5 cm (2 inches) long and 2 to 3 cm (¾ inch to 1 ⅛ inches) wide.
D. The kidneys lie between the 10th and 12th thoracic vertebrae.

QUESTION NUMBER 11.59
Question is about - chronic renal failure
Category of the Question - Physiological Integrity, Reduction of Risk Potential

Jestoni with chronic renal failure (CRF) is admitted to the urology unit. The nurse is aware that the diagnostic test is consistent with CRF if the result is:

A. Increased pH with decreased hydrogen ions.
B. Increased serum levels of potassium, magnesium, and calcium.
C. Blood urea nitrogen (BUN) 100 mg/dl and serum creatinine 6.5 mg/ dl.
D. Uric acid analysis 3.5 mg/dl and phenolsulfonphthalein (PSP) excretion 75%.

QUESTION NUMBER 11.60
Question is about - dysplasia
Category of the Question - Physiological Integrity, Physiological Adaptation

Katrina has an abnormal result on a Papanicolaou test. After admitting that she read her chart while the nurse was out of the room, Katrina asks what dysplasia means. Which definition should the nurse provide?

A. Presence of completely undifferentiated tumor cells that don't resemble cells of the tissues of their origin.
B. Increase in the number of normal cells in a normal arrangement in a tissue or an organ.
C. Replacement of one type of fully differentiated cell by another in tissues where the second type normally isn't found.
D. Alteration in the size, shape, and organization of differentiated cells.

QUESTION NUMBER 11.61
Question is about - AIDS
Category of the Question - Physiological Integrity, Physiological Adaptation

During a routine checkup, Nurse Marianne assesses a male client with acquired immunodeficiency syndrome (AIDS) for signs and symptoms of cancer. What is the most common AIDS-related cancer?

A. Squamous cell carcinoma
B. Multiple myeloma

C. Leukemia
D. Kaposi's sarcoma

QUESTION NUMBER 11.62
Question is about - prostatectomy, subarachnoid block
Category of the Question - Physiological Integrity, Reduction of Risk Potential

Ricardo is scheduled for a prostatectomy, and the anesthesiologist plans to use a spinal (subarachnoid) block during surgery. In the operating room, the nurse positions the client according to the anesthesiologist's instructions. Why does the client require special positioning for this type of anesthesia?

    A. To prevent confusion.
    B. To prevent seizures.
    C. To prevent cerebrospinal fluid (CSF) leakage.
    D. To prevent cardiac arrhythmias.

QUESTION NUMBER 11.63
Question is about - nephrectomy
Category of the Question - Physiological Integrity, Physiological Adaptation

A male client had a nephrectomy 2 days ago and is now complaining of abdominal pressure and nausea. The first nursing action should be to:

    A. Auscultate bowel sounds.   C. Change the client's position.
    B. Palpate the abdomen.   D. Insert a rectal tube.

QUESTION NUMBER 11.64
Question is about - colonoscopy
Category of the Question - Physiological Integrity, Reduction of Risk Potential

Wilfredo with a recent history of rectal bleeding is being prepared for a colonoscopy. How should the nurse Patricia position the client for this test initially?

    A. Lying on the right side with legs straight.
    B. Lying on the left side with knees bent.
    C. Prone with the torso elevated.
    D. Bent over with hands touching the floor.

QUESTION NUMBER 11.65
Question is about - ileostomy
Category of the Question - Physiological Integrity, Reduction of Risk Potential

A male client with inflammatory bowel disease undergoes an ileostomy. On the first day after surgery, Nurse Oliver notes that the client's stoma appears dusky. How should the nurse interpret this finding?

    A. Blood supply to the stoma has been interrupted.
    B. This is a normal finding 1 day after surgery.
    C. The ostomy bag should be adjusted.
    D. An intestinal obstruction has occurred.

QUESTION NUMBER 11.66
Question is about - contractures, burns
Category of the Question - Physiological Integrity, Physiological Adaptation

Anthony suffers burns on the legs, which nursing intervention helps prevent contractures?

A. Applying knee splints.
B. Elevating the foot of the bed.
C. Hyperextending the client's palms.
D. Performing shoulder range-of-motion exercises.

QUESTION NUMBER 11.67
Question is about - burns
Category of the Question - Physiological Integrity, Physiological Adaptation

Nurse Ron is assessing a client admitted with second and third-degree burns on the face, arms, and chest. Which finding indicates a potential problem?

A. Partial pressure of arterial oxygen (PaO2) value of 80 mm Hg.
B. Urine output of 20 ml/hour.
C. White pulmonary secretions.
D. Rectal temperature of 100.6° F (38° C).

QUESTION NUMBER 11.68
Question is about - cerebrovascular accident
Category of the Question - Physiological Integrity, Basic Care and Comfort

Mr. Mendoza who has suffered a cerebrovascular accident (CVA) is too weak to move on his own. To help the client avoid pressure ulcers, Nurse Celia should:

A. Turn him frequently.
B. Perform passive range-of-motion (ROM) exercises.
C. Reduce the client's fluid intake.
D. Encourage the client to use a footboard.

QUESTION NUMBER 11.69
Question is about - dermatitis
Category of the Question - Physiological Integrity, Pharmacological and Parenteral Therapies

Nurse Maria plans to administer dexamethasone cream to a female client who has dermatitis over the anterior chest. How should the nurse apply this topical agent?

A. With a circular motion, to enhance absorption.
B. With an upward motion, to increase blood supply to the affected area.
C. In long, even, outward, and downward strokes in the direction of hair growth.
D. In long, even, outward, and upward strokes in the direction opposite hair growth.

QUESTION NUMBER 11.70
Question is about - beta-blockers
Category of the Question - Physiological Integrity, Pharmacological and Parenteral Therapies

Nurse Kate is aware that one of the following classes of medication protects the ischemic myocardium by blocking catecholamines and sympathetic nerve stimulation is:

A. Beta-adrenergic blockers
B. Calcium channel blocker
C. Narcotics
D. Nitrates

QUESTION NUMBER 11.71
Question is about - jugular distention
Category of the Question - Physiological Integrity, Physiological Adaptation

A male client has jugular distention. In what position should the nurse place the head of the bed to obtain the most accurate reading of jugular vein distention?

A. High Fowler's
B. Raised 10 degrees
C. Raised 30 degrees
D. Supine position

QUESTION NUMBER 11.72
Question is about - inotropics
Category of the Question - Physiological Integrity, Pharmacological and Parenteral Therapies

The nurse is aware that one of the following classes of medications maximizes cardiac performance in clients with heart failure by increasing ventricular contractility?

A. Beta-adrenergic blockers
B. Calcium channel blocker
C. Diuretics
D. Inotropic agents

QUESTION NUMBER 11.73
Question is about - diet
Category of the Question - Physiological Integrity, Reduction of Risk Potential

A male client has a reduced serum high-density lipoprotein (HDL) level and an elevated low-density lipoprotein (LDL) level. Which of the following dietary modifications is not appropriate for this client?

A. Fiber intake of 25 to 30 g daily.
B. Less than 30% of calories from fat.
C. Cholesterol intake of less than 300 mg daily.
D. Less than 10% of calories from saturated fat.

QUESTION NUMBER 11.74
Question is about - acute myocardial infarction
Category of the Question - Management of Care

A 37-year-old male client was admitted to the coronary care unit (CCU) 2 days ago with acute myocardial infarction. Which of the following actions would breach the client's confidentiality?

A. The CCU nurse gives a verbal report to the nurse on the telemetry unit before transferring the client to that unit.
B. The CCU nurse notifies the on-call physician about a change in the client's condition.
C. The emergency department nurse calls up the latest electrocardiogram results to check the client's progress.
D. At the client's request, the CCU nurse updates the client's wife on his condition.

QUESTION NUMBER 11.75
Question is about - cardiopulmonary resuscitation
Category of the Question - Physiological Integrity, Physiological Adaptation

A male client arriving in the emergency department is receiving cardiopulmonary resuscitation from paramedics who are giving ventilation through an endotracheal (ET) tube that they placed in the client's home. During a pause in compressions, the cardiac monitor shows narrow QRS complexes and a heart rate of beats/minute with a palpable pulse. Which of the following actions should the nurse take first?

A. Start an L.V. line and administer amiodarone (Cordarone), 300 mg L.V. over 10 minutes.
B. Check endotracheal tube placement.
C. Obtain an arterial blood gas (ABG) sample.
D. Administer atropine, 1 mg L.V.

Practice Question Set-12

QUESTION NUMBER 12.01
Question is about - hyperparathyroidism
Category of the Question - Physiological Integrity, Reduction of Risk Potential

A patient is admitted to the hospital with a diagnosis of primary hyperparathyroidism. A nurse checking the patient's lab results would expect which of the following changes in laboratory findings?

A. Elevated serum calcium.
B. Low serum parathyroid hormone (PTH)
C. Elevated serum vitamin D
D. Low urine calcium

QUESTION NUMBER 12.02
Question is about - Addison's disease
Category of the Question - Health Promotion and Maintenance

A patient with Addison's disease asks a nurse for nutrition and diet advice. Which of the following diet modifications is not recommended?

A. A diet high in grains.
B. A diet with adequate caloric intake.
C. A high protein diet.
D. A restricted sodium diet.

QUESTION NUMBER 12.03
Question is about - cholecystectomy
Category of the Question - Physiological Integrity, Physiological Adaptation

A patient with a history of diabetes mellitus is in the second postoperative day following cholecystectomy. She has complained of nausea and isn't able to eat solid foods. The nurse enters the room to find the patient confused and shaky. Which of the following is the most likely explanation for the patient's symptoms?

A. Anesthesia reaction

B. Hyperglycemia

C. Hypoglycemia

D. Diabetic ketoacidosis

QUESTION NUMBER 12.04
Question is about - fiberoptic colonoscopy
Category of the Question - Physiological Integrity, Reduction of Risk Potential

A nurse assigned to the emergency department evaluates a patient who underwent fiberoptic colonoscopy 18 hours previously. The patient reports increasing abdominal pain, fever, and chills. Which of the following conditions poses the most immediate concern?

A. Bowel perforation

B. Viral gastroenteritis

C. Colon cancer

D. Diverticulitis

QUESTION NUMBER 12.05
Question is about - liver biopsy, coagulation
Category of the Question - Physiological Integrity, Reduction of Risk Potential

A patient is admitted to the same day surgery unit for liver biopsy. Which of the following laboratory tests assesses coagulation? Select all that apply.

A. Partial thromboplastin time
B. Prothrombin time
C. Platelet count
D. Hemoglobin
E. Complete Blood Count
F. White Blood Cell Count

QUESTION NUMBER 12.06
Question is about - ventricular fibrillation
Category of the Question - Physiological Integrity, Reduction of Risk Potential

A patient on the cardiac telemetry unit unexpectedly goes into ventricular fibrillation. The advanced cardiac life support team prepares to defibrillate. Which of the following choices indicates the correct placement of the conductive gel pads?

A. The left clavicle and right lower sternum.
B. Right of midline below the bottom rib and the left shoulder.
C. The upper and lower halves of the sternum.
D. The right side of the sternum just below the clavicle and left of the precordium.

QUESTION NUMBER 12.07
Question is about - abdominal assessment
Category of the Question - Physiological Integrity, Physiological Adaptation

The nurse performs an initial abdominal assessment on a patient newly admitted for abdominal pain. The nurse hears what she describes as "clicks and gurgles in all four quadrants" as well as "swishing or buzzing sound heard in one or two quadrants." Which of the following statements is correct?

A. The frequency and intensity of bowel sounds varies depending on the phase of digestion.
B. In the presence of intestinal obstruction, bowel sounds will be louder and higher pitched.
C. A swishing or buzzing sound may represent the turbulent blood flow of a bruit and is not normal.
D. All of the above.

QUESTION NUMBER 12.08
Question is about - chemical splash
Category of the Question - Physiological Integrity, Physiological Adaptation

A patient arrives in the emergency department and reports splashing concentrated household cleaner in his eye. Which of the following nursing actions is a priority?

A. Irrigate the eye repeatedly with normal saline solution.
B. Place fluorescein drops in the eye.
C. Patch the eye.
D. Test visual acuity.

QUESTION NUMBER 12.09
Question is about - hip replacement
Category of the Question - Physiological Integrity, Physiological Adaptation

A nurse is caring for a patient who has had hip replacement. The nurse should be most concerned about which of the following findings?

A. Complaints of pain during repositioning.
B. Scant bloody discharge on the surgical dressing.
C. Complaints of pain following physical therapy.
D. Temperature of 101.8° F (38.7° C).

QUESTION NUMBER 12.10
Question is about - seizure disorder
Category of the Question - Physiological Integrity, Physiological Adaptation

A child is admitted to the hospital with an uncontrolled seizure disorder. The admitting physician writes orders for actions to be taken in the event of a seizure. Which of the following actions would not be included?

A. Notify the physician.
B. Restrain the patient's limbs.
C. Position the patient on his/her side with the head flexed forward.
D. Administer rectal diazepam.

QUESTION NUMBER 12.11
Question is about - Epoetin
Category of the Question - Physiological Integrity, Pharmacological and Parenteral Therapies

A patient who has received chemotherapy for cancer treatment is given an injection of Epoetin. Which of the following should reflect the findings in a complete blood count (CBC) drawn several days later?

A. An increase in neutrophil count.
B. An increase in hematocrit.
C. An increase in platelet count.
D. An increase in serum iron.

QUESTION NUMBER 12.12
Question is about - polycythemia vera
Category of the Question - Physiological Integrity, Physiological Adaptation

A patient is admitted to the hospital with suspected polycythemia vera. Which of the following symptoms is consistent with the diagnosis? Select all that apply.

A. Weight loss
B. Increased clotting time
C. Hypertension
D. Headaches
E. Tinnitus

QUESTION NUMBER 12.13
Question is about - platelet count
Category of the Question - Physiological Integrity, Reduction of Risk Potential

A nurse is caring for a patient with a platelet count of 20,000/microliter. Which of the following is an important intervention?

A. Observe for evidence of spontaneous bleeding.
B. Limit visitors to family only.
C. Give aspirin in case of headaches.
D. Impose immune precautions.

QUESTION NUMBER 12.14
Question is about - corticosteroid
Category of the Question - Physiological Integrity, Pharmacological and Parenteral Therapies

A nurse in the emergency department assesses a patient who has been taking long-term corticosteroids to treat renal disease. Which of the following is a typical side effect of corticosteroid treatment? Select all that apply.

A. Hypertension
B. Cushingoid features
C. Hyponatremia
D. Low serum albumin
E. Hypernatremia

QUESTION NUMBER 12.15
Question is about - neutropenia
Category of the Question - Physiological Adaptation, Physiological Adaptation

A nurse is caring for patients in the oncology unit. Which of the following is the most important nursing action when caring for a neutropenic patient?

    A. Change the disposable mask immediately after use.
    B. Change gloves immediately after use.
    C. Minimize patient contact.
    D. Minimize conversation with the patient.

QUESTION NUMBER 12.16
Question is about - immunization
Category of the Question - Health Promotion and Maintenance

A nurse is counseling patients at a health clinic on the importance of immunizations. Which of the following information is the most accurate regarding immunizations?

    A. All infectious diseases can be prevented with proper immunization.
    B. Immunizations provide natural immunity from disease.
    C. Immunizations are risk-free and should be universally administered.
    D. Immunization provides acquired immunity from some specific diseases.

QUESTION NUMBER 12.17
Question is about - allergic reaction
Category of the Question - Physiological Integrity, Physiological Adaptation

A patient is brought to the emergency department after a bee sting. The family reports a history of severe allergic reaction, and the patient appears to have some oral swelling. Which of the following is the most urgent nursing action?

    A. Consult a physician.
    B. Maintain a patent airway.
    C. Administer epinephrine subcutaneously.
    D. Administer diphenhydramine (Benadryl) orally.

QUESTION NUMBER 12.18
Question is about - ADHD
Category of the Question - Physiological Integrity, Pharmacological and Parenteral Therapies

A mother calls the clinic to report that her son has recently started medication to treat attention-deficit/hyperactivity disorder (ADHD). The mother fears her son is experiencing side effects of the medicine. Which of the following side effects are typically related to medications used for ADHD? Select all that apply.

    A. Poor appetite
    B. Insomnia
    C. Sleepiness

    D. Agitation
    E. Decreased attention span

QUESTION NUMBER 12.19
Question is about - schizophrenia, Haldol
Category of the Question - Physiological Integrity, Pharmacological and Parenteral Therapies

A patient at a mental health clinic is taking Haldol (haloperidol) for treatment of schizophrenia. She calls the clinic to report abnormal movements of her face and tongue. The nurse concludes that the patient is experiencing which of the following symptoms:

A. Comorbid depression
B. Psychotic hallucinations

C. Negative symptoms of schizophrenia
D. Tardive dyskinesia

QUESTION NUMBER 12.20
Question is about - hypoglycemia
Category of the Question - Physiological Integrity, Physiological Adaptation

A patient with newly diagnosed diabetes mellitus is learning to recognize the symptoms of hypoglycemia. Which of the following symptoms is indicative of hypoglycemia?

A. Polydipsia
B. Confusion

C. Blurred vision
D. Polyphagia

QUESTION NUMBER 12.21
Question is about - Wilms tumor
Category of the Question - Physiological Integrity, Physiological Adaptation

A child is admitted to the hospital with a diagnosis of Wilms tumor, stage II. Which of the following statements most accurately describes this stage?

A. The tumor is less than 3 cm. in size and requires no chemotherapy.
B. The tumor did not extend beyond the kidney and was completely resected.
C. The tumor extended beyond the kidney but was completely resected.
D. The tumor has spread into the abdominal cavity and cannot be resected.

QUESTION NUMBER 12.22
Question is about - glomerulonephritis
Category of the Question - Physiological Integrity, Physiological Adaptation

A teen patient is admitted to the hospital by his physician who suspects a diagnosis of acute glomerulonephritis. Which of the following findings is consistent with this diagnosis? Select all that apply.

A. Urine specific gravity of 1.040.
B. Urine output of 350 ml in 24 hours.
C. Brown ("tea-colored") urine.
D. Generalized edema.
E. Periorbital swelling.

QUESTION NUMBER 12.23
Question is about - glomerulonephritis
Category of the Question - Physiological Integrity, Physiological Adaptation

Which of the following conditions most commonly causes acute glomerulonephritis?

A. A congenital condition leading to renal dysfunction.
B. Prior infection with group A Streptococcus within the past 10-14 days.
C. Viral infection of the glomeruli.
D. Nephrotic syndrome.

QUESTION NUMBER 12.24
Question is about - hydrocele
Category of the Question - Physiological Integrity, Physiological Adaptation

An infant with hydrocele is seen in the clinic for a follow-up visit at 1 month of age. The scrotum is smaller than it was at birth, but fluid is still visible on illumination. Which of the following actions is the physician likely to recommend?

A. Massaging the groin area twice a day until the fluid is gone.
B. Referral to a surgeon for repair.
C. No treatment is necessary; the fluid is reabsorbing normally.
D. Keeping the infant in a flat, supine position until the fluid is gone.

QUESTION NUMBER 12.25
Question is about - peripheral vascular disease
Category of the Question - Physiological Integrity, Physiological Adaptation

A nurse is caring for a patient with peripheral vascular disease (PVD). The patient complains of burning and tingling of the hands and feet and cannot tolerate touch of any kind. Which of the following is the most likely explanation for these symptoms?

A. Inadequate tissue perfusion leading to nerve damage.
B. Fluid overload leading to compression of nerve tissue.
C. Sensation distortion due to psychiatric disturbance.
D. Inflammation of the skin on the hands and feet.

QUESTION NUMBER 12.26
Question is about - hepatitis A
Category of the Question - Safe and Effective Care Environment, Safety and Infection Control

A nurse is assessing a clinic patient with a diagnosis of hepatitis A. Which of the following is the most likely route of transmission?

A. Sexual contact with an infected partner
B. Contaminated food
C. Blood transfusion
D. Illegal drug use

QUESTION NUMBER 12.27
Question is about - blood transfusion
Category of the Question - Physiological Integrity, Physiological Adaptation

A leukemia patient has a relative who wants to donate blood for transfusion. Which of the following donor medical conditions would prevent this?

    A. A history of hepatitis C five years previously.
    B. Cholecystitis requiring cholecystectomy one year previously.
    C. Asymptomatic diverticulosis.
    D. Crohn's disease in remission.

QUESTION NUMBER 12.28
Question is about - acute gastritis
Category of the Question - Physiological Integrity, Physiological Adaptation

A physician has diagnosed acute gastritis in a clinic patient. Which of the following medications would be contraindicated for this patient?

    A. naproxen sodium (Naprosyn)
    B. calcium carbonate (Tums)
    C. clarithromycin (Biaxin)
    D. furosemide (Lasix)

QUESTION NUMBER 12.29
Question is about - cholecystitis
Category of the Question - Health Promotion and Maintenance

The nurse is conducting nutrition counseling for a patient with cholecystitis. Which of the following information is important to communicate?

    A. The patient must maintain a low calorie diet.
    B. The patient must maintain a high protein/low carbohydrate diet.
    C. The patient should limit sweets and sugary drinks.
    D. The patient should limit fatty foods.

QUESTION NUMBER 12.30
Question is about - myocardial infarction, pulmonary edema
Category of the Question - Physiological Integrity, Physiological Adaptation

A patient admitted to the hospital with myocardial infarction develops severe pulmonary edema. Which of the following symptoms should the nurse expect the patient to exhibit?

    A. Slow, deep respirations
    B. Stridor
    C. Bradycardia
    D. Air hunger

QUESTION NUMBER 12.31
Question is about - postoperative
Category of the Question - Physiological Integrity, Reduction of Risk Potential

A nurse is evaluating a postoperative patient and notes a moderate amount of serous drainage on the dressing 24 hours after surgery. Which of the following is the appropriate nursing action?

A. Notify the surgeon about evidence of infection immediately.
B. Leave the dressing intact to avoid disturbing the wound site.
C. Remove the dressing and leave the wound site open to air.
D. Change the dressing and document the clean appearance of the wound site.

QUESTION NUMBER 12.32
Question is about - fracture, cast
Category of the Question - Physiological Integrity, Reduction of Risk Potential

A patient returns to the emergency department less than 24 hours after having a fiberglass cast applied for a fractured right radius. Which of the following patient complaints would cause the nurse to be concerned about impaired perfusion to the limb?

A. Severe itching under the cast.
B. Severe pain in the right shoulder.
C. Severe pain in the right lower arm.
D. Increased warmth in the fingers.

QUESTION NUMBER 12.33
Question is about - osteoarthritis
Category of the Question - Health Promotion and Maintenance

An older patient with osteoarthritis is preparing for discharge. Which of the following information is correct.

A. Increased physical activity and daily exercise will help decrease discomfort associated with the condition.
B. Joint pain will diminish after a full night of rest.
C. Nonsteroidal anti-inflammatory medications should be taken on an empty stomach.
D. Acetaminophen (Tylenol) is a more effective anti-inflammatory than ibuprofen (Motrin).

QUESTION NUMBER 12.34
Question is about - osteoporosis, alendronate
Category of the Question - Physiologic Integrity, Pharmacological and Parenteral Therapies

Which patient should not be prescribed alendronate (Fosamax) for osteoporosis?

A. A female patient being treated for high blood pressure with an ACE inhibitor.
B. A patient who is allergic to iodine/shellfish.
C. A patient on a calorie restricted diet.
D. A patient on bed rest who must maintain a supine position.

QUESTION NUMBER 12.35

Question is about - Lyme disease

Category of the Question - Physiological Integrity, Physiological Adaptation

Which of the following strategies is not effective for prevention of Lyme disease?

A. Insect repellant on the skin and clothes when in a Lyme endemic area.
B. Long sleeved shirts and long pants.
C. Prophylactic antibiotic therapy prior to anticipated exposure to ticks.
D. Careful examination of skin and hair for ticks following anticipated exposure.

QUESTION NUMBER 12.36

Question is about - IV site

Category of the Question - Physiological Integrity, Pharmacological and Parenteral Therapies

A nurse is performing routine assessment of an IV site in a patient receiving both IV fluids and medications through the line. Which of the following would indicate the need for discontinuation of the IV line as the next nursing action?

A. The patient complains of pain from movement.
B. The area proximal to the insertion site is reddened, warm, and painful.
C. The IV solution is infusing too slowly, particularly when the limb is elevated.
D. A hematoma is visible in the area of the IV insertion site.

QUESTION NUMBER 12.37

Question is about - blood transfusion

Category of the Question - Physiological Integrity, Pharmacological and Parenteral Therapies

A hospitalized patient has received transfusions of 2 units of blood over the past few hours. A nurse enters the room to find the patient sitting up in bed, dyspneic and uncomfortable. On assessment, crackles are heard in the bases of both lungs, probably indicating that the patient is experiencing a complication of transfusion. Which of the following complications is most likely the cause of the patient's symptoms?

A. Febrile non-hemolytic reaction
B. Allergic transfusion reaction
C. Acute hemolytic reaction
D. Fluid overload

QUESTION NUMBER 12.38

Question is about - amniotomy

Category of the Question - Physiological integrity, Physiological Adaptation

ADVERTISEMENTS

A patient in labor and delivery has just received an amniotomy. Which of the following is correct? Select all that apply.

A. Frequent checks for cervical dilation will be needed after the procedure.
B. Contractions may rapidly become stronger and closer together after the procedure.
C. The FHR (fetal heart rate) will be followed closely after the procedure due to the possibility of cord compression.
D. The procedure is usually painless and is followed by a gush of amniotic fluid.
E. The procedure is without pain.

QUESTION NUMBER 12.39
Question is about - hyperbilirubinemia
Category of the Question - Health Promotion and Maintenance

A nurse is counseling the mother of a newborn infant with hyperbilirubinemia. Which of the following instructions by the nurse is not correct?

A. Continue to breastfeed frequently, at least every 2-4 hours.
B. Follow up with the infant's physician within 72 hours of discharge for a recheck of the serum bilirubin and exam.
C. Watch for signs of dehydration, including decreased urinary output and changes in skin turgor.
D. Keep the baby quiet and swaddled, and place the bassinet in a dimly lit area.

QUESTION NUMBER 12.40
Question is about - discharge
Category of the Question - Health Promotion and Maintenance

A nurse is giving discharge instructions to the parents of a healthy newborn. Which of the following instructions should the nurse provide regarding car safety and the trip home from the hospital?

A. The infant should be restrained in an infant car seat, properly secured in the back seat in a rear-facing position.
B. The infant should be restrained in an infant car seat, properly secured in the front passenger seat.
C. The infant should be restrained in an infant car seat facing forward or rearward in the back seat.
D. For the trip home from the hospital, the parent may sit in the back seat and hold the newborn.

QUESTION NUMBER 12.41
Question is about - congestive heart failure
Category of the Question - Physiological Integrity, Pharmacological and Parenteral Therapies

A nurse is administering IV furosemide to a patient admitted with congestive heart failure. After the infusion, which of the following symptoms is not expected?

A. Increased urinary output
B. Decreased edema
C. Decreased pain
D. Decreased blood pressure

QUESTION NUMBER 12.42
Question is about - coronary heart disease
Category of the Question - Health Promotion and Maintenance

There are a number of risk factors associated with coronary artery disease. Which of the following is a modifiable risk factor?

A. Obesity
B. Heredity
C. Gender
D. Age

QUESTION NUMBER 12.43
Question is about - tissue plasminogen activator, myocardial infarction
Category of the Question - Physiological Integrity, Pharmacological and Parenteral Therapies

Tissue plasminogen activator (tPA) is considered for the treatment of a patient who arrives in the emergency department following the onset of symptoms of myocardial infarction. Which of the following is a contraindication for treatment with t-PA?

    A. Worsening chest pain that began earlier in the evening.
    B. History of cerebral hemorrhage.
    C. History of prior myocardial infarction.
    D. Hypertension.

QUESTION NUMBER 12.44
Question is about - myocardial infarction, exercise
Category of the Question - Health Promotion and Maintenance

Following myocardial infarction, a hospitalized patient is encouraged to practice frequent leg exercises and ambulate in the hallway as directed by his physician. Which of the following choices reflects the purpose of exercise for this patient?

    A. Increases fitness and prevents future heart attacks.
    B. Prevents bedsores.
    C. Prevents DVT (deep vein thrombosis).
    D. Prevent constipations.

QUESTION NUMBER 12.45
Question is about - cardiogenic shock
Category of the Question - Physiological Integrity, Reduction of Risk Potential

A patient arrives in the emergency department with symptoms of myocardial infarction, progressing to cardiogenic shock. Which of the following symptoms should the nurse expect the patient to exhibit with cardiogenic shock?

    A. Hypertension
    B. Bradycardia
    C. Bounding pulse
    D. Confusion

QUESTION NUMBER 12.46
Question is about - atherosclerosis
Category of the Question - Health Promotion and Maintenance

A patient in the cardiac unit is concerned about the risk factors associated with atherosclerosis. Which of the following are hereditary risk factors for developing atherosclerosis?

    A. Family history of heart disease
    B. Overweight
    C. Smoking
    D. Age

QUESTION NUMBER 12.47
Question is about - claudication
Category of the Question - Physiological Integrity, Physiological Adaptation

Claudication is a well-known effect of peripheral vascular disease. Which of the following facts about claudication is correct? Select all that apply.

A. It results when oxygen demand is greater than oxygen supply.
B. It is characterized by pain that often occurs during rest.
C. It is a result of tissue hypoxia.
D. It is characterized by cramping and weakness.
E. It is relieved after a short rest.

QUESTION NUMBER 12.48
Question is about - peripheral vascular disease
Category of the Question - Health Promotion and Maintenance

A nurse is providing discharge information to a patient with peripheral vascular disease. Which of the following information should be included in instructions?

A. Walk barefoot whenever possible.
B. Use a heating pad to keep feet warm.
C. Avoid crossing the legs.
D. Use antibacterial ointment to treat skin lesions at risk of infection.

QUESTION NUMBER 12.49
Question is about - Raynaud's disease
Category of the Question - Health Promotion and Maintenance

A patient who has been diagnosed with vasospastic disorder (Raynaud's disease) complains of cold and stiffness in the fingers. Which of the following descriptions is most likely to fit the patient?

A. An adolescent male
B. An elderly woman

C. A young woman
D. An elderly man

QUESTION NUMBER 12.50
Question is about - pregnancy
Category of the Question - Physiological Integrity, Physiological Adaptation

A 23 year old patient in the 27th week of pregnancy has been hospitalized on complete bed rest for 6 days. She experiences sudden shortness of breath, accompanied by chest pain. Which of the following conditions is the most likely cause of her symptoms?

A. Myocardial infarction due to a history of atherosclerosis.
B. Pulmonary embolism due to deep vein thrombosis (DVT).
C. Anxiety attacks due to worries about her baby's health.
D. Congestive heart failure due to fluid overload.

QUESTION NUMBER 12.51
Question is about - thrombolytic therapy
Category of the Question - Physiological Integrity, Pharmacological and Parenteral Therapies

Thrombolytic therapy is frequently used in the treatment of suspected strokes. Which of the following is a significant complication associated with thrombolytic therapy?

A. Air embolism
B. Cerebral hemorrhage
C. Expansion of the clot
D. Resolution of the clot

QUESTION NUMBER 12.52
Question is about - infant
Category of the Question - Physiological Integrity, Physiological Adaptation

An infant is brought to the clinic by his mother, who has noticed that he holds his head in an unusual position and always faces to one side. Which of the following is the most likely explanation?

A. Torticollis, with shortening of the sternocleidomastoid muscle.
B. Craniosynostosis, with premature closure of the cranial sutures.
C. Plagiocephaly, with flattening of one side of the head.
D. Hydrocephalus, with increased head size.

QUESTION NUMBER 12.53
Question is about - Osgood-Schlatter
Category of the Question - Physiological Integrity, Physiological Adaptation

An adolescent brings a physician's note to school stating that he is not to participate in sports due to a diagnosis of Osgood-Schlatter disease. Which of the following statements about the disease is correct?

A. The condition was caused by the student's competitive swimming schedule.
B. The student will most likely require surgical intervention.
C. The student experiences pain in the inferior aspect of the knee.
D. The student is trying to avoid participation in physical education.

QUESTION NUMBER 12.54
Question is about - assessment
Category of the Question - Physiological Integrity, Physiological Adaptation

The clinic nurse asks a 13-year-old female to bend forward at the waist with arms hanging freely. Which of the following assessments is the nurse most likely conducting?

A. Spinal flexibility
B. Leg length disparity
C. Hypostatic blood pressure
D. Scoliosis

QUESTION NUMBER 12.55
Question is about - child abuse
Category of the Question - Psychosocial Integrity

A clinic nurse interviews a parent who is suspected of abusing her child. Which of the following characteristics is the nurse least likely to find in an abusing parent?

A. Low self-esteem
B. Unemployment

C. Self-blame for the injury to the child
D. Single status

QUESTION NUMBER 12.56
Question is about - increased intracranial pressure
Category of the Question - Physiological Integrity, Physiological Adaptation

A nurse in the emergency department is observing a 4-year-old child for signs of increased intracranial pressure after a fall from a bicycle, resulting in head trauma. Which of the following signs or symptoms would be cause for concern?

A. Bulging anterior fontanel.
B. Repeated vomiting.
C. Signs of sleepiness at 10 PM.
D. Inability to read short words from a distance of 18 inches.

QUESTION NUMBER 12.57
Question is about - rubeola
Category of the Question - Physiological Integrity, Physiological Adaptation

A nonimmunized child appears at the clinic with a visible rash. Which of the following observations indicates the child may have rubeola (measles)?

A. Small blue-white spots are visible on the oral mucosa.
B. The rash begins on the trunk and spreads outward.
C. There is low-grade fever.
D. The lesions have a "teardrop on a rose petal" appearance.

QUESTION NUMBER 12.58
Question is about - scarlet fever
Category of the Question - Physiological Integrity, Physiological Adaptation

A child is seen in the emergency department for scarlet fever. Which of the following descriptions of scarlet fever is not correct?

A. Scarlet fever is caused by infection with group A Streptococcus bacteria.
B. "Strawberry tongue" is a characteristic sign.
C. Petechiae occur on the soft palate.
D. The pharynx is red and swollen.

QUESTION NUMBER 12.59
Question is about - allergic reaction, diphenhydramine
Category of the Question - Physiological Integrity, Pharmacological and Parenteral Therapies

A child weighing 30 kg arrives at the clinic with diffuse itching as the result of an allergic reaction to an insect bite. diphenhydramine (Benadryl) 25 mg 3 times a day is prescribed. The correct pediatric dose is 5 mg/kg/day. Which of the following best describes the prescribed drug dose?

    A. It is the correct dose.
    B. The dose is too low.
    C. The dose is too high.
    D. The dose should be increased or decreased, depending on the symptoms.

QUESTION NUMBER 12.60
Question is about - undescended testis
Category of the Question - Physiological Integrity, Physiological Adaptation

The mother of a 2-month-old infant brings the child to the clinic for a well baby check. She is concerned because she feels only one testis in the scrotal sac. Which of the following statements about the undescended testis is the most accurate?

    A. Normally, the testes are descended by birth.
    B. The infant will likely require surgical intervention.
    C. The infant probably has only one testis.
    D. Normally, the testes descend by one year of age.

QUESTION NUMBER 12.61
Question is about - chronic heart failure
Category of the Question - Health Promotion and Maintenance

Mrs. Chua, a 78-year-old client, is admitted with the diagnosis of mild chronic heart failure. The nurse expects to hear when listening to client's lungs indicative of chronic heart failure would be:

    A. Stridor   C. Wheezes
    B. Crackles   D. Friction rubs

QUESTION NUMBER 12.62
Question is about - myocardial infarction, morphine
Category of the Question - Physiological Integrity, Pharmacological and Parenteral Therapies

Patrick who is hospitalized following a myocardial infarction, asks the nurse why he is taking morphine. The nurse explains that morphine:

    A. Decrease anxiety and restlessness
    B. Prevents shock and relieves pain
    C. Dilates coronary blood vessels
    D. Helps prevent fibrillation of the heart

QUESTION NUMBER 12.63
Question is about - digitalis toxicity
Category of the Question - Physiological Integrity, Pharmacological and Parenteral Therapies

Which of the following should the nurse teach the client about the signs of digitalis toxicity?

A. Increased appetite
B. Elevated blood pressure
C. Skin rash over the chest and back
D. Visual disturbances such as seeing yellow spots

QUESTION NUMBER 12.64
Question is about - furosemide
Category of the Question - Physiological Integrity, Pharmacological and Parenteral Therapies

Nurse Trisha teaches a client with heart failure to take oral Furosemide in the morning. The reason for this is to help:

ADVERTISEMENTS

A. Retard rapid drug absorption
B. Excrete excessive fluids accumulated at night
C. Prevents sleep disturbances during night
D. Prevention of electrolyte imbalance

QUESTION NUMBER 12.65
Question is about - pulmonary edema, heart failure
Category of the Question - Physiological Integrity, Physiological Adaptation

What would be the primary goal of therapy for a client with pulmonary edema and heart failure?

A. Enhance comfort
B. Increase cardiac output
C. Improve respiratory status
D. Peripheral edema decreased

QUESTION NUMBER 12.66
Question is about - head injury
Category of the Question - Physiological Integrity, Physiological Adaptation

Nurse Linda is caring for a client with head injury and monitoring the client with decerebrate posturing. Which of the following is a characteristic of this type of posturing?

A. Upper extremity flexion with lower extremity flexion
B. Upper extremity flexion with lower extremity extension
C. Extension of the extremities after a stimulus
D. Flexion of the extremities after stimulus

QUESTION NUMBER 12.67

Question is about - cascara sagrada

Category of the Question - Physiological Integrity, Pharmacological and Parenteral Therapies

A female client is taking Cascara Sagrada. Nurse Betty informs the client that the following may be experienced as side effects of this medication:

A. GI bleeding

B. Peptic ulcer disease

C. Abdominal cramps

D. Partial bowel obstruction

QUESTION NUMBER 12.68

Question is about - intravenous nitroglycerin

Category of the Question - Physiological Integrity, Reduction of Risk Potential

Dr. Marquez orders a continuous intravenous nitroglycerin infusion for the client suffering from myocardial infarction. Which of the following is the most essential nursing action?

A. Monitoring urine output frequently

B. Monitoring blood pressure every 4 hours

C. Obtaining serum potassium levels daily

D. Obtaining infusion pump for the medication

QUESTION NUMBER 12.69

Question is about - myocardial infarction

Category of the Question - Physiological Integrity, Physiological Adaptation

During the second day of hospitalization of the client after a Myocardial Infarction. Which of the following is an expected outcome?

A. Able to perform self-care activities without pain

B. Severe chest pain

C. Can recognize the risk factors of Myocardial Infarction

D. Can Participate in cardiac rehabilitation walking program

QUESTION NUMBER 12.70

Question is about - brain attack

Category of the Question - Physiological Integrity, Basic Care and Comfort

A 68-year-old client is diagnosed with a right-sided brain attack and is admitted to the hospital. In caring for this client, the nurse should plan to:

A. Application of elastic stockings to prevent flaccid by muscle

B. Use hand roll and extend the left upper extremity on a pillow to prevent contractions

C. Use a bed cradle to prevent dorsiflexion of feet

D. Do passive range of motion exercise

QUESTION NUMBER 12.71
Question is about - nephrectomy
Category of the Question - Physiological Integrity, Reduction of Risk Potential

Nurse Liza is assigned to care for a client who has returned to the nursing unit after left nephrectomy. Nurse Liza's highest priority would be:

A. Hourly urine output
B. Temperature

C. Able to turn side to side
D. Able to sips clear liquid

QUESTION NUMBER 12.72
Question is about - cardiac catheterization
Category of the Question - Physiological Integrity, Physiological Adaptation

A 64-year-old male client with a long history of cardiovascular problems including hypertension and angina is to be scheduled for cardiac catheterization. During pre-cardiac catheterization teaching, Nurse Cherry should inform the client that the primary purpose of the procedure is:

A. To determine the existence of CHD.
B. To visualize the disease process in the coronary arteries.
C. To obtain the heart chambers pressure.
D. To measure oxygen content of different heart chambers.

QUESTION NUMBER 12.73
Question is about - cardiac catheterization
Category of the Question - Physiological Integrity, Reduction of Risk Potential

During the first several hours after a cardiac catheterization, it would be most essential for nurse Cherry to...

A. Elevate the client's bed at 45°.
B. Instruct the client to cough and deep breathe every 2 hours.
C. Frequently monitor client's apical pulse and blood pressure.
D. Monitor clients' temperature every hour.

QUESTION NUMBER 12.74
Question is about - mitral valve replacement
Category of the Question - Physiological Integrity, Physiological Adaptation

Kate, who has undergone mitral valve replacement, suddenly experiences continuous bleeding from the surgical incision during the postoperative period. Which of the following pharmaceutical agents should Nurse Aiza prepare to administer to Kate?

A. Protamine Sulfate
B. Quinidine Sulfate
C. Vitamin C
D. Coumadin

QUESTION NUMBER 12.75
Question is about - mitral stenosis

Category of the Question - Health Promotion and Maintenance

In reducing the risk of endocarditis, good dental care is an important measure. To promote good dental care in clients with endocarditis in a teaching plan should include proper use of…

A. Dental floss
B. Electric toothbrush
C. Manual toothbrush
D. Irrigation device

CHAPTER 16:
Answer with Explanation

Answer - Set 1

ANSWER NUMBER 01.01

Solution of the Question - C. 95 mm Hg
Use the following formula to calculate MAP

MAP = systolic + 2 (diastolic)
MAP = 126 mm Hg + 2 (80 mm Hg)
MAP = 286 mm Hg
MAP = 95 mm Hg

ANSWER NUMBER 01.02

Solution of the Question - C. Electrocardiogram, complete blood count, testing for occult blood, comprehensive serum metabolic panel.

An EKG is used to assess chest pain complaints, laboratory tests are used to determine anemia, and a stool test for occult blood is used to detect blood in the stool.

ANSWER NUMBER 01.03

Solution of the Question - D. Heparin-associated thrombosis and thrombocytopenia (HATT)

Due to the use of heparin during surgery, HATT can arise after CABG surgery.

ANSWER NUMBER 01.04

Solution of the Question - B. Corticosteroids

Corticosteroid therapy can reduce antibody synthesis and antibody-coated platelet phagocytosis, allowing more functional platelets to be retained.

ANSWER NUMBER 01.05

Solution of the Question - D. Xenogeneic

A xenogeneic transplant is one in which a person is transplanted into another species.

ANSWER NUMBER 01.06

Solution of the Question - B. Release of tissue thromboplastin

When injured tissue comes into touch with clotting factors, tissue thromboplastin is released.

ANSWER NUMBER 01.07

Solution of the Question - C. Essential thrombocytopenia

Immunologic illnesses including SLE and the human immunodeficiency virus have been related to essential thrombocytopenia.

ANSWER NUMBER 01.08

Solution of the Question - B. Night sweat

A single swollen lymph node (typically), unexplained fever, nocturnal sweats, malaise, and generalized pruritus are among signs of stage 1.

ANSWER NUMBER 01.09

Solution of the Question - D. Breath sounds

Pneumonia, both viral and fungal, is a significant cause of death in neutropenic patients, thus respiratory rate and breath sounds must be monitored often.

ANSWER NUMBER 01.10

Solution of the Question - B. Muscle spasm

Back discomfort or paresthesia in the lower extremities could suggest that a spinal tumor is about to squeeze the spinal cord. This should be discovered and treated as soon as possible, as the tumor may develop and cause paraplegia.

ANSWER NUMBER 01.11

Solution of the Question - C. 10 years

According to epidemiologic research, it takes an average of ten years from first exposure with HIV to the onset of AIDS. The time between HIV infection and AIDS diagnosis can be anything from 9 months to 20 years or more, with a median of 12 years.

ANSWER NUMBER 01.12

Solution of the Question - A. Low platelet count

Platelets and clotting factors are depleted in DIC, which leads to microthrombi and profuse bleeding. Fibrinogen levels fall as clots develop, whereas prothrombin time rises.

ANSWER NUMBER 01.13

Solution of the Question - D. Hodgkin's disease

Fever, night sweats, weight loss, and lymph node enlargement are common symptoms of Hodgkin's disease.

ANSWER NUMBER 01.14

Solution of the Question - C. A Rh-negative

An hereditary D antigen can occasionally be found in human blood. Rh-positive blood is found in people who have the D antigen; Rh-negative blood is found in people who do not have the antigen. It's critical for someone who has Rh-negative blood to obtain Rh-negative blood.

ANSWER NUMBER 01.15

Solution of the Question - B. "I will call my doctor if Stacy has persistent vomiting and diarrhea".

Vomiting, anorexia, and diarrhea that lasts longer than 24 hours are indicators of toxicity, and the patient should cease taking the drug and contact their doctor.

ANSWER NUMBER 01.16

Solution of the Question - D. "This is only temporary; Stacy will re-grow new hair in 3-6 months but may be different in texture".

This is the correct reaction. The nurse should teach the mother how to cope with her own thoughts about the kid's illness so that she does not negatively effect the youngster. When the hair regrows, it is the same color and texture as before.

ANSWER NUMBER 01.17

Solution of the Question - B. Apply viscous Lidocaine to oral ulcers as needed.

Stomatitis can cause pain, which can be alleviated by using topical anesthetics such lidocaine before brushing your teeth.

ANSWER NUMBER 01.18

Solution of the Question - C. Immediately discontinue the infusion

The presence of edema or swelling at the IV site indicates that the needle has been dislodged and the IV fluid is leaking into the tissues, generating the edema. The pressure and IV solution irritate the nerves, causing discomfort in the patient. To avoid more edema and other consequences, the nurse's first move would be to stop the infusion straight away.

ANSWER NUMBER 01.19

Solution of the Question - C. Chronic obstructive bronchitis

Chronic obstructive bronchitis patients seem bloated, with huge barrel chest and peripheral edema, cyanotic nail beds, and, in some cases, circumoral cyanosis.

ANSWER NUMBER 01.20

Solution of the Question - D. Emphysema

Clients with emphysema are typically cachectic due to the huge amount of energy required to breathe. The term "puffer" comes from their pink color and the fact that they frequently breathe through pursed lips.

ANSWER NUMBER 01.21

Solution of the Question - D. 80 mm Hg

When a patient is poised to go into respiratory arrest, their breathing is inefficient, and carbon dioxide is retained. A reading of roughly 80 mm Hg is expected. The rest of the numbers are lower than projected.

ANSWER NUMBER 01.22

Solution of the Question - C. Respiratory acidosis

The client has respiratory acidosis because his Paco2 is high at 80 mm Hg and his metabolic measure, HCO3-, is normal.

ANSWER NUMBER 01.23

Solution of the Question - C. Respiratory failure

The client was reacting to the drug with respiratory signs of impending anaphylaxis, which could lead to eventually respiratory failure.

ANSWER NUMBER 01.24

Solution of the Question - D. Elevated serum aminotransferase

The liver enzymes alanine aminotransferase (ALT), aspartate aminotransferase (AST), and lactate dehydrogenase (LDH) are released into the circulation when hepatic cells die. Cirrhosis of the liver is a chronic, incurable condition characterized by widespread inflammation and fibrosis of the liver tissues.

ANSWER NUMBER 01.25

Solution of the Question - A. Impaired clotting mechanism

Cirrhosis of the liver causes a reduction in Vitamin K absorption and the production of clotting components, resulting in a clotting mechanism that is compromised.

ANSWER NUMBER 01.26

Solution of the Question - B. Altered level of consciousness

The initial indicators of hepatic encephalopathy are changes in behavior and level of consciousness. Hepatic encephalopathy arises when the liver is unable to convert the protein metabolic product ammonia to urea due to liver dysfunction. As a result, ammonia and other harmful substances build up in the blood, causing cell damage.

ANSWER NUMBER 01.27

Solution of the Question - C. "I'll lower the dosage as ordered so the drug causes only 2 to 4 stools a day".

Lactulose is administered to a patient with hepatic encephalopathy to help minimize ammonia absorption in the intestines by binding to it and encouraging more frequent bowel movements. If the patient has diarrhea, it is a sign of overdosage, and the nurse should lessen the amount of medication given to him or her. The feces will be soft or mushy. Lactulose is a sweet substance that can produce cramping and bloating.

ANSWER NUMBER 01.28

Solution of the Question - B. Severe lower back pain, decreased blood pressure, decreased RBC count, increased WBC count.

Aneurysm rupture caused by pressure applied to the abdomen cavity is indicated by severe lower back discomfort. The pain is persistent when an aneurysm ruptures since it can't be relieved until the aneurysm is repaired. Due to the loss of blood, blood pressure drops. Because the vasculature is disrupted and blood volume is lost when an aneurysm ruptures, blood pressure does not rise. The RBC count has declined – not increased – for the same reason. As cells migrate to the injury site, the number of white blood cells (WBCs) rises.

ANSWER NUMBER 01.29

Solution of the Question - D. Apply gloves and assess the groin site.

When dealing with any blood fluid, the primary priority is to follow basic procedures. The second objective is to assess the groin area. This establishes the source of the blood and the amount of blood that has been lost. In this case, the goal is to halt the bleeding.

ANSWER NUMBER 01.30

Solution of the Question - D. Percutaneous transluminal coronary angioplasty (PTCA)

PTCA can alleviate the blockage and restore blood flow and oxygenation.

ANSWER NUMBER 01.31

Solution of the Question - B. Cardiogenic shock

Cardiogenic shock is a type of shock caused by inefficient cardiac pumping.

ANSWER NUMBER 01.32

Solution of the Question - C. Kidneys' excretion of sodium and water.

When blood pressure rises, the kidneys excrete sodium and extra water. By modulating blood volume, this response eventually impacts systolic blood pressure.

ANSWER NUMBER 01.33

Solution of the Question - D. It inhibits reabsorption of sodium and water in the loop of Henle.

Furosemide is a loop diuretic that reduces blood pressure by inhibiting salt and water reabsorption in the loop Henle.

ANSWER NUMBER 01.34

Solution of the Question - C. Pancytopenia, elevated antinuclear antibody (ANA) titer

Pancytopenia, an elevated ANA titer, and a decrease in serum complement levels are common laboratory findings in patients with SLE.

ANSWER NUMBER 01.35

Solution of the Question - C. Narcotics are avoided after a head injury because they may hide a worsening condition.

Changes in state of consciousness that suggest an increase in ICP may be masked by narcotics.

ANSWER NUMBER 01.36

Solution of the Question - A. Appropriate; lowering carbon dioxide (CO_2) reduces intracranial pressure (ICP)

CO_2 has vasodilating characteristics, hence reducing Paco2 through hyperventilation lowers ICP induced by dilated brain arteries.

ANSWER NUMBER 01.37

Solution of the Question - B. A 33-year-old client with a recent diagnosis of Guillain-Barre syndrome

Ascending paralysis and the possibility of respiratory failure characterize Guillain-Barre syndrome. The order of client evaluation should be based on the client's priorities, starting with airway obstruction, breathing, and finally circulation.

ANSWER NUMBER 01.38

Solution of the Question - C. Decreases inflammation.

Colchicines work by preventing leukocyte migration to the synovial fluid, which reduces inflammation.

ANSWER NUMBER 01.39

Solution of the Question - C. Osteoarthritis is the most common form of arthritis

Osteoarthritis is the most prevalent type of arthritis, and it can be very painful. It affects persons of all ages, however the majority are old.

ANSWER NUMBER 01.40

Solution of the Question - C. Myxedema coma

Severe hypothyroidism, also known as myxedema coma, is a life-threatening illness that can occur if thyroid replacement medication is not taken.

ANSWER NUMBER 01.41

Solution of the Question - B. An irregular apical pulse

Cushing's syndrome can cause hypokalemia because it produces aldosterone overproduction, which increases urine potassium loss. As a result, the nurse should immediately notify the physician of any indications or symptoms of hypokalemia, such as an irregular apical pulse.

ANSWER NUMBER 01.42

Solution of the Question - D. Below-normal urine osmolality level, above-normal serum osmolality level

Excessive polyuria generates dilute urine in diabetes insipidus, resulting in a urine osmolality level below normal. At the same time, polyuria depletes the body's water supply, resulting in dehydration and an elevated serum osmolality level.

ANSWER NUMBER 01.43

Solution of the Question - A. "I can avoid getting sick by not becoming dehydrated and by paying attention to my need to urinate, drink, or eat more than usual."

HHNS is frequently caused by insufficient fluid consumption during hyperglycemic episodes. The client can avoid HHNS by detecting the indications of hyperglycemia (polyuria, polydipsia, and polyphagia) and increasing fluid intake.

ANSWER NUMBER 01.44

Solution of the Question - D. Hyperparathyroidism

Hyperparathyroidism, which is characterized by bone pain and weakness due to an excess of parathyroid hormone, is most common in elderly women (PTH). Clients also have polyuria due to hypercalciuria.

ANSWER NUMBER 01.45

Solution of the Question - C. "I'll take two-thirds of the dose when I wake up and one-third in the late afternoon."

Hydrocortisone, a glucocorticoid, should be taken on a schedule that closely mirrors the body's own release of this hormone; two-thirds of the dose should be taken in the morning and one-third in the late afternoon. The undesirable effects are reduced with this dose plan.

ANSWER NUMBER 01.46

Solution of the Question - C. High corticotropin and high cortisol levels

A pituitary tumor that secretes corticotropin would result in high corticotropin and cortisol levels.

ANSWER NUMBER 01.47

Solution of the Question - D. Performing capillary glucose testing every 4 hours.

Because high cortisol might create insulin resistance, putting the client at risk for hyperglycemia, the nurse should test capillary glucose every 4 hours.

ANSWER NUMBER 01.48

Solution of the Question - C. Onset to be at 2:30 p.m. and its peak to be at 4 p.m.

Regular insulin is a short-acting insulin with a 15 to 30 minute start and a 2 to 4 hour peak. Because the insulin was given at 2 p.m., the estimated onset would be between 2:15 and 2:30 p.m., with a peak between 4 and 6 p.m.

ANSWER NUMBER 01.49

Solution of the Question - A. No increase in the thyroid-stimulating hormone (TSH) level after 30 minutes during the TSH stimulation test

When the TSH level does not rise after 30 minutes in the TSH test, hyperthyroidism is confirmed.

ANSWER NUMBER 01.50

Solution of the Question - B. "Rotate injection sites within the same anatomic region, not among different regions."

Within the same anatomic region, the nurse should instruct the client to rotate injection sites. Rotating sites across different regions may create significant day-to-day changes in blood glucose levels; also, insulin absorption varies by region.

ANSWER NUMBER 01.51

Solution of the Question - D. Below-normal serum potassium level.

A client with HHNS has an overall potassium shortfall due to diuresis, which is induced by the hyperosmolar, hyperglycemic state caused by relative insulin deficiency.

ANSWER NUMBER 01.52

Solution of the Question - D. Maintaining room temperature in the low-normal range.

Heat sensitivity, diaphoresis, increased thirst and appetite, and weight loss are all signs and symptoms of Graves' illness, which causes hypermetabolism. The nurse should maintain the client's room temperature in the low-normal range to prevent heat intolerance and diaphoresis.

ANSWER NUMBER 01.53

Solution of the Question - A. Fracture of the distal radius.

Colles' fracture is a distal radius fracture caused by a fall on an outstretched hand. Women are the ones who are most affected.

ANSWER NUMBER 01.54

Solution of the Question - B. Calcium and phosphorous

Osteoporosis causes bones to lose calcium and phosphate salts, causing them to become porous, brittle, and fracture-prone.

ANSWER NUMBER 01.55

Solution of the Question - A. Adult respiratory distress syndrome (ARDS)

ARDS is usually associated with severe hypoxia following smoke inhalation.

ANSWER NUMBER 01.56

Solution of the Question - D. Fat embolism

Fat emboli, which induce shortness of breath and hypoxia, are linked to long bone fractures.

ANSWER NUMBER 01.57

Solution of the Question - D. Spontaneous pneumothorax

A spontaneous pneumothorax happens when the client's lung collapses, resulting in a significant reduction in the amount of functional lung available for oxygenation. His chest pain and shortness of breath were caused by his unexpected collapse.

ANSWER NUMBER 01.58

Solution of the Question - C. Pneumothorax

The presence of air or gas in the pleural cavity, which can impede oxygenation and/or ventilation, is known as pneumothorax.

ANSWER NUMBER 01.59

Solution of the Question - C. Serous fluids fill the space and consolidate the region

The space is filled with serous fluid, which finally congeals, preventing the heart and residual lung from shifting too far into the mediastinum.

ANSWER NUMBER 01.60

Solution of the Question - A. Alveolar damage in the infarcted area.

The infarcted area causes alveolar injury, which might result in the production of bloody sputum in large quantities.

ANSWER NUMBER 01.61

Solution of the Question - D. Respiratory alkalosis

A patient with a big pulmonary embolism will expel a lot of carbon dioxide, which crosses the unaltered alveolar-capillary membrane faster than oxygen and causes respiratory alkalosis.

ANSWER NUMBER 01.62

Solution of the Question - A. Air leak

An air leak causes bubbling in the water seal chamber of a chest drainage system. As air is drawn from the pleural space during pneumothorax, an air leak might occur.

ANSWER NUMBER 01.63

Solution of the Question - B. 21

3000 x 10 divided by 24 x 60.

ANSWER NUMBER 01.64

Solution of the Question - B. 2.4 ml

.05 mg/ 1 ml = .12mg/ x ml, .05x = .12, x = 2.4 ml.

ANSWER NUMBER 01.65

Solution of the Question - D. "I should put on the stockings before getting out of bed in the morning.

External pressure on veins helps to promote venous return.

ANSWER NUMBER 01.66

Solution of the Question - A. Lessen the amount of cellular damage

The primary benefit of rapid, constant rewarming of frostbite is that it reduces cellular damage. The most effective treatment for frostbite is rapid rewarming. Until the skin temperature dips below 0°C, heat conduction and radiation from deeper tissue circulation prevent freezing and ice crystallization.

ANSWER NUMBER 01.67

Solution of the Question - D. Filtering waste through a dialyzing membrane

Hemodialysis filters waste from the blood using a dialyzing membrane. In patients with chronic renal failure, dialysis nearly duplicates the activities of the kidneys. Hemodialysis replaces the kidneys' primary function of eliminating waste, poisons, excess salt, and fluid from the body.

ANSWER NUMBER 01.68

Solution of the Question - B. Contact the physician for an order for immune globulin

If a client is immunocompromised and is exposed to measles, he should be treated with antiviral drugs to strengthen his immunity. If a patient knows he has been exposed to measles and his CD4 count is less than 200, he should consult his doctor to see if post-exposure prophylaxis (PEP) with immunoglobulin is a possibility. If an infection does occur, PEP may give some protection or reduce the severity of the condition. PEP can also include obtaining the MMR vaccine if the CD4 count is 200 or higher. PEP should ideally be given within 72 hours of measles exposure.

ANSWER NUMBER 01.69

Solution of the Question - D. Infection requires skin-to-skin contact and is prevented by hand washing, gloves, and a gown.

The MRSA-infected client should be isolated. When caring for the client, gloves, a gown, and a mask should be worn, and hand cleaning is essential.

ANSWER NUMBER 01.70

Solution of the Question - B. "The pain is due to peripheral nervous system interruptions. I will get you some pain medication."

The pain associated with phantom limb syndrome is caused by a disruption in the peripheral nervous system. According to a recent study, there were around 1.6 million people with limb loss in the United States in 2005, with that figure expected to more than quadruple to 3.6 million by 2050. Among the most prevalent causes of limb loss are vascular issues, trauma, cancer, and congenital limb deficiency. Since the start of the wars in Iraq and Afghanistan, the number of traumatic amputations has also grown. In patients requiring amputation, the prevalence of PLP has been found to range from 42.2 to 78.8%.

ANSWER NUMBER 01.71

Solution of the Question - A. Head of the pancreas

The head of the pancreas, which is a part of the stomach, the jejunum, and a section of the stomach are excised and anastomosed during a Whipple procedure. It is the most common surgery for treating pancreatic cancer that has spread to the pancreas' head. The physician reconnects the remaining organs after conducting the Whipple procedure, allowing the client to digest meals regularly after surgery.

ANSWER NUMBER 01.72

Solution of the Question - C. Fresh raw pepper

Fresh, raw, or whole peppers are not permitted until they have been properly cooked in the food. A low-bacteria diet is intended to limit one's exposure to bacteria and other pathogens that might cause illness. It's frequently prescribed for those who are at a higher risk of infection as a result of a lack of white blood cells caused by illnesses or medical treatments.

ANSWER NUMBER 01.73

Solution of the Question - A. Have a Protime done monthly

Coumadin is a blood thinner. A Protime is one of the bleeding time tests. This test should be performed on a monthly basis. To determine how well the drug is working, the client will need to get his blood tested. The International Normalized Ratio is calculated using a blood test called prothrombin time (PT or protime) (INR). INR tells a doctor how well warfarin is functioning to prevent blood clots and whether or not the dose has to be changed.

ANSWER NUMBER 01.74

Solution of the Question - A. Perform the Valsalva maneuver as the catheter is advanced

If a central venous catheter is being withdrawn, the client should be instructed to hold his breath and bear down. This keeps air from getting into the line.

ANSWER NUMBER 01.75

Solution of the Question - A history of streptococcal infections

Clients who have had streptococcal infections in the past may have antibodies that make streptokinase ineffective. Patients must be monitored for bleeding due to streptokinase's thrombolytic mechanisms of action. The patient's thrombin time, prothrombin time, partial thromboplastin time, complete blood count, and any indications of bleeding must all be monitored carefully. Patients must also be watched for indications and symptoms of a re-infarction or blockage of a vessel.

Option A: There is no reason to test the client for pineapple or banana allergies. Streptokinase can cause an allergic reaction in some people. Fever, shivering, and a rash are some of the symptoms. Rarely, patients have experienced nonfatal anaphylactic responses. In cases of anaphylaxis, patients should be given epinephrine right away and streptokinase therapy should be stopped. Streptokinase's toxicity is thought to be due to the fact that it is a polypeptide derivative.

Answer - Set 2

ANSWER NUMBER 02.01

Solution of the Question - B. Flossing between the teeth

Because platelets are reduced in immune-suppressed and bone marrow-suppressed clients, they should not floss their teeth.

ANSWER NUMBER 02.02

Solution of the Question - A. Apply the new tie before removing the old one.

The tracheostomy tube will not be dislodged inadvertently if the old ties are left in place while the new ties are secured.

ANSWER NUMBER 02.03

Solution of the Question - D. Notifying the physician

300 mL of output indicates hemorrhage and should be reported right away.

ANSWER NUMBER 02.04

Solution of the Question - A. Digoxin

A significant ventricular septal defect (VSD), pulmonary stenosis, right ventricular hypertrophy, and an overriding aorta are all present in a newborn with Tetralogy of Fallot. Digoxin will be used to slow down and strengthen his heart.

ANSWER NUMBER 02.05

Solution of the Question - A.

Spence's Tail can be found at the upper outer quadrant of the breast.

ANSWER NUMBER 02.06

Solution of the Question - A. Tire easily

A child with a ventricular septal defect will become tired quickly. The hole (defect) is in the septum, which separates the heart's lower chambers (ventricles) and permits blood to flow from the left to the right side. The oxygen-rich blood is then pumped back to the lungs rather than out to the body, putting more strain on the heart.

ANSWER NUMBER 02.07

Solution of the Question - B. Measure the fetal activity

The fetus's periodic movement is determined via a nonstress test.

ANSWER NUMBER 02.08

Solution of the Question - C. Turn off the Pitocin infusion

Variable decelerations induced by cord compression are seen on the monitor. If Pitocin is being administered, the nurse should stop it.

ANSWER NUMBER 02.09

Solution of the Question - C. Ventricular tachycardia

Ventricular tachycardia is shown in the graph.

ANSWER NUMBER 02.10

Solution of the Question - B. Be injected into the abdomen.

ANSWER NUMBER 02.11

Solution of the Question - B. Administer the medication separately.

Medications should not be mixed in a single syringe unless the doctor says so.

ANSWER NUMBER 02.12

Solution of the Question - B. Void every 3 hours

Having a bowel movement every three hours keeps stagnant urine from accumulating in the bladder, where bacteria can thrive.

ANSWER NUMBER 02.13

Solution of the Question - C. Feeding the client with dementia

The client with dementia who should be assigned to the nursing assistant's care is the one who is being fed.

ANSWER NUMBER 02.14

Solution of the Question - A. A tracheotomy set

Tracheal edema is a risk for the customer who has recently had a thyroidectomy.

ANSWER NUMBER 02.15

Solution of the Question - D. Birds

Birds carry the fungus that causes histoplasmosis.

ANSWER NUMBER 02.16

Solution of the Question - B. Administer oxygen

The initial step is to provide additional oxygen to the patient. To assist prevent further heart injury, administer oxygen to raise SpO2 to greater than 90%.

ANSWER NUMBER 02.17

Solution of the Question - D. Lower back pain

The growth of an aneurysm causes lower back pain. The pressure in the abdomen is applied by the expansion, and the pain is transferred to the lower back.

ANSWER NUMBER 02.18

Solution of the Question - D. Hypertrophic

The condition hypertrophic cardiomyopathy (HCM) is characterized by significant ventricular hypertrophy and inadequate diastolic filling. It's an autosomal dominant disorder in which the cardiac muscles grow in size and mass asymmetrically along the septum. The size of the cavities of the ventricles shrinks as the thickness of the heart muscles increases, leading them to take longer to relax after systole. Because the size of the ventricle remains basically unaltered, hypertrophic cardiomyopathy has no effect on cardiac output.

ANSWER NUMBER 02.19

Solution of the Question - A. Have the patient sit down.

The first aim is to reduce the patient's oxygen use by seating him down.

ANSWER NUMBER 02.20

Solution of the Question - C. High Fowler's position

By minimizing venous return, the high Fowler's position makes breathing easier. Breathing becomes more difficult in flat and side-lying positions, and the heart's effort increases.

ANSWER NUMBER 02.21

Solution of the Question - D. Disseminated intravascular coagulation (DIC)

Because it initiates the clotting cascade following a bleed, abruptio placentae is a cause of DIC.

ANSWER NUMBER 02.22

Solution of the Question - A. Packed red blood cells

Unmatched (O negative) packed red blood cells are the first blood product given in a trauma emergency.

ANSWER NUMBER 02.23

Solution of the Question - C. Immune response

Corticosteroids restrict the normal inflammatory process in an infected or wounded portion of the body by suppressing eosinophils, lymphocytes, and natural-killer cells. This aids in the resolution of inflammation, stabilizes lysosomal membranes, reduces capillary permeability, and inhibits white blood cell phagocytosis of tissues, preventing the release of further inflammatory chemicals.

ANSWER NUMBER 02.24

Solution of the Question - C. It interferes with viral replication.

In HIV, zidovudine inhibits DNA synthesis, preventing virus replication. The medicine does not kill the virus, activate the immune system, or accelerate the elimination of HIV antibodies.

ANSWER NUMBER 02.25

Solution of the Question - D. "Splint your chest wall with a pillow for comfort."

Showing this patient how to splint his chest wall will help him cough with less discomfort.

ANSWER NUMBER 02.26

Solution of the Question - B. Give a bronchodilator by nebulizer.

More oxygen must be given to the lungs and body of a patient suffering from an acute asthma attack. Bronchodilators inhaled into the lungs expand the airways and increase the amount of oxygen supplied.

ANSWER NUMBER 02.27

Solution of the Question - D. Acute respiratory distress syndrome (ARDS).

ARDS is usually associated with severe hypoxia following smoke inhalation. The other options aren't usually linked with inhaling smoke.

ANSWER NUMBER 02.28

Solution of the Question - D. The water-seal chamber doesn't fluctuate when no suction is applied.

ANSWER NUMBER 02.29

Solution of the Question - A. High-top sneakers.

In patients with neurologic disorders, high-top sneakers are utilized to reduce foot drop and contractures.

ANSWER NUMBER 02.30

Solution of the Question - C. Restlessness and confusion.

A change in mental status is the first indicator of elevated ICP.

ANSWER NUMBER 02.31

Solution of the Question - C. Mix the drug with saline solution only.

Only saline solutions are compatible with phenytoin.

ANSWER NUMBER 02.32

Solution of the Question - A. Abduction

To retain the prosthesis in the acetabulum after surgical hip repair, keep the legs and hips abducted.

ANSWER NUMBER 02.33

Solution of the Question - B. Fluid and electrolyte balance.

Fluid isolation and accumulation in the intestine due to ileus or peripancreatic edema are common complications of acute pancreatitis. Vomiting causes a lot of fluid and electrolyte loss. As a result, managing hypovolemia and restoring electrolyte balance should be your top priority.

ANSWER NUMBER 02.34

Solution of the Question - B. Right side-lying, with the bed flat.

Splinting the biopsy site and minimizing bleeding can be accomplished by placing the patient on his right side with the bed flat.

ANSWER NUMBER 02.35

Correct Answer B. Angina or cardiac arrhythmia

A potentially dangerous consequence of hypothyroidism treatment is the development of angina or heart arrhythmia.

ANSWER NUMBER 02.36

Solution of the Question - B. Diabetes insipidus.

The major goals of treating diabetes insipidus are to maintain proper fluid levels and replace vasopressin.

ANSWER NUMBER 02.37

Solution of the Question - C. More insulin

Patients with Type 1 diabetes may require extra insulin to compensate for higher blood glucose levels during times of infection or illness.

ANSWER NUMBER 02.38

Solution of the Question - A. Hematoma

Hematoma, a delayed consequence after abdominal and vaginal hysterectomy, is indicated by a lower hematocrit level.

ANSWER NUMBER 02.39

Solution of the Question - C. Lactated Ringer's solution

Lactated Ringer's solution replaces sodium and corrects metabolic acidosis, which are both prevalent after a burn.

ANSWER NUMBER 02.40

Solution of the Question - C. Gently roll a sterile swab from the center of the wound outward to collect drainage.

A culture specimen from a wound should be obtained by rolling a swab from the center outward.

ANSWER NUMBER 02.41

Solution of the Question - C. Decreased pain

The loop diuretic furosemide has little effect on pain.

ANSWER NUMBER 02.42

Solution of the Question - C. Obesity

Obesity is a major risk factor for coronary artery disease that can be mitigated with a healthier diet and weight loss.

ANSWER NUMBER 02.43

Solution of the Question - B. History of cerebral hemorrhage

Because tPA increases the risk of bleeding, a history of cerebral hemorrhage is a contraindication. TPA works best when given within 6 hours of the onset of symptoms because it dissolves the clot blocking the coronary artery.

ANSWER NUMBER 02.44

Solution of the Question - C. Prevents DVT (deep vein thrombosis)

To avoid deep vein thrombosis, all hospitalized patients should exercise. In the lower extremities, muscular contraction enhances venous return and prevents hemostasis.

ANSWER NUMBER 02.45

Solution of the Question - D. Confusion

Cardiogenic shock causes a significant reduction in blood flow to the body's organs by impairing the heart muscle's pumping ability. Hypotension, tachycardia, and a weak pulse are all symptoms of this. Cardiogenic shock is a life-threatening consequence of a myocardial infarction.

ANSWER NUMBER 02.46

Solution of the Question - D. Check blood pressure

Pulmonary edema, which can induce severe hypertension, can develop in a patient with congestive heart failure and dyspnea. As a result, the initial step should be to take the patient's blood pressure.

ANSWER NUMBER 02.47

Solution of the Question - C. "Headaches are a frequent side effect of nitroglycerine because it causes vasodilation."

Nitroglycerin is a powerful vasodilator that can cause headaches, dizziness, and hypotension. To reduce these side effects, patients should be educated and doses titrated. Despite the negative side effects, nitroglycerin reduces myocardial oxygen demand and increases blood flow.

ANSWER NUMBER 02.48

Solution of the Question - A. The symptoms may be the result of anemia caused by chemotherapy.

The patient is likely to be experiencing side effects three months following surgery and chemotherapy, which commonly include anemia due to bone marrow suppression.

ANSWER NUMBER 02.49

Solution of the Question - C. The patient should use iron cookware to prepare foods, such as dark green, leafy vegetables and legumes, which are high in iron.

Hemoglobin levels in the normal range are 11.5-15.0. This vegetarian patient has a slight anemia problem. The iron content of food is raised when it is cooked in iron cookware.

ANSWER NUMBER 02.50

Solution of the Question - D. A nurse should remain in the room during the first 15 minutes of infusion.

During the first 15 minutes of infusion, a transfusion reaction is most likely, hence a nurse should be present.

ANSWER NUMBER 02.51

Solution of the Question - B. An increase in hematocrit

Epoetin is a type of erythropoietin that increases hematocrit by stimulating the synthesis of red blood cells. Patients who are anemic, often as a result of chemotherapy, are given epoetin.

ANSWER NUMBER 02.52

Solution of the Question - B, C, D, & F

Polycythemia vera is a disorder in which the bone marrow creates an excessive number of red blood cells. The hematocrit and viscosity of the blood both rise as a result of this. Headaches, dizziness, and vision abnormalities are common side effects. Increased blood pressure and a longer clotting time are two cardiovascular consequences. Histamine is released as a result of an increased number of basophils, causing generalized pruritus. Patients with polycythemia vera are more likely to develop thromboses, which can lead to CVAs (strokes, brain attacks) or myocardial infarctions (MIs); thrombotic complications are the leading cause of death in patients with polycythemia vera. Bleeding is a risk, possibly because platelets are generally big and dysfunctional. The bleeding might be severe and manifest itself as nosebleeds, ulcers, frank GI bleeding, hematuria, and other symptoms.

ANSWER NUMBER 02.53

Solution of the Question - A. Observe for evidence of spontaneous bleeding.

Platelet counts of less than 30,000 per microliter can produce petechiae and bruising, especially in the extremities. When the count goes below 15,000, there is a risk of spontaneous bleeding into the brain and other internal organs. Headaches could be a warning indication, so keep an eye out for them.

ANSWER NUMBER 02.54

Solution of the Question - A, B, D, and E.

Weight gain, fluid retention with hypertension, Cushingoid characteristics, low serum albumin, decreased inflammatory response, and mood changes are among side effects of corticosteroids. Patients are advised to have a low-sodium, high-protein, vitamin, and mineral-rich diet.

ANSWER NUMBER 02.55

Solution of the Question - B. Change gloves immediately after use.

Infection poses a threat to the neutropenic patient. Patients are protected from infection by pathogens picked up on hospital surfaces by changing gloves promptly after usage. For an immunocompromised patient, this pollution can have devastating repercussions.

ANSWER NUMBER 02.56

Solution of the Question - C. We will bring in fresh flowers to brighten the room.

During induction chemotherapy, the leukemia patient's immune system is significantly damaged, putting him or her at danger of infection. Microbes can be carried by fresh flowers, fruit, and plants, so they should be avoided.

ANSWER NUMBER 02.57

Solution of the Question - A. 3-10 years

At the age of four, the incidence of ALL reaches its peak (range 3-10).

ANSWER NUMBER 02.58

Solution of the Question - B. Night sweats and fatigue

Night sweats, tiredness, weakness, and tachycardia are all symptoms of Hodgkin's disease.

ANSWER NUMBER 02.59

Solution of the Question - B. Reed-Sternberg cells

If Reed-Sternberg cells are detected on pathologic inspection of the removed lymph node, a conclusive diagnosis of Hodgkin's disease is made.

ANSWER NUMBER 02.60

Solution of the Question - C. Stay with the patient and focus on slow, deep breathing for relaxation.

The most effective way to reduce anxiety and tension is to breathe slowly and deeply. It increases calm and relaxation by lowering carbon dioxide levels in the brain.

ANSWER NUMBER 02.61

Solution of the Question - D. Capillary refill of < 3 seconds

In a sickle cell anemia patient, it's critical to check the extremities for blood vessel occlusion since a change in capillary refill indicates a shift in circulation.

ANSWER NUMBER 02.62

Solution of the Question - D. Semi-Fowler's with legs extended on the bed

The best oxygenation for this client is achieved by placing him in a semi-position.

ANSWER NUMBER 02.63

Solution of the Question - B. Encouraging fluid intake of at least 200mL per hour

To prevent additional sickling of the blood, it is critical to keep the client in sickle cell crisis hydrated.

ANSWER NUMBER 02.64

Solution of the Question - C. Popsicle

To avoid thrombus formation in sickle cell disease patients, they must stay hydrated. Popsicles, gelatin, juice, and pudding all contain a lot of liquid.

ANSWER NUMBER 02.65

Solution of the Question - C. Start O2

Pain is the most common clinical sign of sickle cell crises. The pulse oximetry, on the other hand, signals that oxygen levels are low, therefore oxygenation takes priority over pain alleviation.

ANSWER NUMBER 02.66

Solution of the Question - C. Egg salad on wheat bread, carrot sticks, lettuce salad, raisin pie

Iron is abundant in egg yolks, wheat bread, carrots, raisins, and green, leafy vegetables, all of which are essential minerals for this client.

ANSWER NUMBER 02.67

Solution of the Question - D. A bus trip to the Museum of Natural History

The only non-threatening solution is to visit a museum.

ANSWER NUMBER 02.68

Solution of the Question - D. Examine the tongue

The tongue of a client with vitamin B12 insufficiency is smooth and meaty red, thus it should be examined as part of the physical examination.

ANSWER NUMBER 02.69

Solution of the Question - C. Roof of the mouth

In dark-skinned people, the oral mucosa and hard palate (mouth roof) are the best markers of jaundice.

ANSWER NUMBER 02.70

Solution of the Question - B. Respirations 28 shallow

There is less hemoglobin and oxygen when there are fewer red blood cells. As a result, the customer is frequently out of breath.

ANSWER NUMBER 02.71

Solution of the Question - A. "I will drink 500mL of fluid or less each day."

Thrombus generation is a risk for the client with polycythemia vera. The advice that the client should drink less than 500mL is inaccurate because hydration with at least 3L of fluid each day is vital in preventing clot formation.

ANSWER NUMBER 02.72

Solution of the Question - C. The client had radiation for treatment of Hodgkin's disease as a teenager.

Leukemia can develop as a result of radiation treatment for other types of cancer. Leukemia has been connected to some chemical-related hobbies and vocations.

ANSWER NUMBER 02.73

Solution of the Question - D. The soles of the feet

Petechiae are rarely visible on dark-skinned people. For assessing the client for petechiae, the soles of the feet and palms of the hands provide a lighter surface.

ANSWER NUMBER 02.74

Solution of the Question - B. "Have you had a respiratory infection in the last 6 months?"

The leukemia patient is susceptible to infection and has had repeated respiratory infections in the last six months.

ANSWER NUMBER 02.75

Solution of the Question - B. Risk for injury related to thrombocytopenia

Due to low platelet counts, the client with acute leukemia has a tendency to bleed, and any accident would compound the condition.

Answer – Set 3

ANSWER NUMBER 03.1

Solution of the Question - A: 45-year-old African American attorney

ANSWER NUMBER 03.2

Solution of the Question - A. African-Americans develop high blood pressure at younger ages than other groups in the US. Researchers have uncovered that African-Americans respond differently to hypertensive drugs than other groups of people. They are also found out to be more sensitive to salt, which increases the risk of developing hypertension.

ANSWER NUMBER 03.3

Solution of the Question - A. Gastric lavage

Option A: Acetaminophen overdose causes hepatotoxicity, which is particularly damaging to the liver. Nausea, vomiting, abdominal pain, and diarrhea are early signs of liver impairment. Hepatic necrosis develops if not treated promptly, and it might lead to death. The initial step in treating an acetaminophen overdose is to remove as much of the medication as possible, which is best accomplished through gastric lavage. Gastric lavage (irrigation) and aspiration involve flushing fluids into the stomach and then aspirating the fluid out. This technique is only performed in life-threatening situations, such as acetaminophen intoxication, and only if the time since intake is less than one (1) hour.

ANSWER NUMBER 03.4

Solution of the Question - C. Manage pain

Pain management is always a priority because it enhances one's overall quality of life. Analgesia is the cornerstone of ureteral colic treatment, which can be accomplished quickly with parenteral opioids or nonsteroidal anti-inflammatory medications (NSAIDs).

ANSWER NUMBER 03.5

Solution of the Question - D. Yearly weight gain of about 5.5 pounds per year

Each year, school-aged youngsters gain roughly 5.5 pounds and grow about 2 inches taller. A child's growth will be constant between the ages of 2 and 10.

ANSWER NUMBER 03.6

Solution of the Question - A. Go get a blood pressure check within the next 15 minutes.

Each year, school-aged youngsters gain roughly 5.5 pounds and grow about 2 inches taller. A child's growth will be constant between the ages of 2 and 10.

ANSWER NUMBER 03.7

Solution of the Question - A. A middle-aged client with a history of being ventilator dependent for over seven (7) years and admitted with bacterial pneumonia five days ago.

A person who has had a chronic ailment and is familiar with their care is the ideal candidate for release. Option A's client is most likely stable and could continue to get medication at home.

ANSWER NUMBER 03.8

Solution of the Question - A. Should be taken in the morning

Option A: Insomnia is an adverse effect of levothyroxine (Synthroid). It's best to take it first thing in the morning to avoid disrupting the client's sleep cycle.

ANSWER NUMBER 03.9

Solution of the Question - D. Notify the healthcare provider of the child's status

These data point to a medical emergency, and epiglottitis could be to blame. Any child who develops an acute inflammatory response in the mouth and throat should seek medical attention very away.

ANSWER NUMBER 03.10

Solution of the Question - C. Bedwetting

Bedwetting is one of the first signs of type 1 diabetes in children. Parents can easily identify bedwetting in a school-aged child.

ANSWER NUMBER 03.11

Solution of the Question - B. Chlamydia

Option B: Chlamydial infections are one of the most common causes of pelvic inflammatory disease or salpingitis. Chlamydial bacteria could enter the reproductive organs through the vaginal or cervix.

ANSWER NUMBER 03.12

Solution of the Question - C. An adolescent who has been on pain medications terminal cancer with an initial assessment finding pupils and a relaxed respiratory rate of 10.

Nurses who are transferred to other units should be allocated to a client with the fewest possible immediate complications. This customer has pinpoint pupils, indicating opioid poisoning, and has the lowest likelihood of complications in the near future.

ANSWER NUMBER 03.13

Solution of the Question - C. Avoiding very heavy meals

For the client with coronary artery disease, eating large, heavy meals might move blood away from the heart for digestion, which is harmful. A buildup of plaque in the arteries can obstruct the delivery of blood and oxygen to the body's primary organs.

ANSWER NUMBER 03.14

Solution of the Question - C. The level of the drug is 100 ml at 8 AM and is 80 ml at noon

The minimum dose is 10 milliliters per hour, or 40 milliliters in a four-hour period. At noon, only 60 mL should be left. When more medicine is left in the container than intended, the pump stops working.

ANSWER NUMBER 03.15

Solution of the Question - B. Spinal column manipulation

The premise behind chiropractic is that ailments are caused by disruptions in the passage of mental signals between the brain and body organs. Misalignment of the vertebrae causes such obstruction. The subluxation is reduced by manipulation.

ANSWER NUMBER 03.16

Solution of the Question - A. Decrease in level of consciousness

A subsequent drop in consciousness could suggest an increase in intracranial pressure, resulting in insufficient brain oxygenation. A decrease in LOC could indicate the presence of a transient ischemic event, which could signal the onset of thrombotic CVA.

ANSWER NUMBER 03.17

Solution of the Question - C. Moist, productive cough

Noisy breathing and a dry, non-productive cough are often the first respiratory symptoms to show in a newly diagnosed cystic fibrosis patient (CF). The first findings are the other alternatives. The cells that create mucus, perspiration, saliva, and digestive fluids are affected by CF, which is an inherited (genetic) condition. These secretions are normally thin and slick, but in people with CF, a faulty gene causes them to thicken and cling together. The secretions, rather than functioning as lubricants, clog tubes, ducts, and passages, particularly in the pancreas and lungs. The most deadly complication of CF is respiratory failure.

ANSWER NUMBER 03.18

Solution of the Question - B. Send him to the emergency room for evaluation

This client needs to be assessed right now. Delaying therapy may cause further deterioration and injury. Home care nurses must prioritize interventions that are in the best interests of the client based on assessment findings.

ANSWER NUMBER 03.19

Solution of the Question - D. No special orders are necessary for this examination

The client must be informed of the general guideline during radiography tests: remove any clothing, jewelry, or things that may interfere with the exam.

ANSWER NUMBER 03.20

Solution of the Question - B. "When you can climb 2 flights of stairs without problems, it is generally safe."

For roughly six (6) weeks after the myocardial infarction, there is a risk of heart rupture. Around that time, scar tissue should begin to grow. The standard suggestion offered by healthcare practitioners is to wait until the client can tolerate climbing stairs.

ANSWER NUMBER 03.21

Solution of the Question - B. A teenager who got a singed beard while camping

This client is at the most danger, as he or she may experience respiratory distress. Any client with charred facial hair has been exposed to heat or fire at close range, which could have resulted in catastrophic lung injury. Because the lungs' internal lining lacks nerve fibers, the client will be unaware of any swelling.

ANSWER NUMBER 03.22

Solution of the Question - C. "I understand the need to use those new skills."

The toddler stage, according to Erikson, is characterized by a gradual growth in autonomy. To explore the surroundings and acquire autonomy, the toddler must employ motor skills.

ANSWER NUMBER 03.23

Solution of the Question - A. Verify correct placement of the tube

Aspiration and food content entering the lungs are prevented by properly positioning the tube. The most accurate approach to determine the position of the nasogastric tube is to use an x-ray to visualize it. Another way is to aspirate the contents of the stomach and measure the pH. (usually pH 1 to 5). The presence of bilirubin in aspirated stomach contents can be used to confirm that it was placed in the stomach.

ANSWER NUMBER 03.24

Solution of the Question - C. Tall peaked "T" waves

Hyperkalemia is indicated by a tall peaked T wave. The healthcare provider should be contacted if the medicine is to be stopped.

ANSWER NUMBER 03.25

Solution of the Question - A. All striated muscles

Rhabdomyosarcoma is the most prevalent soft tissue sarcoma in children. It is present throughout the body and originates in striated (skeletal) muscles. If the cancer is in the head or neck area, rhabdomyosarcoma symptoms include rapid bulging or swelling of the eyes, conjunctival chemosis, and headache. It can also have a negative impact on the urinary and reproductive systems. The lung is a common location of metastasis.

ANSWER NUMBER 03.26

Solution of the Question - D. Restore yin and yang

Health is maintained for Chinese medicine practitioners by balancing the forces of yin and yang. Traditional Chinese medicine is a medical system that originated in China some 5000 years ago, making it the world's oldest continuously operating medical system.

ANSWER NUMBER 03.27

Solution of the Question - C. Force fluids and reassess blood pressure

Orthostatic hypotension, defined as a drop in systolic blood pressure of more than 15 mmHg and an increase in heart rate of more than 15% with dizziness, indicates volume depletion, insufficient vasoconstrictor mechanisms, and autonomic insufficiency.

ANSWER NUMBER 03.28

Solution of the Question - D. Left ventricular functioning

In the pulmonary artery, the catheter is inserted. When the catheter balloon is inflated, information about left ventricular function is received.

ANSWER NUMBER 03.29

Solution of the Question - B. Initiate high-quality chest compressions

CPR should be started with chest compressions, according to new guidelines from the American Heart Association (rather than checking for the airway first). Before examining the airway and administering rescue breaths, start CPR with 30 chest compressions. Adults, children, and infants needing CPR should start with chest compressions first, but newborns should not. CPR can maintain oxygenated blood flowing to the brain and other essential organs until a more permanent medical solution can restore a normal cardiac rhythm.

ANSWER NUMBER 03.30

Solution of the Question - A. Blood pressure 94/60 mm Hg

The heart rate is slowed by both drugs. Blood pressure is affected by metoprolol. To properly take both drugs, the heart rate and blood pressure must be within normal ranges (HR 60-100; systolic BP ≥ 100).

ANSWER NUMBER 03.31

Solution of the Question - C, E, F, & G

Grunting occurs when an infant uses partial glottic closure to maintain a functional residual capacity tolerable in the face of poorly compliant lungs. While the baby prolongs the expiratory phase against this partially closed glottis, there is a longer and greater residual volume that keeps the airway open, as well as an audible expiratory sound.

Nasal flare, when the nostrils open when inhaling, is a sign of trouble breathing or respiratory pain.

Option F: Cyanosis is a bluish tinge to the skin that indicates a decrease in the amount of oxygen in the bloodstream connecting to red blood cells.

Option G: Asymmetric chest movement occurs when the aberrant side of the lungs expands less and lags behind the normal side.

ANSWER NUMBER 03.32

Solution of the Question - D. Progressive placental insufficiency

A prolonged pregnancy that lasts longer than 38 to 42 weeks is known as a postmature or postterm pregnancy (normal term pregnancy). If there is evidence that placental insufficiency has occurred and interfered with fetal growth, the infants of such a pregnancy are labeled postmature or dysmature. It affects about 12% of all pregnancies. After 42 weeks, the placenta loses its ability to function, and calcium deposits form, reducing blood perfusion, oxygen supply, and food supply to the fetus.

ANSWER NUMBER 03.33

Solution of the Question - B. "I just can't 'catch my breath' over the past few minutes and I think I am in grave danger."

All of these comments would make the nurse nervous, but Option B is the most dangerous. Postoperative pulmonary embolism is more likely to occur in patients who have had hip or knee surgery. Pneumococcal embolism is characterized by sudden dyspnea and tachycardia. Deep vein thrombosis can develop within 7 to 14 days after surgery without prophylaxis (e.g., anticoagulant drugs) and lead to pulmonary embolism if not treated. Other symptoms of DVT include discomfort and tenderness near or below the clot, skin discoloration, swelling, or tightness in the afflicted leg, which the nurse should be aware of. Dyspnea, tachycardia, disorientation, and pleuritic chest discomfort are all symptoms of pulmonary embolism.

ANSWER NUMBER 03.34

Solution of the Question - D. Decreased appetite

Furosemide is a loop diuretic used to treat pulmonary edema, heart failure-related edema, nephrotic syndrome, and hypertension. Unless you take a potassium supplement or eat a potassium-rich diet, furosemide promotes potassium loss. Hypokalemia causes a decrease in appetite. Anorexia, weariness, nausea, decreased GI motility, muscle weakness, dysrhythmias, decreased urine osmolality, and altered level of consciousness are all signs and symptoms of hypokalemia.

ANSWER NUMBER 03.35

Solution of the Question - Gravida 3 para 1

Gravida refers to the number of confirmed pregnancies, and each pregnancy is recorded only once, even if it is a multiple pregnancy (i.e., twins, triplets). The total number of pregnancies that have achieved viability (20 weeks) regardless of whether the babies were born alive is referred to as parity. As a result, this woman is presently pregnant, has had two previous pregnancies, and one viable birth (twins).

ANSWER NUMBER 03.36

Solution of the Question - B. Improve the client's nutrition status

Due to defective venous valves, venous blood gathers and stagnates in the lower leg, causing venous stasis. The cells of the lower extremities eventually run out of oxygen and nutrients, causing them to die or necrose. Venous stasis ulcers, which are shallow but big brown sores with uneven edges that commonly occur on the lower leg or ankle, result as a result of this. In a client with venous stasis ulcers, the goal of clinical care is to facilitate healing. Only appropriate nutrition will allow you to do this. Venous ulcers are frequently caused by nutritional deficits. To enhance wound healing, dietary changes that include meals strong in protein, iron, zinc, and vitamins C and A are recommended.

ANSWER NUMBER 03.37

Correct order is shown above.

1. Ask the client to empty his or her bladder. Before delivering the pre-operative medication, the client must first void. If the client does not have a catheter, it is critical to empty the bladder prior to administering preoperative drugs to avoid bladder injury (especially in pelvic surgeries). If the bladder is not empty, a straight catheter or an indwelling catheter may be required.

2. Tell the client that he or she should stay in bed. Drowsiness and lightheadedness are common side effects of preoperative medicines, putting the client at risk for damage.

3. Raise the bed's side rails. When a client decides to get out of bed without assistance, raising the bed's side rails helps to prevent falls and injuries.

4. Make sure the call bell is within easy reach. Clients should always be able to reach call bells.

ANSWER NUMBER 03.38

Solution of the Question - A. Specific feedback is given as close to the event as possible

ANSWER NUMBER 03.39

Solution of the Question - B & E.

Option B: Patients with multiple sclerosis should avoid exercising until they are exhausted since vigorous physical activity elevates body temperature and can exacerbate symptoms.

Option E: For people with multiple sclerosis who desire to exercise, continuous exercise with no rest periods is not recommended. Short rest times, preferably lying down, should be recommended to the patient. Excessive fatigue may contribute to the worsening of symptoms once again.

ANSWER NUMBER 03.40

Solution of the Question - C. We have safety bars installed in the bathroom and have 24-hour alarms on the doors.

It's worth noting that all of the possibilities are correct statements. However, it is critical to emphasize the importance of safety.

Option C: A priority of home care is to ensure the safety of the client with increasing memory loss. In order to prevent falls and other injuries, any evident risks should be removed in addition to installing safety bars. A safe home setting helps the patient to be as independent and autonomous as possible.

ANSWER NUMBER 03.41

Solution of the Question - A. Warfarin (Coumadin); B. Finasteride (Propecia, Proscar)

Warfarin is Option A. (Coumadin). When administered at any point during pregnancy, it is linked to central nervous system problems, spontaneous abortion, stillbirth, preterm, bleeding, and ocular malformations, as well as fetal warfarin syndrome if given during the first trimester.

ANSWER NUMBER 03.42

Solution of the Question - A, B, C, D, and E.

Extreme sensitivity to ultraviolet (UV) rays from the sun and other light sources is known as photosensitivity. When drugs in the body interact with UV radiation from the sun, a type of photosensitivity known as Phototoxic responses occurs. The most common cause of this reaction is anti-infectives.

Option A: Ciprofloxacin is a bacterial antibiotic that is used to treat a number of ailments. Ciprofloxacin is a quinolone antibiotic, which means it belongs to a group of antibiotics known as quinolones. It works by preventing bacteria from growing. This antibiotic is solely used to treat bacterial infections. It won't work if you have a viral infection (such as common cold, flu). Antibiotics might lose their potency if they are used excessively or unnecessarily.

Option B: Sulfonamides are synthetic bacteriostatic antibiotics that compete with each other to prevent bacteria from converting p-aminobenzoic acid to dihydropteroate, which is required for folate synthesis and, eventually, purine and DNA synthesis. Because humans do not produce folate but instead obtain it from their diet, their DNA synthesis is unaffected.

Option C: Norfloxacin is an antibiotic that belongs to the fluoroquinolone class of medicines. Norfloxacin is an antibiotic that fights germs in the body. Norfloxacin is a prescription antibiotic that is used to treat bacterial infections of the prostate and urinary tract (bladder and kidneys). Norfloxacin is also prescribed for the treatment of gonorrhea.

Option D: A combination of sulfamethoxazole and trimethoprim is used to treat infections such urinary tract infections, otitis media (middle ear infections), bronchitis, traveler's diarrhea, and shigellosis (bacillary dysentery). This medication is also used to prevent or treat Pneumocystis jiroveci pneumonia, often known as Pneumocystis carinii pneumonia (PCP). The antibiotic sulfamethoxazole trimethoprim is a combination of sulfamethoxazole and trimethoprim. It works by eradicating the microorganisms responsible for a wide range of diseases.

Isotretinoin is a medication that is used to treat severe acne that has not responded to other therapies. It may also be recommended for other reasons, such as various skin issues or some types of cancer. Because this medication is a vitamin A derivative (retinoid), your body reacts to it in the same way that it does to vitamin A.

ANSWER NUMBER 03.43

Solution of the Question - D. Aspirin

Aspirin is not known to induce urine discolouration. A stroke induced by a ruptured blood artery is one of the side effects and dangers of taking aspirin. The FDA does not suggest aspirin therapy for the prevention of heart attacks in adults who haven't had a heart attack, stroke, or another cardiovascular ailment.

ANSWER NUMBER 03.44

Solution of the Question - A. Corgard

Nadolol (Corgard) should be kept at room temperature, between 59 and 86 degrees Fahrenheit (15 and 30 degrees Celsius), away from heat, moisture, and light. Keep the bottle well wrapped and do not store it in the bathroom.

ANSWER NUMBER 03.45

Solution of the Question - D. IgG

The only immunoglobulin that can pass through the placental barrier is IgG. IgG immunoglobulins account for 70-80% of all immunoglobulins in the blood. Specific IgG antibodies are created during the first few weeks following an infection or other antigen exposure, then decrease and stabilize. When exposed to the same antigen, the body stores a database of IgG antibodies that can be quickly replicated. Long-term defense against germs is based on IgG antibodies.

ANSWER NUMBER 03.46

Solution of the Question - B. Start prophylactic AZT treatment

Treatment with azidothymidine (AZT) is the most important intervention. It's an antiretroviral drug that works by preventing and treating HIV/AIDS by slowing the virus's reproduction. PEP (post-exposure prophylaxis) is an HIV therapy that suppresses the virus and prevents infection after it has been exposed. PEP should be started within 72 hours of possible HIV exposure, therefore it's critical to get help right away.

ANSWER NUMBER 03.47

Solution of the Question - C. Autonomic neuropathy

The autonomic nerves, which govern the bladder, intestinal tract, and genitals, among other organs, are affected by autonomic neuropathy (also known as Diabetic Autonomic Neuropathy). Bladder paralysis, evidenced by bladder urgency and inability to begin urine, is a frequent sign of this form of neuropathy.

ANSWER NUMBER 03.48

Solution of the Question - B. Anorexia nervosa

Anorexia nervosa is indicated by all of the clinical signs and symptoms. Anorexia nervosa is characterized by self-imposed starvation as a result of a distorted body image and an extreme, illogical fear of gaining weight, even when the patient is severely underweight. Anorexia nervosa can manifest itself as a refusal to eat, as well as excessive exercising, self-induced vomiting, or the overuse of laxatives or diuretics.

ANSWER NUMBER 03.49

Solution of the Question - B. Hypercalcemia

Polyuria, severe stomach discomfort, and confusion are all symptoms of hypercalcemia.

ANSWER NUMBER 03.50

Solution of the Question - C. RH negative, RH positive

Rhogam inhibits the generation of anti-RH antibodies in Rh-positive fetuses' mothers.

ANSWER NUMBER 03.51

Solution of the Question - D. The effects of PKU are reversible.

Phenylketonuria (PKU) is a hereditary condition in which the blood level of phenylalanine (a protein building block) rises. If PKU is not treated, phenylalanine levels in the body can rise to dangerous levels, resulting in intellectual impairment and other major health issues. PKU manifests itself in a variety of ways, from moderate to severe. Classic PKU is the most severe form of this illness. Until they are a few months old, infants with classic PKU appear normal. These youngsters will develop a persistent intellectual handicap if they are not treated. Seizures, developmental delays, behavioral issues, and psychiatric illnesses are all frequent. Excess phenylalanine in the body can cause a musty or mouse-like stench in untreated persons. Children with classic PKU have lighter skin and hair than their unaffected relatives, and they are more likely to develop skin problems like eczema. PKU's effects last for the rest of the child's life (via Genetic Home Reference).

ANSWER NUMBER 03.52

Solution of the Question - A. Onset of pulmonary edema

Overdosing on aspirin can result in metabolic acidosis and pulmonary edema. Tinnitus, hyperventilation, vomiting, dehydration, and fever are all early signs of aspirin toxicity. Drowsiness, strange behavior, shaky walking, and coma are all late indicators. Aspirin overdose causes abnormal breathing that is frequently fast and deep. Pulmonary edema is thought to be caused by an increase in permeability inside the lung's capillaries, resulting in "protein leakage" and fluid transudation in both the renal and pulmonary tissues. Changes in renal tubule permeability can cause a shift in colloid osmotic pressure, which can make pulmonary edema worse (via Medscape).

ANSWER NUMBER 03.53

Solution of the Question - D. Provide a secure environment for the patient.

The safety of this patient is your first concern. Patient safety protocols can aid in the reduction of medical errors and the prevention of negative patient outcomes. When the purpose is to aid people, it seems self-evident that working to safeguard them from unwanted or unanticipated harm is critical.

ANSWER NUMBER 03.54

Solution of the Question - C. Cough following bronchodilator utilization

The bronchodilator will help you cough more effectively.

ANSWER NUMBER 03.55

Solution of the Question - B. Weight gain

Heart failure and congenital heart abnormalities are linked to weight increase caused by fluid accumulation. The kidneys absorb less blood and filter less fluid out of the circulation into the urine when the heart does not circulate blood properly. Extra fluid in the circulatory system collects in the lungs, liver, around the eyes, and occasionally in the legs.

ANSWER NUMBER 03.56

Solution of the Question - C. Oily skin

The skin would not be oily and would be dry.

ANSWER NUMBER 03.57

Solution of the Question - D. Observe for signs of bleeding.

A customer using thrombolytic medicine is most concerned about bleeding. The conversion of plasminogen to the active form, plasmin, which ultimately degrades fibrin, is the basic mechanism of all thrombolytics. On the surface of thrombi, fibrin-bound plasminogen can be proteolyzed, as can the unbound form in the plasma. Unbound plasmin destroys fibrin, fibrinogen, factor V, and factor VIII, among other things.

ANSWER NUMBER 03.58

Solution of the Question - A. Green vegetables and liver

Folic acid is abundant in green vegetables and liver.

ANSWER NUMBER 03.59

Solution of the Question - D. Cl. difficile

Meningitis has not been connected to C. difficile. Clostridium difficile (C. diff) is a life-threatening bacteria that causes diarrhea. It's frequently a side effect of antibiotic treatment.

ANSWER NUMBER 03.60

Solution of the Question - D. The life span of RBC is 120 days.

In the body, red blood cells have a lifespan of 120 days. RBC population studies are now carried out using an ex vivo label that allows researchers to investigate both donor and autologous RBC.

ANSWER NUMBER 03.61

Solution of the Question - B. Upon admission

Admission triggers the start of discharge education. It should ideally include the client and his or her family, as well as hospital personnel. Effective discharge planning can reduce the likelihood of the client being readmitted to the hospital, as well as aid in rehabilitation, ensuring that drugs are supplied and administered correctly, and adequately prepare those who will be responsible for the client's care.

ANSWER NUMBER 03.62

Solution of the Question - B. Initiative vs. guilt

The third stage of psychosocial development, focusing on initiative versus guilt, begins as children enter the preschool years (3-6 years old). It is critical for children of this age to understand that they have control over themselves and the world.

ANSWER NUMBER 03.63

Solution of the Question - C. Autonomy vs. shame and doubt

The second stage of Erik Erikson's stages of psychosocial development is autonomy vs. shame and doubt. Between the ages of 18 months and three years, this stage occurs. Children at this age, according to Erikson, are focused on establishing a better sense of control.

ANSWER NUMBER 03.64

Solution of the Question - D. Intimacy vs. isolation

Between the ages of 19 and 40, Intimacy vs Isolation takes place during young adulthood. The main source of tension at this period of life is building close, loving relationships with others.

ANSWER NUMBER 03.65

Solution of the Question - B. 13-year-old female: 105 BPM, 22 RPM, 105/50 mmHg

For 11 to 14-year-olds, a normal range of vital signs is: 60-105 BPM heart rate; 12-20 CPM respiratory rate Body temperature: 98.0 degrees Fahrenheit (36.6 degrees Celsius) to 98.6 degrees Fahrenheit; blood pressure: systolic-85-120, diastolic-55-80 mmHg; (37 degrees Celsius). The diastolic pressure of the customer is below the usual level. Her respiratory and cardiac rates have both climbed slightly.

ANSWER NUMBER 03.66

Solution of the Question - A. Amitriptyline (Elavil)

Elavil (amitriptyline) is a tricyclic antidepressant that is used to treat depression symptoms.

ANSWER NUMBER 03.67

Solution of the Question - D. Multiple Sclerosis

Multiple sclerosis (MS) is a brain and spinal cord illness that can be devastating (central nervous system). Antibiotics are ineffective in treating it.

ANSWER NUMBER 03.68

Solution of the Question - D. Migraines

Hyperkalemia does not cause migraines. When hyperkalemia is present, the symptoms are nonspecific and primarily related to muscle or cardiac function.

ANSWER NUMBER 03.69

Solution of the Question - C. Weight gain

Patients newly diagnosed with type 1 diabetes experience rapid weight loss. In persons with diabetes, a lack of insulin stops the body from transporting glucose from the bloodstream to the cells, where it can be used as energy. When this happens, the body begins to burn fat and muscle for energy, resulting in a loss of overall body weight.

ANSWER NUMBER 03.70

Solution of the Question - A. Increased appetite

Appetite loss is to be expected. The most common cause of meningitis is an infectious pathogen that has colonized or established a localized infection elsewhere in the host. The skin, the nasopharynx, the respiratory tract, the gastrointestinal (GI) tract, and the genitourinary tract are all potential sites of colonization or infection. By evading host defenses, the bacteria infects the submucosa at these locations (eg, physical barriers, local immunity, and phagocytes or macrophages).

ANSWER NUMBER 03.71

Solution of the Question - D. Haemophilus aegyptius

Haemophilus influenzae biogroup aegyptius (Hae) is the cause of pink eye, which is an acute and often purulent conjunctivitis.

ANSWER NUMBER 03.72

Solution of the Question - A. Borrelia burgdorferi

In the United States, Lyme disease is the most frequent vector-borne disease. Borrelia burgdorferi and, in rare cases, Borrelia mayonii are the bacteria that cause Lyme disease.

ANSWER NUMBER 03.73

Solution of the Question - D. CT scan

A CT scan would be used to investigate the hemiparesis further. In the immediate examination of patients with apparent acute stroke, noncontrast CT scanning is the most often used technique of neuroimaging.

ANSWER NUMBER 03.74

Solution of the Question - C. Thyroid function tests

Weight gain and a low temperature tolerance are signs that your thyroid isn't working properly. Thyroid function tests are used to differentiate between hyperthyroidism and hypothyroidism and euthyroidism. Direct measurements of the serum concentrations of the two thyroid hormones, triiodothyronine (T3) and tetraiodothyronine (T4), also known as thyroxine, are often used to achieve this task.

ANSWER NUMBER 03.75

Solution of the Question - C. Blood cultures

To explore the fever and rash symptoms, blood cultures would be taken. A blood culture is a test that looks for foreign invaders in the blood, such as bacteria, yeast, and other microbes. The presence of these bacteria in the bloodstream can indicate a blood infection, known as bacteremia. A positive blood culture indicates the presence of microorganisms in the bloodstream.

Answer - Set 4

ANSWER NUMBER 04.01

Solution of the Question - A. Sexual dysfunction related to radiation therapy

Radiation therapy is known to cause sterility in male customers, which would be a major concern for this client. In light of the client's age and life choices, it's critical to address his or her psychosocial requirements. When discovered early, Hodgkin's disease, on the other hand, has a fair prognosis. Recognize the significance of sex in a person's, partner's, or patient's incentive for change. Because lymphomas are more common among the relatively young and in their productive years, these people may be more affected by these issues and less aware of the options for treatment.

ANSWER NUMBER 04.02

Solution of the Question - A. Platelet count

Answer A is correct because patients with autoimmune thrombocytopenic purpura (ATP) have low platelet counts. For over three months, laboratory testing will reveal a low platelet count, usually 40109/L. Large platelets and microscopic platelet fragments can be seen on the blood film. The number of megakaryocytes in the bone marrow has grown.

ANSWER NUMBER 04.03

Solution of the Question - A. Bleeding precautions

Bleeding occurs in patients with low platelet counts, which range from 120,000 to 400. The goal is to keep bleeding to a minimum. Review the following laboratory results for coagulation status as needed: platelet count, prothrombin time/international normalized ratio (PT/INR), activated partial thromboplastin time (aPTT), fibrinogen, bleeding time, fibrin degradation products, vitamin K, activated coagulation time (ACT); and educate the at-risk patient and caregivers on how to avoid tissue trauma or disruption of normal clotting mechanisms.

ANSWER NUMBER 04.04

Solution of the Question - C. Elevate the head of the bed 30°

Pressure on the sella turcica is avoided by elevating the head of the bed 30 degrees, which relieves headaches. A, B, and D are all wrong. Patients are monitored in an intensive care unit for neurological deterioration, epistaxis, visual impairment, diabetes insipidus (DI), and hypotension secondary to acute hypocortisolism in the immediate postoperative period.

ANSWER NUMBER 04.05

Solution of the Question - B. Check the vital signs

A substantial amount of fluid loss can result in a fluid and electrolyte imbalance that has to be addressed. The vital signs would show the depletion of electrolytes. Keep an eye out for symptoms of hypovolemic shock (e.g., tachycardia, tachypnea, hypotension). Frequent evaluations can uncover abnormalities early on, allowing for quick response. Polyuria reduces the volume of blood in the circulatory system.

ANSWER NUMBER 04.06

Solution of the Question - C. Pinch the soft lower part of the nose for a minimum of 5 minutes

To avoid blood aspiration, the client should be positioned erect and leaning forward. External bleeding can occur in the mouth as a result of a cut, bite, or cutting or losing a tooth; nosebleeds for no apparent reason; significant bleeding from a little cut, or bleeding from a cut that restarts after a brief break. Hemophiliacs do not bleed quicker or more frequently than the general population. Instead, they bleed for longer due to a clotting factor deficit. Clients are frequently aware of bleeding before it manifests clinically. For certain customers, bleeding can be life-threatening.

ANSWER NUMBER 04.07

Solution of the Question - A. Blood pressure

In a client who has had an adrenal gland removed, blood pressure is the best sign of cardiovascular collapse. Because of the tumor activity, the residual gland may have been inhibited. After bilateral adrenalectomy, primary adrenal insufficiency develops. Volume depletion, hypotension, hyponatremia, hyperkalemia, fever, and stomach pain are signs and symptoms. In cases of verified corticosteroid or aldosterone deficit, patients are treated with replacement medication based on glucocorticoids (hydrocortisone or cortisone) or mineralocorticoids (fludrocortisone).

ANSWER NUMBER 04.08

Solution of the Question - D. Glucometer readings as ordered

IV glucocorticoids elevate blood glucose levels, which typically necessitates the use of insulin. Cortisone and prednisone compensate for cortisol deficiency, allowing salt reabsorption to occur. Fludrocortisone is a mineralocorticoid that promotes sodium and water replacement in patients who require aldosterone replacement. Acute adrenal insufficiency is a medical emergency that necessitates the administration of fluids and corticosteroids very away. If you're being treated for adrenal crisis, you'll need IV hydrocortisone at first, but by the second day, you should be able to switch to an oral type of replacement.

ANSWER NUMBER 04.09

Solution of the Question - B. Check the calcium level

Calcium production is controlled by the parathyroid glands, which might be injured during a thyroidectomy. The sensation is caused by a lack of calcium in the body. Reflexes should be checked on a regular basis. Twitching, numbness, paresthesias, positive Chvostek's and Trousseau's signs, and seizure activity are all symptoms of neuromuscular irritability.

ANSWER NUMBER 04.10

Solution of the Question - D. Decreased cardiac output r/t bradycardia

The drop in pulse can reduce cardiac output and cause shock, so it should be prioritized over the other options. Protect yourself from the cold. Provide extra blankets or layers of clothing. External heat sources should be avoided at all costs. Keep an eye on the patient's temperature.

ANSWER NUMBER 04.11

Solution of the Question - Answer: B. "That feeling of warmth is normal when the dye is injected."

When dye is injected, it is common for the client to feel heated. A needle stick may cause discomfort to the customer. When the dye is injected, he or she may experience symptoms such as flushing in the face or other parts of the body. The specific symptoms will vary depending on the body part being evaluated.

ANSWER NUMBER 04.12

Solution of the Question - D. The nurse wears gloves to take the client's vital signs.

Taking the client's vital signs does not necessitate the use of gloves. Gloves should be worn if the client has a current infection with methicillin-resistant Staphylococcus aureus. Before making touch with the patient, wash your hands or conduct hand hygiene. Assign these responsibilities to the sufferer and their significant others as well. Know when to wash your hands and when not to wash your hands, also known as the "5 moments for hand hygiene."

ANSWER NUMBER 04.13

Solution of the Question - D. The client has a grand mal seizure.

The client will have a grand mal seizure while receiving ECT. This implies that the electroconvulsive therapy has been completed. During the primary treatment session, the seizure threshold is established through trial and error with increasingly increased current dosages. Following the initial dosage calculation, the dose for subsequent ECT sessions is 1.5 to 2 times the seizure threshold for bilateral ECT and six times the seizure threshold for right unilateral ECT. The seizure threshold typically rises with ECT treatment as the patient builds tolerance.

ANSWER NUMBER 04.14

Solution of the Question - A. Examine the perianal area with a flashlight 2 or 3 hours after the child is asleep

Pinworm infection develops when the eggs are eaten or inhaled. In 2–8 weeks, the eggs hatch in the upper intestine and mature. Females mate and then move out of the anus, where they can deposit up to 17,000 eggs. It is quite itchy as a result of this. The mother should be instructed to examine the rectal area with a flashlight 2–3 hours after the child has fallen sleeping. The eggs will stick to clear tape if it is placed on a tongue blade. After that, the specimen should be brought in for evaluation.

ANSWER NUMBER 04.15

Solution of the Question - B. The entire family should be treated.

Vermox (mebendazole) or Antiminth are used to treat enterobiasis, or pinworms (pyrantel pamoate). To ensure that no eggs remain, the entire family should be treated. Because a single treatment is usually enough, compliance is usually high. After that, the family should be tested again in two weeks to check that no eggs are still present. Because enterobiasis can lead to recurring reinfection, treating the entire household, whether or not they are symptomatic, is recommended to avoid a recurrence.

ANSWER NUMBER 04.16

Solution of the Question - A. The client receiving linear accelerator radiation therapy for lung cancer

Any client with radioactivity should not be allocated to the pregnant nurse. The patient who is having linear accelerator therapy visits the radium department. Because the radiation is contained within the department, the client is not exposed to it. These patients are radioactive in extremely modest amounts, especially after the treatments are completed. Clients should dispose of pee and feces in specific containers and use plastic spoons and forks for 72 hours.

ANSWER NUMBER 04.17

Solution of the Question - A. The client with Cushing's disease

Cushing's illness is characterized by adrenocortical hypersecretion. The client's immune system is inhibited as a result of the increase in cortisone levels. High cortisol levels also disturb the immune system, as this hormone causes lymphocytes to decrease and neutrophils to increase. It induces the marginating pool of neutrophils in the bloodstream to detach, resulting in an increase in circulating neutrophil numbers despite no increase in neutrophil production.

ANSWER NUMBER 04.18

Solution of the Question - D. Malpractice

The nurse could be charged with malpractice, which is when they fail to perform or do anything that harms the customer. Giving an overdose to an infant comes into this category. In the United States, a patient can sue a clinician for medical malpractice, which is commonly characterized as failing to give the level of care that another clinician in the same position with the same credentials would have provided, resulting in the patient's injury.

ANSWER NUMBER 04.19

Solution of the Question - D. Starting a blood transfusion

A blood transfusion should not be started by a licensed practical nurse. An LPN performs tasks such as recording vital signs, collecting samples, giving medication, maintaining patient comfort, and reporting the state of their patients to the nurses under the supervision of doctors and RNs.

ANSWER NUMBER 04.20

Solution of the Question - B. Contacting the physician

The vital indicators are out of the ordinary and should be reported right once. Early detection of changes in vital signs is usually associated with speedier detection of changes in the patient's cardiopulmonary status as well as, if necessary, an upgrade in service level. Patient safety is a top priority for every healthcare institution, and detecting any clinical deterioration as soon as possible, whether the patient is in the emergency room or on the hospital floor, is critical.

ANSWER NUMBER 04.21

Solution of the Question - B. The RN with 3 years of experience in labor and delivery

The nurse with three years of labor and delivery experience is the most knowledgeable about preeclampsia problems. When evaluating a patient assignment, registered nurses should be aware of their rights and duties. The charge nurse must filter through various choice factors in a short period of time during the nurse-patient assignment process, which is generally a manual process.

ANSWER NUMBER 04.22

Solution of the Question - B. The narcotic count has been incorrect on the unit for the past 3 days.

The Department of Health recommends that controlled drug inventories be kept to a bare minimum in order to meet patients' therapeutic needs. To prevent unauthorised access, they should be kept in a locked cabinet or safe, with the keys kept somewhere safe.

ANSWER NUMBER 04.23

Solution of the Question - B. File a formal reprimand

After discussing the issue with the nurse, the next step is to memorialize the occurrence by filing a formal reprimand. When nurses observe gaps or missing information in a patient's treatment paperwork, they should avoid making conclusions. Despite the fact that healthcare professionals have extremely busy schedules, it's always best to take the time to double-check the details rather than making assumptions and being wrong.

ANSWER NUMBER 04.24

Solution of the Question - Answer: D. The 30-year-old with an exacerbation of multiple sclerosis being treated with cortisone via a centrally placed venous catheter

Clients with multiple sclerosis who are receiving cortisone through a central line are at the greatest risk of problems. Multiple sclerosis is a difficult disease to understand. Weakness, coordination issues, or spasticity can occur in addition to sensory and visual alterations. Bladder and bowel dysfunction, depression, cognitive impairment, exhaustion, sexual dysfunction, sleep difficulties, and vertigo are some of the other health issues. The others, on the other hand, are more stable.

ANSWER NUMBER 04.25

Solution of the Question - B. The client who is 6 months pregnant with abdominal pain and the client with facial lacerations and a broken arm

The ideal candidates for placing in the same room are the pregnant client and the client with a broken arm and facial lacerations. Patient cohorting based on the presence or absence of specific pathogens, combined with standard hygienic precautions, has been shown to reduce the incidence and prevalence of chronic infections in these two species. As a result, patient cohorting has become an important part of infection control in patients.

ANSWER NUMBER 04.26

Solution of the Question - A. The eye should be cleansed with warm water, removing any exudate, before instilling the eyedrops.

The nurse should wipe the region with water before administering eye drops. Use cotton balls or gauze pledgets wet with regular saline or water to clean the eyes and lashes. When the conjunctival sac is uncovered, material is not transported into the eye.

ANSWER NUMBER 04.27

Solution of the Question - C. "We are going on a camping trip this weekend, and I have bought hot dogs to grill for his lunch."

When answering this question, keep in mind the ABCs (airway, breathing, and circulation). Because a hotdog is the same size and shape as a child's trachea, it offers an aspiration risk. Foods that can induce choking, such as entire grapes, large pieces of meat, poultry, and hot dogs, candies, and cough drops, should be avoided.

ANSWER NUMBER 04.28

Solution of the Question - C. Ask the parent/guardian to room-in with the child.

To foster parent-child bonding, the nurse should urge rooming-in. It is OK for parents to be present in the room throughout the child's evaluation. Toddlers have a strong aversion to strangers and may feel as if they are losing control and autonomy while in the hospital. To reduce fear, explain the procedures to them at their level of comprehension.

ANSWER NUMBER 04.29

Solution of the Question - B. Store the hearing aid in a warm place.

The hearing aid should be kept in a cool, dry location. The life of your hearing aid can be extended with proper maintenance and care. Keep your hearing aids away from heat and moisture as much as possible. When wearing hearing aids, avoid applying hairspray or other hair care products. It can be severely damaged if it is exposed to moisture. Although some hearing aids are now water resistant, it is still recommended that you remove them before showering or swimming. If they come into contact with water, quickly dry them with a towel. Never use a hair dryer or other heated instrument to dry them since the excessive heat can damage them.

ANSWER NUMBER 04.30

Solution of the Question - C. Risk for aspiration

When choosing an answer, always remember your ABCs (airway, breathing, and circulation). Place the youngster on his or her side in a prone or side-lying position. Encourages the outflow of blood and unswallowed saliva from the mouth, which could be inhaled.

ANSWER NUMBER 04.31

Solution of the Question - A. High fever

A high temperature is frequently present when a child has bacterial pneumonia. A fever with tachycardia and/or chills and sweats (typically greater than 38° C or 100.4° F) is a serious clinical finding. The severity of lung consolidation, the kind of organism, the extent of the infection, host variables, and the presence or absence of pleural effusion all influence physical findings.

ANSWER NUMBER 04.32

Solution of the Question - B. A tracheostomy set

Emergency tracheostomy equipment should always be kept at the bedside of a kid with epiglottitis and the likelihood of full obstruction of the airway. Prepare for tracheostomy or intubation; anticipate the necessity for a mechanical airway. To enhance oxygenation and ventilation while avoiding aspiration, an artificial airway is required.

ANSWER NUMBER 04.33

Solution of the Question - C. Exophthalmos

Exophthalmos (eyeball protrusion) is a common side effect of hyperthyroidism. Graves' orbitopathy (ophthalmopathy) is caused by the effects of thyroid stimulating antibodies and cytokines generated by cytotoxic T lymphocytes, which cause inflammation, cellular proliferation, and accelerated growth of extraocular muscles and retro-orbital connective and adipose tissues (killer cells). Thyroid stimulating antibodies and cytokines activate periorbital fibroblasts and preadipocytes, generating excess hydrophilic glycosaminoglycans (GAG) synthesis and retro-orbital fat accumulation.

ANSWER NUMBER 04.34

Solution of the Question - D. Cheese omelet

A gluten-free diet should be followed by the youngster with celiac disease. Gluten causes the immune system to harm or kill villi in children with celiac disease. The small intestine is lined with villi, which are microscopic tubules that resemble fingers. The villi's purpose is to transport food nutrients to the bloodstream through the small intestine's walls. If villi are lost, the youngster may become malnourished, regardless of how much food he consumes. This is due to their inability to absorb nutrition. Anemia, convulsions, joint discomfort, weakening bones, and malignancy are all complications of the condition.

ANSWER NUMBER 04.35

Solution of the Question - C. Apply oxygen by mask

When answering this question, keep in mind the ABCs (airway, breathing, and circulation). To raise the O2 saturation level, start with oxygen. As directed, provide humidified oxygen. Humidified oxygen stops the airways from drying out, reduces convective moisture losses, and enhances compliance.

ANSWER NUMBER 04.36

Solution of the Question - B. A moderate amount of straw-colored fluid

Normal amniotic fluid is straw-colored and odorless, while an amniotomy is an artificial breach of membranes. The quick return of amniotic fluid from the vaginal canal is the most prevalent indicator of a successful rupture of membranes. This substance is normally transparent and odorless.

ANSWER NUMBER 04.37

Solution of the Question - D. "When can I get my epidural?"

The end of the latent phase of labor is marked by a 2 cm dilation. The cervix steadily dilates to about 6 cm during the latent phase. In comparison to the active phase, the latent phase is often much longer and less predictable in terms of cervical change rate. A normal latent phase in nulliparous and multiparous women can extend up to 20 hours and 14 hours, respectively, without being considered excessive.

ANSWER NUMBER 04.38

Solution of the Question - B. Turn the client to her left side

The typical fetal heart rate is 120–160 beats per minute; bradycardia is 100–110 beats per minute. The initial step is to turn the client to the left and administer oxygen. A sluggish heart rate, also known as bradycardia, can signal that the baby isn't getting enough oxygen to the brain. Tachycardia, or a rapid heart rate, can indicate oxygen depletion. During contractions and labor, there is an appropriate range of fetal heart rate acceleration and deceleration – or speeding up and slowing down.

ANSWER NUMBER 04.39

Solution of the Question - D. Progressive cervical dilation

Pitocin is thought to cause cervical dilatation. In the obstetric realm, oxytocin is prescribed and approved by the FDA for two distinct time frames: antepartum and postpartum. Exogenous oxytocin is FDA-approved for enhancing uterine contractions in the antepartum period with the goal of a successful vaginal birth of the fetus.

ANSWER NUMBER 04.40

Solution of the Question - B. Apply the fetal heart monitor

At this moment, using a fetal heart monitor is the best course of action. In breech presentation, fetal heart beats can be heard high in the belly. To detect fetal distress early and provide rapid assistance, keep a constant eye on the FHR and uterine contractions.

ANSWER NUMBER 04.41

Solution of the Question - B. The membranes are still intact.

Because the membranes are intact, the nurse decides to utilize an external monitor. The test is done to see if a fetus is at danger for intrauterine death or newborn problems, which is mainly due to high-risk pregnancies or fetal hypoxemia. The frequency of usage is determined by clinical judgment, but it is widespread because it is non-invasive and poses little danger to the mother and fetus; nonetheless, the test has no predictive value and only detects fetal hypoxia at the time of testing.

ANSWER NUMBER 04.42

Solution of the Question - D. Potential fluid volume deficit related to decreased fluid intake

To avoid nausea and vomiting, clients admitted to labor are advised not to eat throughout the process. Although ice chips are permitted, the amount of liquids consumed may not be adequate to prevent a fluid volume deficit. Provide clear drinks and ice chips as needed (e.g., clear broth, tea, cranberry juice, jell-O, popsicles). It aids in hydration and may supply some calories for energy generation.

ANSWER NUMBER 04.43

Solution of the Question - D. There is uteroplacental insufficiency.

This data points to a late deceleration. The shortage of oxygen in the uteroplacental space causes this form of deceleration. Late decelerations are the most dangerous of the three forms of fetal heart rate decelerations that occur during labor. Reduced blood flow to the placenta causes them, and they can indicate impending fetal acidemia.

ANSWER NUMBER 04.44

Solution of the Question - C. Reposition the client

When a nurse notices a late deceleration, the first thing she should do is turn the client to the side—preferably the left side. It's also a good idea to give oxygen. The goal of initial treatment for repeated varied decelerations should be to alleviate possible cord compression. Repositioning the mother is a good first step. If the fetus is early, variable decelerations might be detected as a result of fetal movement.

ANSWER NUMBER 04.45

Solution of the Question - D. Acceleration of FHR with fetal movements

Accelerations are to be expected when moving. Accelerations are small rises in the FHR that last only a few seconds. Fetal movement, vaginal examinations, uterine contractions, umbilical vein compression, fetal scalp stimulation, and even external audio stimulation are all common causes. Accelerations are thought to be a reassuring sign of fetal well-being.

ANSWER NUMBER 04.46

Solution of the Question - C. The sensation of the bladder filling is diminished or lost.

The urge to void and the sensation of a full bladder are reduced with epidural anesthesia. The course of labor will be slowed if your bladder is full. Patients who are given epidural analgesia may not feel the need to urinate, resulting in urine retention and bladder overdistension. The detrusor muscle can be stretched and damaged if the bladder is overfilled. The use of lumbar epidural analgesia for labor and delivery, for example, has been linked to postpartum urine retention on numerous occasions. The fact that these patients have trouble voiding supports this theory.

ANSWER NUMBER 04.47

Solution of the Question - B. Luteinizing hormone is high.

Ovulation is caused by the pituitary's production of luteinizing hormone. The release of luteinizing hormone from the anterior pituitary is stimulated by the continuing increase in estrogen around day 14. Ovulation, or the discharge of the dominant follicle in preparation for conception, happens within 10–12 hours after LH levels peak.

ANSWER NUMBER 04.48

Solution of the Question - C. Regularity of the menses

The regularity of the client's menses is required for the rhythm technique of birth control to work. Each month, women are only fertile (have an egg) for a few days. Women who use the rhythm method keep track of their bodies and examine their previous menstrual cycles in order to figure out when their fertile days are. They can either refrain from having sex on those days or use a "barrier" method of birth control, such as condoms or spermicide.

ANSWER NUMBER 04.49

Solution of the Question - C. Diaphragm

The diaphragm is the finest technique of birth control for a diabetic client. The diaphragm is a contraceptive (birth control) device that keeps sperm from entering the uterus. The diaphragm is a tiny, reusable rubber or silicone cup that covers the cervix and has a flexible rim. The diaphragm is put deep into the vaginal canal before sex, with a portion of the rim fitting securely behind the pubic bone. Only when combined with spermicide is the diaphragm effective in preventing conception.

ANSWER NUMBER 04.50

Solution of the Question - D. Sudden, stabbing pain in the lower quadrant

Until the fallopian tube ruptures, the symptoms of an ectopic pregnancy are difficult to detect. A quick, stabbing pain in the bottom region extends down the leg or up into the chest, according to the client. Patients who come with vaginal bleeding should have a pelvic exam performed to check for infections and the cervical os. Palpation of the bilateral adnexa to assess for any abnormal masses/structures or elicit adnexal discomfort is also possible with bimanual pelvic exams.

ANSWER NUMBER 04.51

Solution of the Question - C. Baked chicken, fruit cup, potato salad, coleslaw, yogurt, and iced tea

All of the options are delicious, but the pregnant customer requires a well-balanced diet with plenty of calcium. Meat, fruit, potato salad, and yogurt, which offers 360 mg of calcium, are all included in this food item. Each day, about 300 additional calories are required to support a healthy pregnancy. Protein, fruits, vegetables, and whole grains should all be part of a well-balanced diet. Sweets and fats should be consumed in moderation.

ANSWER NUMBER 04.52

Solution of the Question - B. Metabolic acidosis with dehydration

Hyperemesis is characterized by persistent nausea and vomiting. Dehydration is a side effect of vomiting. Metabolic acidosis will occur if the client is dehydrated. If not handled properly, severe cases of hyperemesis can lead to vitamin shortage, dehydration, and malnutrition. If left untreated, Wernicke's encephalopathy, which is caused by a vitamin B1 shortage, can result in death and severe disability.

ANSWER NUMBER 04.53

Solution of the Question - B. The presence of fetal heart tones

The existence of fetal heart tones is the most conclusive indicator of pregnancy. Answers A, C, and D are all subjective indications that could be related to different medical issues. Between six and eight weeks of pregnancy, fetal heart tones can be heard. The provider can acquire essential information regarding the pregnancy between eight and ten weeks of gestation, including placental location, fetal position and anatomy, amniotic fluid volume, and maternal anatomy, including cervix and uterus measurements.

ANSWER NUMBER 04.54

Solution of the Question - C. Hypoglycemic, large for gestational age

A diabetic mother's child is frequently large for gestational age. Due to the absence of glucose from the mother, glucose levels drop immediately after birth. Hyperinsulinemia generated by hyperplasia of embryonic pancreatic beta cells as a result of maternal-fetal hyperglycemia causes hypoglycemia. The newborn experiences hypoglycemia due to a lack of substrate once the continuous supply of glucose is cut off after birth.

ANSWER NUMBER 04.55

Solution of the Question - B. An alternate method of birth control is needed when taking antibiotics.

Another type of birth control should be utilized if the client is using oral contraceptives and is starting antibiotics. Oral contraceptive effectiveness is affected by antibiotics. Antibiotics are thought to reduce oral contraceptive efficacy by inducing the cytochrome P450 group of hepatic microsomal enzymes and interfering with ethinylestradiol enterohepatic cycle.

ANSWER NUMBER 04.56

Solution of the Question - B. Positive HIV

Breastfeeding is not recommended for HIV patients since the virus might be passed to the infant through breast milk. Breastfeeding is the best strategy to prevent HIV transmission to a newborn through breast milk. In the United States, where women have access to clean water and cheap replacement feeding (infant formula), the CDC and the American Academy of Pediatrics recommend that HIV-positive mothers, regardless of ART or maternal viral load, absolutely forego nursing their infants.

ANSWER NUMBER 04.57

Solution of the Question - A. Assess the fetal heart tones

The signs and symptoms of placenta previa include painless vaginal bleeding. Assess fetal heart sounds so that the mother is aware of her baby's health. Assess any bleeding or spotting that may occur so that appropriate steps can be taken. The majority of instances are detected with sonography early in pregnancy, although others may arrive to the emergency room with painless vaginal bleeding in the second trimester.

ANSWER NUMBER 04.58

Solution of the Question - D. Her contractions are 5 minutes apart.

When the client's contractions are every 5 minutes and consistent, the client should be directed to the labor and delivery unit. She should also be told to go to the hospital if she has a ruptured membrane or is bleeding profusely. True labor is characterized by regular contractions. These contractions become stronger as labor continues, and the time between them decreases.

ANSWER NUMBER 04.59

Solution of the Question - A. Low birth weight

Smoking mothers' infants have a tendency to be underweight at delivery. Preterm birth, low birth weight, and birth abnormalities of the mouth and lip are all increased risks for growing kids when mothers smoke during pregnancy. Smoking raises the risk of sudden infant death syndrome both during and after pregnancy (SIDS).

ANSWER NUMBER 04.60

Solution of the Question - A. Within 72 hours of delivery

RhoGam should be given within 72 hours to guard against antibody formation. RhoGAM is normally administered at week 28 of pregnancy and lasts for around 12 weeks. If the fetus is Rh-positive, RhoGAM will be administered to the mother within 72 hours of delivery. After birth, cord blood samples can be used to determine the baby's blood type.

ANSWER NUMBER 04.61

Solution of the Question - B. Fetal heart tones

When the membranes tear, the fetal heart tones often dip temporarily. The heart tones should rapidly revert to normal. It's important to record any changes in fetal heart tones, such as bradycardia or tachycardia. During the process, the nurse is responsible for monitoring both the mother and the fetus, as well as noting the color of the draining amniotic fluid and documenting the findings in the medical file.

ANSWER NUMBER 04.62

Solution of the Question - A. Active

When the client is 4–7cm dilated, she enters the active phase of labor. Around 6 cm of cervical dilation, active labor with faster cervical dilatation begins. The cervix dilates at a rate of 1.2 to 1.5 centimeters per hour during the active phase. Multiparas, or women who have had a previous vaginal delivery, had a higher rate of cervical dilatation. The absence of cervical change for more than 4 hours in the presence of adequate contractions or for more than 6 hours in the absence of adequate contractions is considered labor arrest and may require medical intervention.

ANSWER NUMBER 04.63

Solution of the Question - B. Wrapping the newborn snugly in a blanket

An addicted mother's child will go through withdrawal. Wrapping the baby in a blanket will help avoid muscle irritation, which is common in these babies. The first clinical management strategy is non-pharmacological care, such as rooming-in and environmental control, which should be continued even after discharge from the hospital. Unless there is mother polysubstance addiction or a medical contraindication, breastfeeding should be vigorously promoted.

ANSWER NUMBER 04.64

Solution of the Question - C. Checking the client's blood pressure

The client should be monitored for hypotension and indications of shock every 5 minutes for 15 minutes after epidural anesthesia. It's critical to keep track of the patient's hemodynamic condition both during and after the procedure. Pulse oximeter for pulse and oxygen saturation, as well as blood pressure cuff and continuous EKG to check cardiovascular state, are the bare minimum of monitors necessary.

ANSWER NUMBER 04.65

Solution of the Question - B. Wash her hands for 2 minutes before care

Hand washing is the most effective approach to avoid postoperative wound infection. SSI can be averted in up to 60% of cases. Before, during, and after surgery, adequate general hygiene, operative sterility, and strong barriers against infection transmission are used to prevent postoperative wound infection.

ANSWER NUMBER 04.66

Solution of the Question - B. Misalignment

A misalignment is very likely in a client with a hip fracture. Most hip fractures can be diagnosed, or at least suspected, based on the patient's medical history. Traditionally, a fall results in a sore hip and incapacity to walk. Clinicians should look into the possibility that the fall was caused by anything more serious, such as syncope, stroke, or myocardial infarction.

ANSWER NUMBER 04.67

Solution of the Question - B. Hormonal disturbances

Women lose the hormones needed to absorb and use calcium after menopause. Primary osteoporosis is linked to the aging process and the reduction of sex hormones. The microarchitecture of the bones has deteriorated, resulting in a loss of bone mineral density and an increased risk of fracture. Osteoporosis is described as a low bone mineral density produced by a change in bone microstructure, which puts patients at risk for low-impact, fragility fractures. Osteoporotic fractures are associated with a considerable reduction in quality of life, as well as an increase in morbidity, mortality, and disability.

ANSWER NUMBER 04.68

Solution of the Question - B. The buttocks are 15° off the bed.

In Bryant's traction, the infant's hips should be around 15 degrees off the bed. Bryant's traction is an orthopedic traction technique. It is mostly utilized in young children with femur fractures or congenital hip deformities. Both of the patient's limbs are vertically held in the air at a ninety degree angle, with the hips and knees slightly bent. Using a pulley system, the hips are gradually moved outward from the body over a number of days. The patient's body acts as a counter-traction device.

ANSWER NUMBER 04.69

Solution of the Question - A. Utilizes a Steinmann pin

Pins and screws are used in balanced skeletal traction. A Steinman pin is a big bone stabilizer that passes into huge bones like the femur. A pin is inserted into the child's damaged bone and attached to the weights for some forms of femur fractures. "Balanced skeletal traction" is the term for this. The weights hold the various sections of the bone in their appropriate positions, allowing the bone to recover properly.

ANSWER NUMBER 04.70

Solution of the Question - A. Serum collection (Davol) drain

During orthopedic surgery, bleeding is a typical complication. To ensure that the client is not hemorrhaging, the blood-collection equipment should be monitored on a regular basis. When drainage mechanisms are present, keep them open. Take note of the wound drainage characteristics. By limiting the collection of blood and fluids in the joint area, it lowers the risk of infection (medium for bacterial growth). Purulent, non-serious, odorous discharge is a sign of infection, and continual drainage from an incision could indicate a forming skin tract, which could speed up the infectious process.

ANSWER NUMBER 04.71

Solution of the Question - A. "I must flush the tube with water after feedings and clamp the tube."

After each feeding, the client's family member should be taught to flush the tube and clamp it. Percutaneous endoscopic gastrostomy (PEG) is a procedure that involves inserting a flexible feeding tube through the abdominal wall and into the stomach. PEG bypasses the mouth and esophagus, allowing nutrition, fluids, and/or drugs to be delivered straight to the stomach.

ANSWER NUMBER 04.72

Solution of the Question - C. The client's hematocrit is 26%.

Anemia should be checked on a client who has had a total knee replacement. A hematocrit of 26% is dangerously low and may necessitate a blood transfusion. The percentage of blood cells that are red blood cells is reported as the result of a hematocrit test. The normal ranges differ significantly depending on ethnicity, age, and gender. The percentage of normal red blood cells is also defined differently in different medical practices.

ANSWER NUMBER 04.73

Solution of the Question - B. The client's parents are skilled stained-glass artists.

Plumbism is the medical term for lead poisoning. Eating unfired ceramics created in Central America or Mexico is one of the factors linked to lead ingestion. The child lives in a home that was built after 1976 (when lead was removed from paint) and whose parents enjoy making stained glass. Stained glass is made with lead, which can fall on the work surface, causing the youngster to eat the lead beads.

ANSWER NUMBER 04.74

Solution of the Question - A. High-seat commode

The high-seat commode is a piece of equipment that can assist with daily duties. It's best to keep the hips higher than the knees. Patients can also use equipment to assist them in adhering to their newly prescription hip precautions. To avoid bending more than 90 degrees at the hip, some patients purchase elevated toilet seats and chairs.

ANSWER NUMBER 04.75

Solution of the Question - B. Have narcan (naloxone) available

Narcan is a narcotic overdose antidote. Naloxone is used to treat opioid toxicity and, more particularly, to reverse respiratory depression caused by opioid use. It can be used in cases of accidental or intentional overdose, as well as acute and chronic toxicity. Heroin, fentanyl, carfentanil, hydrocodone, oxycodone, methadone, and other opioids are commonly treated with naloxone.

Answer - Set 5

ANSWER NUMBER 05.01

Solution of the Question - A. Blood sugar check

When someone has a history of diabetes, the first thing they should do is check their blood sugar levels.

ANSWER NUMBER 05.02

Solution of the Question - C. The overall mental and physical abilities of the child.

When it comes to potty training, age isn't the most important aspect. The most significant component is the child's overall mental and physical abilities.

ANSWER NUMBER 05.03

Solution of the Question - C. Contact the Poison Control Center quickly.

For this youngster, the poison control center will have a specific plan of action.

ANSWER NUMBER 05.04

Solution of the Question - C. Vastus lateralis.

The bulkiest region of the vastus lateralis thigh muscle, which connects the top and middle thirds of the muscle, is where medications are injected.

ANSWER NUMBER 05.05

Solution of the Question - D. Ask the father who is in the room the child's name.

The child's name can be deduced from the father's statement in this situation. After the medication has been identified, you should not withhold it from the child.

ANSWER NUMBER 05.06

Solution of the Question - A. Elevated serum calcium.

The calcium level in the blood is controlled by the parathyroid glands. The serum calcium level will be raised in hyperparathyroidism. Osteopenia is characterized by the persistent excessive resorption of calcium from bone induced by too much parathyroid hormone.

ANSWER NUMBER 05.07

Solution of the Question - D. A restricted sodium diet.

To avoid excessive fluid loss, a patient with Addison's disease requires adequate dietary salt. Patients should eat as much as they want. Because of the salt wasting that occurs if primary adrenal insufficiency (Addison disease) is left untreated, those with primary adrenal insufficiency (Addison disease) should have plenty of salt. Primary adrenal insufficiency frequently necessitates 2-4 g of sodium chloride each day for infants.

ANSWER NUMBER 05.08

Solution of the Question - C. Hypoglycemia

Hypoglycemia is likely to be present in a diabetic patient who is unable to eat after surgery. The symptoms of confusion and shakiness are common. Confusion, difficulty concentrating, irritability, hallucinations, focal impairments (eg, hemiplegia), and, eventually, coma and death can result from a reduction in cerebral glucose availability (ie, neuroglycopenia).

ANSWER NUMBER 05.09

Solution of the Question - A. Bowel perforation.

The most serious consequence of fiberoptic colonoscopy is bowel perforation. Progressive abdominal pain, fever, chills, and tachycardia are all warning indications of developing peritonitis. Endoscopic perforation of the colon is one of the most significant consequences of colonoscopy, with rates ranging from 0.03 percent to 0.7 percent. Despite the fact that colonoscopic perforation (CP) is a rare occurrence, it is associated with high mortality and morbidity rates.

ANSWER NUMBER 05.10

Solution of the Question - A, B, and C.

Coagulation tests look at prothrombin time, partial thromboplastin time, and platelet count.

Option A: The partial thromboplastin time (PTT; also known as activated partial thromboplastin time (aPTT)) is a screening test that determines a person's capacity to form blood clots appropriately. It counts how long it takes for a clot to develop in a blood sample when drugs (reagents) are added.

Option B: A prothrombin time (PT) test is a blood test that determines how long blood takes to clot. To screen for bleeding issues, a prothrombin time test might be utilized. PT is also used to see if blood clot-prevention medication is effective.

Option C: Platelets, also known as thrombocytes, are microscopic cell fragments that are required for normal blood coagulation. They are generated in the bone marrow from very large cells called megakaryocytes and then discharged into the bloodstream to circulate. The platelet count is a test that determines how many platelets are present in a blood sample.

ANSWER NUMBER 05.11

Solution of the Question - B. Contaminated food.

Hepatitis A is the only form that spreads through contaminated food via the fecal-oral pathway. HAV is a Picornaviridae enterovirus with a single-stranded, positive-sense, linear RNA genome. In humans, viral replication is reliant on hepatocyte uptake and synthesis, and viral assembly is limited to liver cells. Viruses are nearly entirely acquired through eating (eg, fecal-oral transmission)

ANSWER NUMBER 05.12

Solution of the Question - A. A history of hepatitis C five years previously

Hepatitis C is a viral infection that causes liver inflammation and is transferred by bodily fluids such as blood. Due to the increased risk of infection in the recipient, patients with hepatitis C should not donate blood for transfusion.

ANSWER NUMBER 05.13

Solution of the Question - A. Naproxen sodium (Naprosyn).

The nonsteroidal anti-inflammatory medicine naproxen sodium can cause inflammation of the upper gastrointestinal system. As a result, it's not recommended for people who have gastritis. Naproxen is a pain reliever that is used to treat a variety of ailments including headaches, muscle pains, tendonitis, tooth pain, and menstrual cramps. It also helps to relieve the pain, swelling, and stiffness associated with arthritis, bursitis, and gout episodes.

ANSWER NUMBER 05.14

Solution of the Question - D. The patient should limit fatty foods.

Cholecystitis, or gallbladder inflammation, is most usually caused by gallstones, which can prevent bile (essential for fat absorption) from entering the intestines. To avoid gallbladder discomfort, patients should limit dietary fat by avoiding fatty meats, fried foods, and creamy desserts.

ANSWER NUMBER 05.15

Solution of the Question - D. Air hunger.

Air hunger, anxiety, and agitation are common symptoms of pulmonary edema. Coughing up blood or bloody froth; difficulty breathing while lying down (orthopnea); feeling of "air hunger" or "drowning" (if you wake up 1 to 2 hours after falling asleep and fight to recover your breath, this is called "paroxysmal nocturnal dyspnea").

ANSWER NUMBER 05.16

Solution of the Question - C. A patient with a history of ventricular tachycardia and syncopal episodes.

To stop ventricular tachycardia and ventricular fibrillation, an automated internal cardioverter-defibrillator provides an electric shock to the heart. For a patient with substantial ventricular symptoms, such as tachycardia resulting in syncope, this is required.

ANSWER NUMBER 05.17

Solution of the Question - B. The patient has a pacemaker.

An automated internal cardioverter-defibrillator (AICD) shocks the heart to stop ventricular tachycardia and ventricular fibrillation events. For a patient with substantial ventricular symptoms, such as tachycardia leading to syncope, this is required.

ANSWER NUMBER 05.18

Solution of the Question - B. The patient suddenly complains of chest pain and shortness of breath.

Chest pain, shortness of breath, and extreme anxiety are common pulmonary embolism symptoms. The doctor should be notified right away. Patients suspected of having pulmonary embolism—due to unexplained dyspnea, tachypnea, or chest discomfort, or the presence of pulmonary embolism risk factors—must undergo diagnostic tests until the diagnosis is established or excluded, or an alternative diagnosis is proven.

Option B: In individuals who have respiratory symptoms that aren't explained by other diagnoses, pulmonary embolism should be suspected. Symptoms include productive cough and wheezing.

ANSWER NUMBER 05.19

Solution of the Question - C. The patient will be admitted to the surgical unit and resection will be scheduled.

An abdominal aortic aneurysm that is quickly expanding poses a substantial risk of rupture and should be removed as soon as possible. There are currently no other viable therapy choices.

ANSWER NUMBER 05.20

Solution of the Question - D. Check for signs of bleeding, including examination of urine and stool for blood.

A platelet count of 25,000/microliter indicates severe thrombocytopenia and should urge the use of bleeding measures, such as checking urine and stool for signs of bleeding.

ANSWER NUMBER 05.21

Solution of the Question - B. Repeated vomiting.

Increased pressure within the skull produced by bleeding or swelling can harm fragile brain tissue and be life-threatening. Because the vomiting area within the medulla is triggered, repeated vomiting might be an early symptom of hypertension.

ANSWER NUMBER 05.22

Solution of the Question - A. Small blue-white spots are visible on the oral mucosa.

Koplik's spots, which appear as little blue-white dots on the oral mucosa, are a symptom of measles infection. Koplik spots (bluish-gray specks or "grains of sand" on a red base) emerge on the buccal mucosa opposing the second molars near the conclusion of the prodrome. The Koplik dots usually emerge 1-2 days before the rash appears and persist for 2 days after the rash has appeared. As the rash emerges, this enanthem begins to slough. Although this is the measles' pathognomonic anthem, its absence does not rule out the diagnosis.

ANSWER NUMBER 05.23

Solution of the Question - C. Petechiae occur on the soft palate.

The presence of Petechiae on the soft palate is a sign of rubella infection.

ANSWER NUMBER 05.24

Solution of the Question - B. The dose is too low.

The pediatric dose of diphenhydramine is 5 mg/kg/day (5 X 30 = 150 mg/day) for this child, who weighs 30 kg. As a result, the recommended daily intake is 150 mg. The youngster should be given 50 mg three times a day rather than 25 mg three times a day, divided into three dosages each day. Without contacting a physician, dosing should not be titrated based on symptoms.

ANSWER NUMBER 05.25

Solution of the Question - D. Normally, the testes descend by one year of age.

By the age of one year, the testes should have descended. When the environment is chilly or the cremasteric reflex is triggered, it is usual for the testes to retract into the inguinal canal in young newborns. The examination should be carried out in a warm environment with warm hands. Both testes are most likely present and will drop within a year. If not, a thorough examination will be conducted to decide the best course of action.

ANSWER NUMBER 05.26

Solution of the Question - C. The tumor extended beyond the kidney but was completely resected.

Wilms tumor staging is validated during surgery as follows: Stage I: The tumor is limited to the kidney and is completely resected; stage II: The tumor extends beyond the kidney but is completely resected; stage III: The non-hematogenous tumor is confined to the abdomen; stage IV: Hematogenous metastasis has occurred with spread beyond the abdomen; and stage V: Bilateral renal involvement is present at the time of diagnosis.

ANSWER NUMBER 05.27

Solution of the Question - A, B, & C

Acute glomerulonephritis is marked by a high urine specific gravity due to oliguria, as well as a dark "tea-colored" urine due to a large volume of red blood cells.

Option A: The urine is a dark brown color. It has a specific gravity of over 1.020. RBCs and RBC casts can be found.

Proteinuria, hematuria, a decrease in GFR (ie, oliguria or anuria), and active urine sediment with RBCs and RBC casts are examples of functional alterations. Increased intravascular volume, edema, and, in many cases, systemic hypertension occur from lower GFR and avid distal nephron salt and water retention.

Option C: Even if it's minuscule, this is a universal discovery. 30 percent of pediatric patients have gross hematuria, which appears as smoky, coffee, or cola-colored urine.

ANSWER NUMBER 05.28

Solution of the Question - B. Prior infection with group A Streptococcus within the past 10-14 days.

The immunological response to a previous upper respiratory infection with group A Streptococcus is the most common cause of acute glomerulonephritis. Glomerular inflammation develops 10-14 days after infection, resulting in dark urine and body fluid retention. At the time of diagnosis, periorbital edema and hypertension are common symptoms.

ANSWER NUMBER 05.29

Solution of the Question - C. No treatment is necessary; the fluid is reabsorbing normally.

A hydrocele is a fluid buildup in the scrotum caused by a patent tunica vaginalis. The transparent fluid is visible when the scrotum is illuminated with a pocket light. The fluid usually resorbs within the first few months of life, and no treatment is required.

ANSWER NUMBER 05.30

Solution of the Question - A. Inadequate tissue perfusion leading to nerve damage.

Nerve injury is common in patients with peripheral vascular disease due to insufficient tissue perfusion. Ischemic rest pain, on the other hand, is more concerning; it relates to discomfort in the extremity caused by a combination of PVD and poor perfusion. Poor cardiac output frequently exacerbates ischemic rest discomfort. Placing the extremities in a dependent position, where perfusion is improved by gravity's actions, will often partially or completely alleviate the disease.

ANSWER NUMBER 05.31

Solution of the Question - A. Family history of heart disease.

A family history of heart disease is a hereditary risk factor that cannot be changed by changing one's lifestyle. It's been proven that having a first-degree relative with heart disease raises your risk.

ANSWER NUMBER 05.32

Solution of the Question - A, C, and D.

Claudication is the pain a patient with peripheral vascular disease feels when the demand for oxygen in the leg muscles exceeds the supply. Cramping, weakness, and discomfort occur as the tissue becomes hypoxic.

Claudication is muscle pain caused by a lack of oxygen, which is initiated by exercise and eased by rest.

Option C: Because the discomfort isn't always persistent, the disorder is also known as intermittent claudication. It starts with workout and concludes with relaxation. However, if claudication progresses, discomfort may persist even when you're resting.

Claudication is pain caused by insufficient blood supply to muscles during exercising. This pain is most commonly felt in the legs after walking at a specific pace and for a certain period of time — depending on the severity of the discomfort.

ANSWER NUMBER 05.33

Solution of the Question - C. Avoid crossing the legs.

Crossing the legs should be avoided by patients with peripheral vascular disease because it can obstruct blood flow. Atherosclerosis causes PVD, which is also known as arteriosclerosis obliterans. The atheroma is made up of a cholesterol core that is connected to proteins by a fibrous intravascular coating. The atherosclerotic process can lead to full obstruction of medium and large arteries over time. The condition is usually segmental, with a lot of diversity from one patient to the next.

ANSWER NUMBER 05.34

Solution of the Question - C. young woman.

Raynaud's illness is most common in young women, and it's often linked to rheumatic diseases like lupus and rheumatoid arthritis. The blood supply to the fingers and toes is reduced due to artery spasm. Raynaud's disease commonly affects the fingers in persons who have it. Raynaud's disease affects the toes in approximately 40% of persons. The condition can affect the nose, ears, nipples, and lips in rare cases.

ANSWER NUMBER 05.35

Solution of the Question - B. Pulmonary embolism due to deep vein thrombosis (DVT).

Pulmonary embolism is the most common cause of rapid onset shortness of breath and chest discomfort in a hospitalized patient on prolonged bed rest. Both pregnancy and extended inactivity raise the risk of clot development in the legs' deep veins. After that, the clots can break free and migrate to the lungs.

ANSWER NUMBER 05.36

Solution of the Question - B. Cerebral hemorrhage.

When treating a stroke victim with thrombolytic therapy to dissolve a suspected clot, cerebral bleeding is a considerable concern. The treatment's efficacy necessitates its implementation as quickly as feasible, typically before the etiology of the stroke has been discovered.

ANSWER NUMBER 05.37

Solution of the Question - A. Torticollis, with shortening of the sternocleidomastoid muscle.

The sternocleidomastoid muscle contracts in torticollis, reducing neck range of motion and causing the chin to point to the opposite side.

ANSWER NUMBER 05.38

Solution of the Question - C. The student experiences pain in the inferior aspect of the knee.

When the infrapatellar ligament of the quadriceps muscle presses on the tibial tubercle, causing pain and swelling in the inferior side of the knee, it is known as Osgood-Schlatter disease. Activities that involve repeated use of the quadriceps, such as track and soccer, are common causes of Osgood-Schlatter disease.

ANSWER NUMBER 05.39

Solution of the Question - D. Scoliosis.

A typical teenage exam should include a check for scoliosis, which is a lateral deviation of the spine. It's determined by bending the teen's waist with arms dangling and looking for lateral curvature and unequal rib level. Female teenagers are more likely to develop scoliosis.

ANSWER NUMBER 05.40

Solution of the Question - C. Self-blame for the injury to the child.

A tendency to blame the kid or others for the injury received is part of the profile of a parent at risk of abusive behavior. Abusers frequently blame others for their faults, particularly their spouses. This is similar to hypersensitivity, but they aren't the same. This arises because the majority of abusive persons do not hold themselves accountable for their behavior. Instead, they'll try to place blame on the person they've assaulted, claiming that they "deserved it" or were pushed into a corner.

ANSWER NUMBER 05.41

Solution of the Question - C. Nonsteroidal anti-inflammatory drugs are the first choice in treatment.

For juvenile idiopathic arthritis, nonsteroidal anti-inflammatory medications (NSAIDs) are an important first-line treatment (formerly known as juvenile rheumatoid arthritis). The therapeutic anti-inflammatory benefits of NSAIDs take 3-4 weeks to manifest.

ANSWER NUMBER 05.42

Solution of the Question - B. A blood culture is drawn.

Because antibiotics may interfere with the identification of the causal organism, they must be started after the blood culture is drawn.

ANSWER NUMBER 05.43

Solution of the Question - A. Possible fracture of the tibia.

The child's inability to walk, combined with limb swelling, raises the possibility of a fracture.

ANSWER NUMBER 05.44

Solution of the Question - A, B, and D.

Cerebral palsy is characterized by delayed developmental milestones, hence regular assessment and treatments are critical. Children may experience visual and speech impairments as a result of upper motor neuron damage. Parent support groups assist families in sharing and coping with their problems. Physical therapy and other interventions can help to reduce the level of developmental milestone delays.

Option A: A short test is administered during developmental screening to see if the child has specific developmental delays, such as motor or movement delays. If the screening test findings are concerning, the doctor will refer the patient for developmental and medical examinations.

Option B: Cerebral palsy (CP) is a collection of conditions that impact a person's ability to move, balance, and maintain posture. The most prevalent motor disability in children is cerebral palsy. Cerebral refers to something that has to do with the brain. Palsy refers to muscle weakness or difficulty using muscles. A person's capacity to regulate his or her muscles is harmed by CP, which is caused by faulty brain development or damage to the growing brain.

Option D: The Individuals with Disabilities Education Act (IDEA) makes both early intervention and school-aged programs available (IDEA). Part C of IDEA covers early intervention services (from birth to 36 months of age), while Part B covers school-aged children's services (3 through 21 years of age). Regardless of whether

ANSWER NUMBER 05.45

Solution of the Question - A. Duchenne's is an X-linked recessive disorder, so daughters have a 50% chance of being carriers and sons a 50% chance of developing the disease.

The recessive Duchenne gene is found on one of a female carrier's two X chromosomes. Her youngster will be affected if he inherits the gene from his father. As a result, there is a 50% risk that a son may be afflicted. Daughters are unaffected, but 50% become carriers after receiving one copy of the faulty gene from their mother. The father, who cannot be a carrier, provides the other X chromosome.

ANSWER NUMBER 05.46

Solution of the Question - C. Procedure that compresses plaque against the wall of the diseased coronary artery to improve blood flow

A PTCA procedure is used to enhance blood flow in a damaged coronary artery. It's done during a heart catheterization procedure. The surgical operation to treat a damaged coronary artery is known as an aorta coronary bypass graft.

ANSWER NUMBER 05.47

Solution of the Question - B. Administration of thyroid hormone will prevent problems.

This problem can be corrected with early detection and ongoing hormone replacement therapy.

ANSWER NUMBER 05.48

Solution of the Question - C. Protection from self-harm and harm to others.

Involuntary hospitalization may be required for those who are deemed harmful to themselves or others, or who are profoundly incapacitated.

ANSWER NUMBER 05.49

Solution of the Question - A. "I don't remember anything about what happened to me."

Suppression is the deliberate removal of an undesirable thought or feeling from one's consciousness. The term "voluntary forgetfulness" refers to an intentional exclusion employed to protect one's own self-esteem.

ANSWER NUMBER 05.50

Solution of the Question - D. Risk for infection

Membranes ruptured more than 24 hours before birth increase the risk of infection for both the mother and the baby. Membrane rupture is caused by a multitude of circumstances that eventually contribute to increased membrane deterioration. Increased intrauterine pressure is generated by an increase in local cytokines, an imbalance in the interaction between matrix metalloproteinases and tissue inhibitors of matrix metalloproteinases, increased collagenase and protease activity, and other variables.

ANSWER NUMBER 05.51

Solution of the Question - A. Expose the cast to air and turn the child frequently

Every two hours, the infant should be turned with the exposed surface to the air. The bones are held in place by casts and splints while they recover. They also help with muscle spasms, edema, and pain.

ANSWER NUMBER 05.52

Solution of the Question - C. Administer a laxative to the client the evening before the examination

The importance of bowel preparation is that it allows for better vision of the bladder and ureters. An intravenous pyelogram (IVP) is an x-ray exam that employs a contrast substance injection to check the kidneys, ureters, and bladder in order to identify blood in the urine or side or lower back pain. An IVP may provide enough information for the clinician to treat the patient with medicine rather than surgery.

ANSWER NUMBER 05.53

Solution of the Question - D. It is not "caught" but is a response to a previous B-hemolytic strep infection.

AGN is considered a noninfectious kidney illness and is classified as an immune-complex disease in relation to an antecedent streptococcal infection that occurred 4 to 6 weeks before.

ANSWER NUMBER 05.54

Solution of the Question - D. No measurable voiding in 4 hours.

Because potassium is eliminated through the kidneys, there is a risk of hyperkalemia with sustained potassium treatment and a decrease in urine output. A successful treatment for acute hyperkalemia comprises administering calcium to protect the heart from arrhythmias, moving potassium (K+) into the cells, and improving K+ removal from the body.

ANSWER NUMBER 05.55

Solution of the Question - B. Massage the fundus

Because uterine atony is the most common source of bleeding in the first hour after delivery, the nurse should massage the fundus until it is firm. Postpartum hemorrhage affects between 3% and 5% of obstetric patients. These preventable occurrences are responsible for one-quarter of all maternal fatalities worldwide and 12% of maternal deaths in the United States each year.

ANSWER NUMBER 05.56

Solution of the Question - A. Unequal leg length

Leg shortening is a symptom of hip developmental dysplasia. A "ball-and-socket" joint, the hip is made up of two halves. The ball at the top of the thigh bone (femur) fits snugly into the socket, which is part of the big pelvis bone, in a normal hip. The hip joint has not formed normally in newborns and children with developmental dysplasia (dislocation) of the hip (DDH). The ball is loose in the socket and could dislocate easily.

ANSWER NUMBER 05.57

Solution of the Question - B. Administer stool softeners every day as ordered.

Using stool softeners on a daily basis will prevent defecation strain and the Valsalva maneuver. If constipation develops, laxatives will be required to avoid straining. Antidysrhythmics would be appropriate if straining on defecation resulted in the Valsalva maneuver and rhythm abnormalities.

ANSWER NUMBER 05.58

Solution of the Question - B. Introduce him/herself and accompany the client to the client's room.

Change that affects an individual's sense of security causes anxiety. When a client is anxious, the nurse should remain cool, reduce stimuli, and shift the client to a more quiet, secure/safe environment.

ANSWER NUMBER 05.59

Solution of the Question - C. "I have to turn my head to see my room."

The intraocular pressure rises, resulting in a progressive loss of peripheral vision in the affected eye as well as rainbow halos surrounding lights. The microscopic blockage of the trabecular meshwork causes an increase in intraocular pressure. Blindness develops in the damaged eye if left untreated or undiscovered.

ANSWER NUMBER 05.60

Solution of the Question - A. Has increased airway obstruction.

The narrower the airway, the higher the pitch of the sound. As a result, the obstruction has grown or worsened. There is no sign of secretions, thus there is no reason for suctioning.

ANSWER NUMBER 05.61

Solution of the Question - D. Low self-esteem

Batterers have typically been physically or psychologically abused as children or have experienced parental violence histories. Batterers are also manipulative, have low self-esteem, and have a strong desire to control or dominate their partners.

ANSWER NUMBER 05.62

Solution of the Question - A. Isometric

The nurse should teach the client isometric exercises for the muscles of the casted extremity, which require the client to contract and relax muscles alternately without moving the affected portion.

ANSWER NUMBER 05.63

Solution of the Question - A. Counsel the woman to consent to HIV screening

The client's actions put her at a significant risk of contracting HIV. The first step is to test. If the lady tests positive for HIV, the sooner she begins treatment, the better.

ANSWER NUMBER 05.64

Solution of the Question - B. Explain that this behavior is expected.

Fear of strangers emerges around the age of 6-8 months during normal development. Clinging to parents, sobbing, and shrinking away from strangers are examples of such behaviors. These fears/behaviors can last well into toddlerhood and even into preschool.

ANSWER NUMBER 05.65

Solution of the Question - B. Separation from parents

Separation anxiety is most noticeable between the ages of 6 and 30 months. It is the most stressful experience a toddler can have while in the hospital. If separation is prevented, young children have an incredible ability to cope with different types of stress.

ANSWER NUMBER 05.66

Solution of the Question - B. They are able to think logically in organizing facts.

When given the opportunity to control and organize objects, the child in the concrete operational stage, according to Piaget, is capable of mature thought.

ANSWER NUMBER 05.67

Solution of the Question - D. Safety

For the depressed client, safety is a top priority. Suicide prevention measures must be included in the plan. Depression can be effectively treated in primary care settings with an evidence-based collaborative strategy in which primary care practitioners are routinely supported in caring for a caseload of patients by mental health providers.

ANSWER NUMBER 05.68

Solution of the Question - A. Sports and games with rules

Cooperation is the goal of play for a 7-year-old. It's critical to follow the rules. Play promotes the development of logical reasoning and social skills.

ANSWER NUMBER 05.69

Solution of the Question - A. High Fowler's

The heart workload is reduced and breathing is made easier by sitting in a chair or lying in a bed in a high Fowler's position.

ANSWER NUMBER 05.70

Solution of the Question - A. Urinary output of 30 ml per hour

This is adequate production for a youngster of this age, but it does not indicate overload. When sodium-ATPase activity is disrupted, an intracellular sodium shift occurs, contributing to hypovolemia and cellular edema. Inflammatory and vasoactive mediators are released in response to heat injury. Local vasoconstriction, systemic vasodilation, and enhanced transcapillary permeability are all caused by these mediators. Water, inorganic solutes, and plasma proteins are rapidly transferred between the intravascular and interstitial compartments as transcapillary permeability increases.

ANSWER NUMBER 05.71

Solution of the Question - A. Acute pain related to biologic and chemical factors

Pain control is the top goal for interdisciplinary care for patients with migraine headaches.

ANSWER NUMBER 05.72

Solution of the Question - A, B, C, D, & E.

The customer should be advised on the foods and medications that are permissible. He should also be informed about the potential negative effects of the medications he has been prescribed. Pain-distracting techniques should also be included in the lesson plan.

Option A: It may induce the chemical norepinephrine to be released by nerve cells in the brain. Higher levels of tyramine in the system, combined with unusually high levels of brain chemicals, can produce brain alterations that result in headaches.

Option B: Oral contraceptives and vasodilators like nitroglycerin can make migraines worse. The widely documented adverse effect of migraine type headache is dilation of cerebral arteries.

Option C: Abortive therapy should be used as soon as feasible once a migraine has started. Aspirin, caffeine, and acetaminophen-containing combination analgesics are an effective first-line migraine abortive treatment. Ibuprofen in regular doses is beneficial in the treatment of acute migraines.

Option D: Medication overuse headaches, also known as rebound headaches, are caused by long-term use of headache medications, such as migraine medications. Pain medicines might help with headaches that occur from time to time. However, if used more than a couple of times each week, they can cause drug overuse headaches.

Option E: According to the National Center for Complementary and Integrative Health, complementary therapies are "add-on therapies" that are used in addition to established treatments (NCCIH). Complementary therapies include massage, spinal manipulation, and acupuncture, to name a few.

ANSWER NUMBER 05.73

Solution of the Question - C. Take the patient's vital signs.

A nursing assistant's education and area of work include taking vital signs.

ANSWER NUMBER 05.74

Solution of the Question - B. Set up oxygen and suction equipment.

The LPN/LVN can set up the oxygen and suctioning equipment.

ANSWER NUMBER 05.75

Solution of the Question - D. "It's OK to take over-the-counter medications."

Patients with seizure disorders should not take over-the-counter drugs without first consulting their doctor.

Answer - Set 6

ANSWER NUMBER 06.01

Question is about - room assignments

Solution of the Question - B. 12-year-old male with a fractured femur

The 6-year-old should have a roommate who is at least his or her age, thus the 12-year-old is the best choice. There is a bed available, and the patient is assigned to it. Sex, semi-private versus private, isolation concerns, acuity, telemetry, and speciality demands are all factors to consider. All of this must be considered in order to guarantee that each patient is directed to the appropriate location and receives the appropriate care. However, proper capacity management necessitates careful consideration and execution of bed assignments.

ANSWER NUMBER 06.02

Solution of the Question - B. Report chest pain.

Heart attacks and strokes have been linked to Cox II inhibitors. Because bleeding has been connected to the use of Cox II inhibitors, any changes in cardiac status or indicators of a stroke should be reported immediately, as should any changes in bowel or bladder habits. Celecoxib, like all NSAIDs, comes with a boxed warning from the FDA about cardiovascular risk, including an increased risk of heart attacks and strokes. Celecoxib is being investigated for increased cardiovascular risk as a selective COX-2 inhibitor, after another selective COX-2 inhibitor, rofecoxib, was pulled from the market in 2004 due to cardiovascular risk concerns.

ANSWER NUMBER 06.03

Solution of the Question - D. Allows 24 hours before bearing weight

It takes 24 hours for a plaster-of-Paris cast to dry, and the client should not bear weight during that time. The casting material will begin to dry in about 10 to 15 minutes after the application process is completed. Because of a chemical reaction that happens when the plaster dries, the temperature of the skin may rise. When plaster is used, the cast might take anywhere from 1 to 2 days to harden entirely.

ANSWER NUMBER 06.04

Solution of the Question - A. "It will be alright for your friends to autograph the cast."

Answers B, C, and D are erroneous since there is no reason why the client's friends should not be permitted to autograph the cast; it will not affect the cast in any way. When opposed to plaster, fiberglass provides a number of advantages. Because it is lighter, the cast created from it will be lighter as well. Fiberglass is more robust and porous, allowing air to flow in and out. If the limb needs to be X-rayed during the healing process, fiberglass is the superior option. It comes in a range of hues as well.

ANSWER NUMBER 06.05

Solution of the Question - A. Assisting the LPN with opening sterile packages and peroxide

When the nurse wears sterile gloves and Q-tips to care for the pins, she is doing it right. Every day, all pins and wire sites must be cleaned. Prior to release from the hospital, the hospital nursing staff will undertake basic pin care once a day. Following discharge, the patient and his or her family will visit the clinic for pin care education and training.

ANSWER NUMBER 06.06

Solution of the Question - A. Check the bowel sounds

A body cast, also known as a spica cast, covers the entire body from the upper abdomen to the knees or lower. To make sure the client isn't suffering from a paralytic ileus, listen to their bowel noises. If bowel noises are present, or if the patient reports passing flatus, clear fluids can be started and aperiments can be given. If no bowel noises are heard, patients should not begin oral fluids because this signals an ileus.

ANSWER NUMBER 06.07

Solution of the Question - C. Halo traction

For the client with a cervical fracture, halo traction will be prescribed. Halo-gravity traction is a technique for gently pulling the head and spine upward and stretching the spine. A halo (a metal ring that surrounds the head) is attached to a pulley system by doctors. Weights are gradually added to the pulley system over several weeks to progressively pull the head forward. Traction is the term for this pulling. During halo-gravity traction, children are admitted to the hospital.

ANSWER NUMBER 06.08

Solution of the Question - B. "The CPM machine controls should be positioned distal to the site."

The continuous-passive-motion device's controller should be situated distant from the client. Many clients complain of pain during CPM treatments, prompting them to switch the unit off. The leg is flexed and extended by the CPM. Continuous passive motion (CPM) is a therapy that involves the use of a machine to move a joint without the patient exerting any effort. The physical therapist can vary the amount of movement and speed of a motorized device that gently bends the joint back and forth to a specific number of degrees. CPM machines are most typically utilized on knee joints (following certain types of knee surgery), although they are also available for other joints.

ANSWER NUMBER 06.09

Solution of the Question - A. Palms rest lightly on the handles

The palms of the client's hands should be lightly resting on the handles. The elbows should be flexed to a maximum of 30 degrees but not extended. Following the selection of a walker model, the "fit" of the walker becomes critical. The elbows should be bent in a comfortable and natural position when holding on to the walker. When the arms are relaxed at the side, the top of the walker should be even with the crease on the bottom of the wrist.

ANSWER NUMBER 06.10

Solution of the Question - C. Elevate the client's hips.

Elevating the hips and wrapping the chord with moist, sterile saline gauze should be used to treat the client with a prolapsed cord. Until a cesarean section can be performed, the nurse should push up on the presenting region with her fingers. The cord will slide down the vagina if the cesarean section is not performed before the membrane ruptures.

ANSWER NUMBER 06.11

Solution of the Question - A. Report muscle weakness to the physician.

Muscle weakness is an indication of rhabdomyolysis, thus clients using antilipidemics should be urged to report it. Myalgia is the most common harmful side effect of rosuvastatin. If the patient is experiencing mild to moderate muscle pain, the medicine should be stopped to rule out other possible causes of myalgia. If the underlying cause is resolved, the patient can resume the original or lower dose of rosuvastatin; however, if symptoms recur, rosuvastatin should be discontinued indefinitely. Switching to a lower-dose statin prescription may help with muscle aches and pains.

ANSWER NUMBER 06.12

Solution of the Question - B. Check the blood glucose level

Hyperstat is an IV push used to treat hypertensive crises, however it can also cause hyperglycemia. When you stop using the medication, your blood glucose level will drop quickly. This drug is used to treat extremely low blood sugar levels (hypoglycemia). The secretion of too much insulin can be caused by a variety of circumstances (such as a pancreatic tumor, cancer, or leucine sensitivity). Insulin is a naturally occurring chemical that helps to reduce blood sugar levels. This medication works by blocking the release of insulin from the pancreas, allowing blood sugar levels to return to normal. Diazoxide is a thiazide medication, however unlike other thiazides, it has no diuretic ("water pill") effects.

ANSWER NUMBER 06.13

Solution of the Question - C. Heart rate of 60 bpm

A baby's heart rate of 60 should be reported right away. If the heart rate is less than 100 beats per minute, the dose should be maintained. On the AV node, digoxin has vagomimetic actions. The parasympathetic nervous system is stimulated, which slows electrical conduction in the atrioventricular node and lowers heart rate. The AV node's refractory time is lengthened as calcium levels rise because phase 4 and phase 0 of the cardiac action potential are both prolonged. A lower ventricular response is associated with slower AV node conduction.

ANSWER NUMBER 06.14

Solution of the Question - C. Leave the medication in the brown bottle

Because of its instability and tendency to become less potent when exposed to air, light, or water, nitroglycerine should be kept in a brown bottle (or even a specific air- and water-tight, solid or plated silver or gold container). Keep nitroglycerin pills in an airtight, dark-colored (brown) glass container that you can't see through. Keep the container closed tightly. Keep nitroglycerin tablets and liquid spray out of direct sunlight and away from heat and moisture.

ANSWER NUMBER 06.15

Solution of the Question - C. Turkey breast

Turkey has the lowest fat and cholesterol content. Turkey and chicken both have a lot of high-quality protein. Turkey thigh is somewhat higher in protein than chicken thigh, whereas chicken thigh is slightly higher in protein than turkey thigh. The protein content of the other beef cuts is comparable.

ANSWER NUMBER 06.16

Solution of the Question - B. Neck

Distension of the jugular veins in the neck should be checked. Increased blood volume, which can occur with right-sided heart failure, or anything that prevents the right atrium from filling or blood from moving into the right ventricle, can raise central venous pressure and jugular vein distention.

ANSWER NUMBER 06.17

Solution of the Question - A. Phlebostatic axis

The manometer should be placed on the phlebostatic axis, which is located at the fifth intercostal space midaxillary line. The phlebostatic axis can be found by drawing an imaginary line from the sternum's fourth intercostal space and intersecting it with an imaginary line drawn along the middle of the chest below the axillae.

ANSWER NUMBER 06.18

Solution of the Question - B. Administer the medications

Zestril is an ACE inhibitor that is commonly used in conjunction with a diuretic like Lasix to treat hypertension. ACE inhibitors appear to augment the antihypertensive effects of diuretics in hypertension studies, albeit the interaction appears to be additive rather than synergistic. Diuretics in combination with ACE inhibitors appear to be no more efficacious than diuretics in combination with beta blockers.

ANSWER NUMBER 06.19

Solution of the Question - B. Measuring the extremity

Measuring the extremities is the best indicator of peripheral edema. A paper tape measure, rather than a plastic or cloth one, should be used, and the area should be marked with a pen for the most objective assessment. One of the girth measurement procedures is the circumferential method. Each upper or lower extremity is marked with a semi-permanent marker at a specific location with reference to the bony prominences for consistent measurements.

ANSWER NUMBER 06.20

Solution of the Question - D. Visitation is limited to 30 minutes when the implant is in place.

Close interaction with clients who have radium implants should be limited to 30 minutes every visit. The basic rule is to restrict the amount of time individuals are exposed to radium, keep a safe distance between them and the radium source, and use lead as a radium shield. It is critical to instill these values in family members. Internal radiation therapy involves putting radiation inside the body to kill cancer cells using a pill, liquid, implant, or temporary source, and may necessitate certain safety precautions for staff and family while the patient is in the hospital or at home, according to the National Cancer Institute.

ANSWER NUMBER 06.21

Solution of the Question - B. Split pea soup, mashed potatoes, pudding, milk

A client who has had a face stroke will have trouble swallowing and chewing, and these foods need the least amount of chewing. Consult a speech therapist to assess gag reflexes; aid in the teaching of alternate swallowing strategies, encourage the patient to eat smaller boluses of food, and tell the patient of foods that are easier to swallow; supply thicker liquids or a pureed diet as needed.

ANSWER NUMBER 06.22

Solution of the Question - A. "I will make sure I eat breakfast within 10 minutes of taking my insulin."

Because NovoLog insulin takes effect quickly, food should be ready within 10–15 minutes following injection. It takes 1 to 3 hours for the medication to take effect. Subcutaneous injection of crystalline NPH insulin is used. There is no intramuscular or intravenous administration. NPH insulin comes in a two-phase solution, which means it contains a solvent or a rapid-acting insulin solution in addition to NPH. It comes in the form of a suspension pen-injector or a subcutaneous suspension.

ANSWER NUMBER 06.23

Solution of the Question - B. The umbilical cord needs time to separate.

Food should be ready within 10–15 minutes of taking NovoLog insulin because it onsets quickly. It takes 1 to 3 hours for the effects to kick in. Subcutaneous delivery of crystalline NPH insulin is used. Intramuscular or intravenous administration is not an option. NPH insulin comes as a two-phase solution that includes a solvent or a rapid-acting insulin solution in addition to NPH. It's available as a suspension pen-injector or a subcutaneous suspension.

ANSWER NUMBER 06.24

Solution of the Question - D. Reverse drug toxicity and prevent tissue damage

Methotrexate and Trimetrexate, both folic acid antagonists, have an antidote in the form of leucovorin. Leucovorin is a form of folic acid. The FDA has approved leucovorin for use after high-dose methotrexate therapy in osteosarcoma to reduce methotrexate toxicity or to counteract the toxicity of folate antagonists. When oral folic acid intake is not possible, leucovorin is occasionally used as an alternate treatment for megaloblastic anemia.

ANSWER NUMBER 06.25

Solution of the Question - A. HibTITER

With the polio vaccine, the Haemophilus influenza vaccine is administered at 4 months. It protects the child from Hib disease, which can be fatal and cause lifelong disability; it protects the child from the most common type of Hib disease, meningitis (an infection of the lining surrounding the brain and spinal cord); and it prevents the child from missing school or child care, as well as the parents from missing work.

ANSWER NUMBER 06.26

Solution of the Question - A. 30 minutes before meals.

Proton pump inhibitors stop the stomach from producing acid. The optimal time to take proton pump inhibitors is 30 minutes before your first meal of the day. Take each dose with a full glass of water (8 ounces). Esomeprazole is commonly prescribed for a period of 4 to 8 weeks. If the client requires more time to heal, the doctor may suggest a second course of treatment.

ANSWER NUMBER 06.27

Solution of the Question - A. Call security for assistance and prepare to sedate the client.

If the client poses a threat to the staff or other clients, the nurse should seek assistance and prepare to sedate him with a medicine like Haldol. If seclusion appears to be a possibility, notify personnel. The usual order of priority for interventions is strict limitations, chemical restraints (tranquilizers), then seclusion. Seclusion may be necessary if nursing treatments (calm atmosphere and strong limit setting) and pharmaceutical restraints (tranquilizers–e.g., haloperidol [Haldol]) have failed to control escalating manic behaviors.

ANSWER NUMBER 06.28

Solution of the Question - A. Check the client for bladder distention

A full bladder could be indicated by the client's fundus being shifted to the side. The nurse should then examine for bladder distention and, if required, catheterize the patient. After delivery, the uterus continues to contract and shrinks rapidly as estrogen and progesterone levels fall. The top section of the uterus, known as the fundus, is midline and palpable halfway between the symphysis pubis and the umbilicus immediately after delivery.

ANSWER NUMBER 06.29

Solution of the Question - C. Tuberculosis

Tuberculosis symptoms include a low-grade temperature, blood-tinged sputum, tiredness, and night sweats. Some of the most frequent physical symptoms of pulmonary tuberculosis are a chronic cough, hemoptysis, weight loss, low-grade fever, and night sweats. The clinical appearance of secondary tuberculosis differs from that of original progressive tuberculosis. The tissue reaction and hypersensitivity are more severe in secondary illness, and patients frequently develop cavities in the upper lungs.

ANSWER NUMBER 06.30

Solution of the Question - B. Prinzmetal's angina

Triptan products should not be prescribed if the customer has a history of Prinzmetal's angina since they promote vasoconstriction and coronary spasms. If you have or have ever had heart disease, a heart attack, angina (chest pain), irregular heartbeats, stroke or'mini-stroke,' or circulation problems like varicose veins, blood clots in the legs, Raynaud's disease (blood flow problems in the fingers, toes, ears, and nose), or ischemic bowel disease, tell your doctor (bloody diarrhea and stomach pain caused by decreased blood flow to the intestines). It's possible that your doctor will urge you not to take sumatriptan.

ANSWER NUMBER 06.31

Solution of the Question - A. Pain on flexion of the hip and knee

Kernig's sign is present when discomfort arises when the hip and knee are flexed. Kernig's sign is one of the meningitis symptoms that can be seen physically. When the hip is bent to 90 degrees, severe hamstring stiffness prevents the leg from straightening.

ANSWER NUMBER 06.32

Solution of the Question - A. Agnosia

Agnosia is a term that refers to the inability to recognize what objects are and what they are used for. For example, a person with agnosia would try to eat with a fork rather than a spoon, drink from a shoe rather than a cup, or write with a knife rather than a pencil. In the case of humans, this could mean failing to recognize who they are due to the brain's inability to puzzle out a person's identity based on the information provided by the eyes, rather than due to memory loss.

ANSWER NUMBER 06.33

Solution of the Question - C. Sundowning

The "sundowning" phenomenon is characterized by an increase in perplexity at night. When the sun begins to set, there is an increase in perplexity that lasts through the night. The phrase "sundowning" refers to a period of bewilderment that begins late in the afternoon and lasts into the evening. Sundowning can result in a number of behaviors, including bewilderment, anxiety, anger, and disobedience. Pacing or roaming might occur as the sun sets.

ANSWER NUMBER 06.34

Solution of the Question - C. "I'll get you some juice and toast. Would you like something else?"

The befuddled client may forget that he ate earlier. Don't squabble with the customer. Get him something to eat that will keep him satisfied until lunchtime. Irrational thinking should not be challenged. Challenges to the patient's thinking can be interpreted as dangerous, leading to a defensive response. Maintain normal fluid and electrolyte balance; establish/ maintain normal nutrition, body temperature, oxygenation (use supplementary oxygen if patients have low oxygen saturation), blood glucose levels, and blood pressure.

ANSWER NUMBER 06.35

Solution of the Question - D. Nausea

Clients on acetylcholinesterase inhibitors like Exelon frequently experience nausea and gastrointestinal distress. Dizziness, unsteadiness, and clumsiness are some of the other negative symptoms. The most common side effects linked with rivastigmine use are gastrointestinal. Nausea and vomiting are the most common symptoms. These acute symptoms are most common during the initial dose-escalation phase of therapy, when the medication is titrated higher to reach a therapeutic level. If providing an oral formulation, these incidents can be reduced by adopting a moderate titration schedule and taking the prescription with food.

ANSWER NUMBER 06.36

Solution of the Question - B. Report the finding to the doctor

Any lesion should be brought to the attention of the doctor. This could be a sign of a herpes infection. Clients with open herpes lesions are delivered via Cesarean section since there is a risk of infection spreading to the fetus through direct contact with the sores. Primary HSV infection has a higher risk of perinatal transmission than recurrent infection during pregnancy. If a primary HSV outbreak is discovered during pregnancy, oral antiviral therapy may be used to help lessen the length and intensity of symptoms as well as viral shedding.

ANSWER NUMBER 06.37

Solution of the Question - B. Cervical cancer

The client who has HPV is more likely to get cervical and vaginal cancer as a result of this STI. Multiple epithelial lesions and malignancies, mostly of the cutaneous and mucosal surfaces, are caused by the Human Papillomavirus (HPV). HPV is now thought to be a cause of laryngeal, oral, lung, and anogenital cancers. Low-risk subtypes 6 and 11 are characterized by the production of condylomata and low-grade precancerous lesions. HPV subtypes 16 and 18 are high-risk, causing high-grade intraepithelial lesions that can develop to cancer.

ANSWER NUMBER 06.38

Solution of the Question - B. Herpes

A painful lesion is most likely a herpetic lesion. Herpes genitalis can be caused by either type 1 or type 2 herpes simplex viruses, and it can be a primary or recurring infection. Viruses replicate in epithelial tissue and then go dormant in sensory neurons, reactivating as localized recurrent lesions on a regular basis. It is still one of the most common sexually transmitted diseases (STI), but due to the ambiguous nature of its symptoms, it is often overlooked.

ANSWER NUMBER 06.39

Solution of the Question - C. Fluorescent treponemal antibody (FTA)

The test for treponema pallidum is fluorescent treponemal antibody (FTA). The fluorescent treponemal antibody absorption (FTA-ABS) test is a blood test that detects antibodies to the microorganisms Treponema pallidum. Syphilis is caused by these microorganisms. Syphilis is a sexually transmitted infection (STI) disseminated by contact with syphilitic sores.

ANSWER NUMBER 06.40

Solution of the Question - D. Elevated hepatic enzymes

Hemolysis, increased liver enzymes, and a low platelet count are all symptoms of HELLP. Hemolysis, increased liver enzymes, and low platelets syndrome, or HELLP syndrome, has traditionally been thought to be a consequence or development of severe preeclampsia. The inheritability of propensity to preeclampsia and/or HELLP syndrome in pregnancy has also been investigated by genetic analysis. Both genetic and immunological variables play a role in pathogenesis, according to the findings.

ANSWER NUMBER 06.41

Solution of the Question - A. The nurse places her thumb on the muscle inset in the antecubital space and taps the thumb briskly with the reflex hammer.

The biceps reflex is triggered by pressing your thumb against the biceps tendon and striking it with the reflex hammer while watching your arm move. Rep with the other arm and compare. Deep tendon reflexes are evoked in all four extremities using a reflex hammer. Visually and by palpating the tendon or muscle in issue, note the amount or power of the response.

ANSWER NUMBER 06.42

Solution of the Question - B. Brethine 10 mcg IV

Because it elevates blood glucose levels, brethine should be used with caution. Terbutaline can induce an increase in the baby's heart rate and blood sugar levels for a short period of time. These side effects are usually minor and can be treated easily after delivery if they occur. Long-term usage of this medicine is causing worry since the risk of harm to the infant increases.

ANSWER NUMBER 06.43

Solution of the Question - C. The infant is at high risk for respiratory distress syndrome.

The lungs are considered mature when the L/S ratio hits 2:1. One of numerous measures used by doctors to determine fetal lung development is the Lecithin-to-Sphingomyelin Ratio (L/S ratio). This biochemical test, which collects a sample of amniotic fluid via amniocentesis to determine the risk of the newborn having respiratory distress syndrome, was originally developed in the 1970s (RDS). After that, the sample was analyzed using thin-layer chromatography to determine the size of lecithin in comparison to sphingomyelin.

ANSWER NUMBER 06.44

Solution of the Question - C. Jitteriness

In a neonate, jitteriness is an indication of a seizure. Treatment for babies with clinical indications of hypoglycemia, such as apnea, hypotonia, jitteriness, apathy, hypothermia, tremors, and seizures, must keep blood glucose levels above 0.45 g/L (2.5 mmol/L). Urgently deliver an IV bolus dose of glucose (150-200 mg/kg), followed by a constant rate infusion.

ANSWER NUMBER 06.45

Solution of the Question - B. Hypersomnolence

The customer should become drowsy, have heat flushes, and be sluggish. Minor facial flushing and warmth are the most common side effects of the medication, but they usually go away on their own. Neuromuscular illness, such as myasthenia gravis, can cause neuromuscular function to deteriorate at lower drug dosages.

ANSWER NUMBER 06.46

Solution of the Question - D. Increase the rate of the IV infusion

If the client's blood pressure drops following an epidural anesthesia injection, the nurse should turn her to the left side, give her oxygen through a mask, and speed up the IV infusion. If your blood pressure does not return to normal, you should see a doctor. Epinephrine should be kept on hand in case of an emergency.

ANSWER NUMBER 06.47

Solution of the Question - A. Alteration in nutrition

Pancreatic cancer is associated with severe nausea and vomiting, as well as a change in diet. In around 90% of patients, weight loss occurs. Around 75% of individuals experience abdominal pain. Anorexia, palpable, non-tender, enlarged gallbladder, acholic stools, and dark urine are all symptoms of bile salts in the skin.

ANSWER NUMBER 06.48

Solution of the Question - C. Daily measurement of abdominal girth

The most objective approach of determining ascites is to use a paper tape measure and mark the region that is measured. The pathologic accumulation of fluid within the peritoneal cavity is known as ascites. It is the most frequent cirrhosis consequence, affecting nearly half of all patients with decompensated cirrhosis within ten years. The transition from compensated to decompensated cirrhosis is marked by the appearance of ascites.

ANSWER NUMBER 06.49

Solution of the Question - B. Fluid volume deficit

Hypovolemic shock is indicated by the vital signs. Monitor and record vital indicators, notably blood pressure and heart rate. Hypotension and tachycardia can be caused by a decrease in circulating blood volume. HR fluctuation is a compensatory mechanism that keeps cardiac output constant. The pulse is usually weak and erratic, especially if an electrolyte imbalance is present. Hypovolemia results in hypotension.

ANSWER NUMBER 06.50

Solution of the Question - A. Likes to play football

Pathological fractures are a concern for the client with osteogenesis imperfecta, and these fractures are more likely to occur if he participates in contact sports. If the client becomes dehydrated or deoxygenated, he may develop hypoxia symptoms; strenuous exertion, especially in hot conditions, might aggravate the issue.

ANSWER NUMBER 06.51

Solution of the Question - D. Tell the family members to take the fruit home

Fresh fruit should not be given to a neutropenic client since it must be peeled and/or cooked before consumption. He should also avoid eating items that have been cultivated on or in the ground, as well as salads from the salad bar. Potted or cut flowers should also be removed from the room by the nurse. If at all feasible, any source of bacteria should be eradicated.

ANSWER NUMBER 06.52

Solution of the Question - B. Increase the infusion of Dextrose in normal saline

The use of dextrose in normal saline as a source of water, electrolytes, and calories is recommended. Bleeding, postoperative edema, and airway impairment are early problems after total laryngectomy, and these should be closely watched, especially in the immediate postoperative period.

ANSWER NUMBER 06.53

Solution of the Question - C. Cover the insertion site with a Vaseline gauze

If the client pulls the chest tube out of the chest, the nurse should immediately apply an occlusive bandage to the insertion site. The nurse should then contact the doctor, who will likely request a chest x-ray and potentially reinsert the tube. At the bedside, in the procedure room, or in the surgical suite, a chest tube can be implanted. In the insertion and removal of a closed chest tube drainage system, health care providers frequently help physicians.

ANSWER NUMBER 06.54

Solution of the Question - A. Assess for signs of abnormal bleeding

The average Protime is between 12 and 20 seconds. A Protime of 120 seconds suggests an exceptionally lengthy Protime, which can cause spontaneous bleeding. Patients who are taking warfarin should be closely monitored to ensure the medication's safety and efficacy. Periodic blood testing is advised to determine the patient's prothrombin time (PT) and international normalized ratio (INR) (INR).

ANSWER NUMBER 06.55

Solution of the Question - C. A cup of yogurt

The most calcium-rich food is yogurt, which contains about 400 mg of calcium. A growing baby requires a lot of calcium to develop properly. If a mother does not ingest enough calcium to meet her baby's needs, the body will draw calcium from her bones, reducing bone mass and placing her at risk for osteoporosis. Osteoporosis causes significant bone loss, resulting in brittle, weak bones that are readily fractured.

ANSWER NUMBER 06.56

Solution of the Question - C. The nurse inserts a Foley catheter.

A Foley catheter should be placed in the client receiving magnesium sulfate, and intake and output should be evaluated hourly. Throughout the magnesium sulfate infusion, strict intake and outflow will be monitored. If a Foley catheter is in place, record urine output at least once every hour. Otherwise, make a list of all voids and measure them. While taking magnesium sulfate, urine output should be at least 30 mL/hour. Notify the provider if the urine output is less than normal.

ANSWER NUMBER 06.57

Solution of the Question - D. Notify the physician of the mother's refusal

The doctor should be notified if the client's mother refuses the blood transfusion. The court may require treatment because the client is a juvenile. Understanding the ethical and legal concerns involved, providing precise medical management, using prohemostatic drugs, and other key interventions and strategies to limit blood loss and hence lessen the likelihood of needing a blood transfusion are all part of proper management of such patients.

ANSWER NUMBER 06.58

Solution of the Question - B. Laryngeal edema

Because of the burn region, the nurse should be primarily concerned with laryngeal edema. Fluid resuscitation should be started for severe burns (> 20% TBSA) in order to keep urine production > 0.5 mL/kg/hour. The Parkland formula is a popular fluid resuscitation formula. 4 ml of LR x patient's weight (kg) x percent TBSA = total amount of fluid to be given over the first 24 hours.

ANSWER NUMBER 06.59

Solution of the Question - D. The client gains weight.

The customer suffering from anorexia benefits the most from weight increase. To determine the success of the treatment plan, expect to gain roughly 1 pound (0.5 kg) per week. Set a minimum weight goal and daily dietary requirements. Malnutrition affects mood by causing despair and agitation, as well as reducing cognitive function and decision-making. Improved dietary status improves cognitive abilities, allowing psychological work to begin.

ANSWER NUMBER 06.60

Solution of the Question - D. Paresthesia of the toes

Paresthesia is unusual and could be a sign of compartment syndrome. Acute compartment syndrome develops when pressure builds up inside a closed osteofascial compartment, impairing local circulation. Acute compartment syndrome is considered a surgical emergency since it might progress to ischemia and finally necrosis if not treated properly.

ANSWER NUMBER 06.61

Solution of the Question - B. Tachycardia and diarrhea

Barbiturates have sedative properties. Tachycardia, diarrhea, and tachypnea will occur when the client stops using barbiturates. Barbiturates cause a decrease in blood pressure and an increase in heart rate when used with IV anesthetics. Respiratory depression and apnea are possible side effects. Given the risk of serious side effects, including death, a pharmacist should double-check the dosing and conduct a complete medication reconciliation to ensure there are no drug interactions, especially additive CNS depressive effects.

ANSWER NUMBER 06.62

Solution of the Question - A. Right breech presentation

The newborn is in breech presentation if the fetal heart tones may be heard in the right upper abdomen. The position of the baby in the womb is not optimum for birth. Though most breech babies are healthy when they are delivered, they are at a higher risk of birth abnormalities or trauma during delivery. This position can also be troublesome since it raises the possibility of producing a loop in the umbilical cord, which could harm the infant if delivered vaginally.

ANSWER NUMBER 06.63

Solution of the Question - D. Spasm of bronchial smooth muscle

Bronchial spasms are a symptom of asthma. Allergies or worry might cause a spasm like this. Asthma is a disorder characterized by acute, fully reversible airway inflammation that commonly occurs as a result of exposure to a trigger. The pathogenic process begins with the inhalation of an irritant (e.g., cold air) or allergen (e.g., pollen), which causes airway inflammation and increased mucus production due to bronchial hypersensitivity.

ANSWER NUMBER 06.64

Solution of the Question - A. Serve high-calorie foods she can carry with her

Maniac patients rarely sit long enough to eat and burn a lot of calories to stay awake. The best options for improving nutrition are finger foods or foods that a client can eat while moving about. Reduced environmental stimulation may help the client relax; however, the nurse must provide a peaceful area free of noise, television, and other distractions.

ANSWER NUMBER 06.65

Solution of the Question - B. Hips are slightly elevated above the bed and the legs are suspended at a right angle to the bed

For broken femurs and dislocated hips, Bryant's traction is employed. Hips should be raised 15 degrees off the bed. Bryant's traction is used to treat dislocated hips in children (DDH). The child's body and the weights are used to retain the end of the femur (the big bone that runs from the knee to the hip) in the hip socket in Bryant's traction. Traction will assist in properly positioning the top of the femur into the hip socket.

ANSWER NUMBER 06.66

Solution of the Question - B. The nurse wears gloves when providing care.

Shingles is caused by the herpes zoster virus. If a client has shingles, they should be put on contact precautions. Using gloves when providing care will prevent the virus from spreading. To prevent disease transmission to yourself or other clients, use universal precautions when caring for the client. VZV can be passed on to others and induce chickenpox in those who have never had it before.

ANSWER NUMBER 06.67

Solution of the Question - B. 30 minutes before the infusion

30 minutes before the third or fourth dose, take a trough level. Draw through specimens as soon as possible (30 minutes) before the next dose. Do not begin drawing specimens until the steady condition has been reached (ie, before the fourth dose). Draw peak specimens 1-2 hours after the intravenous dose has been completed.

ANSWER NUMBER 06.68

Solution of the Question - B. Keep the diaphragm in a cool location

The client who uses a diaphragm should keep it in a cool place. The diaphragm is a contraceptive (birth control) device that keeps sperm from entering the uterus. The diaphragm is a tiny, reusable rubber or silicone cup that covers the cervix and has a flexible rim. The diaphragm is put deep into the vaginal canal before sex, with a portion of the rim fitting securely behind the pubic bone.

ANSWER NUMBER 06.69

Solution of the Question - C. "I'm drinking four glasses of fluid during a 24-hour period."

Breastfeeding mothers should consume enough of liquids, and four glasses in a 24-hour period is insufficient. Breastfeeding mothers require more assistance, encouragement, and reassurance. Breastfeeding is a skill that must be acquired, despite the fact that it is a natural procedure. Breastfeeding can appear difficult at first since the baby may want to feed/suck constantly. Babies, on the other hand, develop their own patterns with time, and the mother becomes more comfortable and at ease.

ANSWER NUMBER 06.70

Solution of the Question - A. Facial pain

The face nerve is the seventh cranial nerve. The client will endure facial pain if there is injury. The sensory part, also known as the intermediate nerve, is made up of the following elements: (3) cutaneous sensory impulses from the external auditory meatus and region behind of the ear; (1) taste to the anterior two-thirds of the tongue; (2) secretory and vasomotor fibers to the lacrimal gland, mucous membranes of the nose and mouth, and the submandibular and sublingual salivary glands;

ANSWER NUMBER 06.71

Solution of the Question - B. Change the color of her urine

Pyridium users should be informed that the medicine causes their urine to turn orange or crimson. Pyridium can also turn your skin and sclera yellow if you take too much of it. Urinary tract pain, burning, irritation, and discomfort, as well as urgent and frequent urination caused by urinary tract infections, surgery, injury, or examination procedures, can all be relieved with phenazopyridine. Phenazopyridine, on the other hand, is not an antibiotic and does not treat infections.

ANSWER NUMBER 06.72

Solution of the Question - B. Perform a pregnancy test

Because of its teratogenic properties, Accutane is not recommended for use by pregnant women. Under the former FDA system, isotretinoin was classified as a pregnancy category X medicine, and it is not recommended for women who are pregnant or may become pregnant. When pregnant women take isotretinoin, there have been recorded cases of severe congenital defects.

ANSWER NUMBER 06.73

Solution of the Question - D. Encourage fluids

Because renal impairment can occur when taking Acyclovir, clients should be encouraged to drink enough of fluids. The most serious side effect of parenteral acyclovir treatment is acute kidney damage (AKI). The rate of AKI is equivalent to that of other nephrotoxic drugs like aminoglycosides. Patients with chronic kidney disease (CKD) are at a higher risk. Acyclovir dosage must be adjusted for optimal body weight and baseline renal function.

ANSWER NUMBER 06.74

Solution of the Question - A. Pregnancy

Although there is no evidence that MRI scans represent a risk during pregnancy, it is recommended that MRI scans be avoided during this time, especially in the first three months. This is especially true during the first trimester of pregnancy, as this is when organogenesis occurs. The same problems apply to MRI in general during pregnancy, but the fetus may be more sensitive to the effects, particularly to heat and noise.

ANSWER NUMBER 06.75

Solution of the Question - D. Changes in skin color

Because Amphotericin B is toxic to the kidneys and liver, and induces bone marrow suppression, it should be evaluated for hepatic, renal, and bone marrow function. Jaundice is a symptom of liver damage that is not caused by Amphotericin B. Amphotericin B can cause cellular toxicity due to the similarities of mammalian and fungal membranes, which both contain sterols (the therapeutic target for amphotericin B).

Answer - Set 7

ANSWER NUMBER 07.01

Solution of the Question - C. The NA performs the patient's complete bath and oral care.

The nursing assistant should help the patient with morning care as needed, but the goal is to keep this patient as mobile and independent as possible.

ANSWER NUMBER 07.02

Solution of the Question - A. "I will avoid exercise because the pain gets worse."

Back exercises help to strengthen the back, reduce strain on compressed nerves, and prevent re-injury. Lower back strengthening exercises can help relieve and prevent lower back discomfort. It can also help to strengthen the muscles of the core, legs, and arms. Exercise also boosts blood flow to the lower back, which may help to alleviate stiffness and speed up the healing process, according to studies.

ANSWER NUMBER 07.03

Solution of the Question - B. Check the Foley tubing for kinks or obstruction.

These symptoms are indicative of autonomic dysreflexia, a neurologic emergency that requires immediate treatment to avoid a hypertensive stroke. The origin of this syndrome is unpleasant stimuli, most commonly a distended bladder or constipation, thus the first step should be to check for inadequate catheter drainage, bladder distention, or fecal impaction.

ANSWER NUMBER 07.04

Solution of the Question - B. A 67-year-old patient with stroke 3 days ago and left-sided weakness.

Stable, non-complex patients, such as the stroke patient, should be assigned to the new graduate RN who is being orientated to the unit.

ANSWER NUMBER 07.05

Solution of the Question - D. Monitor respiratory effort and oxygen saturation level.

Assessing breathing patterns and providing a sufficient airway are the first priorities for a patient with a SCI. Because the spinal nerves (C3–5) innervate the phrenic nerve, which controls the diaphragm, a patient with a high cervical injury is at risk for respiratory compromise.

ANSWER NUMBER 07.06

Solution of the Question - B. Take a patient's vital signs and record them every 4 hours.

Taking and recording a patient's vital signs is part of the nursing assistant's training and education.

ANSWER NUMBER 07.07

Solution of the Question - A, B, D, and E

Except for direct catheterization, all of the techniques have the potential to trigger voiding in patients with SCI.

ANSWER NUMBER 07.08

Solution of the Question - A, C, and D

Option A: Within the area of practice of the LPN/LVN, checking for indicators of pressure.

Option C: The LPN/scope LVN's of practice includes looking for indicators of infection.

Option D: The LPN/LVN also has the necessary abilities to use hydrogen peroxide to clean the halo insertion sites.

ANSWER NUMBER 07.09

Solution of the Question - C. Impaired Adjustment to Spinal Cord Injury

The patient's statement shows that he or she is having trouble adjusting to the restrictions of the disability and that further counseling, training, and assistance is needed.

ANSWER NUMBER 07.10

Solution of the Question - B. A 68-year-old patient with chronic amyotrophic lateral sclerosis (ALS)

The traveling nurse is new to neurology nursing and should be allocated to patients with stable, non-complex diseases.

ANSWER NUMBER 07.11

Solution of the Question - D. Self-care Deficit related to fatigue and neuromuscular weakness

The priority at this moment, according to the patient's remark, is Self-Care Deficit as a result of weariness following physical treatment. Fatigue is defined as an overwhelming sense of lassitude or a lack of physical or mental energy that prevents you from doing things you want to do.

ANSWER NUMBER 07.12

Solution of the Question - D. Shallow respirations and decreased breath sounds

The primary goal of treatment for a GBS patient is to maintain good respiratory function. These individuals are in danger of developing respiratory failure, which is a life-threatening condition. 40% of individuals exhibit respiratory or oropharyngeal weakness when they first arrive. Up to one-third of patients experience respiratory failure and require breathing support at some point throughout their illness.

ANSWER NUMBER 07.13

Solution of the Question - B. Notify the physician immediately.

The alterations that the nursing assistant is describing are typical of a myasthenia crisis, which occurs frequently after an illness. The patient's respiratory function may be compromised. In addition to alerting the physician, the nurse should keep a close eye on the patient's breathing. Intubation and mechanical ventilation may be required.

ANSWER NUMBER 07.14

Solution of the Question - C. "Alteplase dissolves clots and may cause more bleeding into your wife's brain."

Alteplase is a clot-busting medication. There is already bleeding into the brain in a patient who has had a hemorrhagic stroke. Alteplase, for example, can make the bleeding worse.

ANSWER NUMBER 07.15

Solution of the Question - A. The student instructs the patient to sit up straight, resulting in the patient's puzzled expression.

Neglect syndrome is common in patients who have had a stroke in the right hemisphere of the brain. When questioned why they lean to the left, many say they think they're sitting up straight. They frequently overlook food on the left side of their food trays and the left side of their body. The nurse would need to remind the pupil about this occurrence and go over the best course of action.

ANSWER NUMBER 07.16

Solution of the Question - C. Left anterior descending artery

The left anterior descending artery provides the main blood supply for the heart's anterior wall. The left anterior descending artery is a branch of the left coronary artery that provides blood to the heart's front side.

ANSWER NUMBER 07.17

Solution of the Question - B. During diastole

Although the coronary arteries receive a small amount of blood during systole, diastole provides the majority of the blood flow to the arteries.

ANSWER NUMBER 07.18

Solution of the Question - B. Coronary artery disease

Coronary artery disease is responsible for more than half of all deaths in the United States.

ANSWER NUMBER 07.19

Solution of the Question - A. Atherosclerosis

The most common cause of CAD is atherosclerosis, or plaque formation.

ANSWER NUMBER 07.20

Solution of the Question - B. Plaques obstruct the artery.

The coronary arteries are supplied with oxygen and other nutrients by arteries rather than veins. Atherosclerosis is a lipoprotein-driven disease that causes intimal inflammation, necrosis, fibrosis, and calcification at specific points in the arterial tree.

ANSWER NUMBER 07.21

Solution of the Question - C. Heredity

It is impossible to change our genetic makeup, which is referred to as "heredity."

ANSWER NUMBER 07.22

Solution of the Question - D. 200 mg/dl

Cholesterol levels greater than 200 mg/dl are considered high. They may necessitate dietary restrictions as well as medication. Exercise also aids in the reduction of cholesterol levels. The other levels are all below the officially acceptable cholesterol levels and entail a lower risk of coronary artery disease. Serum cholesterol levels should be between 125 and 200 mg/dl.

ANSWER NUMBER 07.23

Solution of the Question - B. Enhance myocardial oxygenation

When a client shows indications and symptoms of cardiac compromise, the first aim is always to improve myocardial oxygenation. The myocardial experiences damage if it does not receive enough oxygen.

ANSWER NUMBER 07.24

Solution of the Question - C. Oral medication administration.

Oral drug administration is a medical treatment for coronary artery disease that is noninvasive. For acute cases of angina, the most common vasodilator is nitroglycerin. It works by widening or dilating the coronary arteries, increasing blood flow to the heart muscle, and relaxing the veins, reducing the volume of blood returning to the heart from the rest of the body. The amount of effort the heart has to do is reduced as a result of this combination of actions.

ANSWER NUMBER 07.25

Solution of the Question - C. Inferior

The right coronary artery delivers blood to the right ventricle, which is the heart's lower chamber. As a result, a prolonged obstruction in that location could result in myocardial infarction.

ANSWER NUMBER 07.26

Solution of the Question - A. Chest pain

The most frequent sign of a heart attack is chest discomfort, which is caused by a lack of oxygen to the heart. Ischemia is characterized by a heavy chest pressure or squeezing, a "burning" sensation, or trouble breathing. Discomfort or pain in the left shoulder, neck, or arm is common. In a few circumstances, chest pain may be unusual. Over the course of a few minutes, the intensity increases.

ANSWER NUMBER 07.27

Solution of the Question - B. Left fifth intercostal space, midclavicular line

The left intercostal space in the midclavicular line is the correct landmark for getting an apical pulse. This is the position of the left ventricular apex and the point of greatest impulse.

ANSWER NUMBER 07.28

Solution of the Question - D. Pulmonary

These symptoms are commonly used to describe pulmonary discomfort. The skin, ribs, intercostal muscles, pleura, esophagus, heart, aorta, diaphragm, or thoracic vertebrae are only few of the structures in the chest that can cause pain. Intercostal, sympathetic, vagus, and phrenic nerves can all transmit pain. The deep tissues of the thorax have shared innervations that lead to the central nervous system, making it difficult to pinpoint the source of pain.

ANSWER NUMBER 07.29

Solution of the Question - C. Pulmonic

At the second left intercostal space along the left sternal border, abnormalities of the pulmonic valve are auscultated. The cardiac system develops murmurs as a result of changes in blood flow or mechanical operation. Murmurs are caused by a variety of mechanisms. Low blood viscosity caused by anemia, septal defects, inability of the ductus arteriosus to close in infants, high hydrostatic pressure on heart valves producing valve failure, hypertrophic obstructive cardiomyopathy, and valvular specific diseases are all examples of common conditions.

ANSWER NUMBER 07.30

Solution of the Question - C. Troponin I

Troponin I levels rise quickly after myocardial infarction and can be detected within an hour. Troponin I levels are undetectable in those who haven't had a heart attack. Troponin C, troponin I, and troponin T are three subunits of the troponin complex, which is found on the myofibrillar thin (actin) filament of striated (skeletal and cardiac) muscle. Troponin T and I are cardiac isoforms that are solely found in heart muscle. As a result, cardiac troponin T (cTnT) and I (cTnI) levels are more selective for myocardial damage than creatine kinase (CK) levels, and because of their great sensitivity, they may even be increased when CKMB levels are not.

ANSWER NUMBER 07.31

Solution of the Question - D. To decrease oxygen demand on the client's heart

Morphine is given because it lowers the demand for oxygen in the heart. Morphine has been used to ease pain during a myocardial infarction (MI) since the early 1900s. An observational research published in 2005 indicated some concerns, yet there are few viable alternatives. Morphine is a powerful opioid that reduces pain and, as a result, reduces the activation of the autonomic nervous system. When a patient is undergoing a MI, these are good benefits.

ANSWER NUMBER 07.32

Solution of the Question - C. Coronary artery thrombosis

Coronary artery thrombosis causes the artery to become occluded, resulting in myocardial death. A myocardial infarction happens when a coronary artery becomes so badly clogged that the blood flow to a section of the myocardium is significantly reduced or interrupted, causing injury or death (heart muscle).

ANSWER NUMBER 07.33

Solution of the Question - C. Potassium

Furosemide is taken with potassium supplementation because of the potassium loss caused by this diuretic. When the heart is unable to completely pump blood throughout the body, loop diuretics act on the ascending loop of Henle in the kidney, helping the body push out extra fluid that could accumulate in the lungs, legs, and ankles. However, they may cause the body to excrete an excessive amount of potassium, thus increasing the risk of death from heart arrhythmias. As a precaution, many doctors prescribe potassium supplements to their loop diuretic patients as a precaution.

ANSWER NUMBER 07.34

Solution of the Question - D. Metabolic

Glucose and fatty acids are two metabolites whose levels rise after a heart attack. Acute myocardial infarction causes a distinct neurohumoral response, with increased catecholamine release, raised plasma levels of free fatty acids and glucose, and decreased glucose tolerance.

ANSWER NUMBER 07.35

Solution of the Question - A. Ventricular dilation

S3 is auscultated since rapid filling of the ventricles induces vasodilation. The third heart sound (S3) is a low-frequency, transient vibration heard at the end of the right or left ventricle's rapid diastolic filling cycle in early diastole.

ANSWER NUMBER 07.36

Solution of the Question - A. Left-sided heart failure

The left ventricle produces the greatest amount of cardiac output. Left ventricular function may be reduced as a result of an anterior wall MI. Fluid collects in the interstitial and alveolar spaces of the lungs when the left ventricle fails to function properly, resulting in left-sided heart failure. This generates crackles.

ANSWER NUMBER 07.37

Solution of the Question - D. Electrocardiogram

The ECG is the most used instrument for determining the location of a myocardial infarction since it is the quickest, most accurate, and most extensively utilized.

ANSWER NUMBER 07.38

Solution of the Question - B. Administer oxygen

The initial priority of care is to provide supplemental oxygen to the client. During an infarction, the myocardium is deprived of oxygen, thus extra oxygen is given to help oxygenate it and avoid further damage.

ANSWER NUMBER 07.39

Solution of the Question - A. "Tell me about your feelings right now."

The most suitable answer is to validate the client's feelings. It gives the client a sense of security and comfort.

ANSWER NUMBER 07.40

Solution of the Question - A. Beta-adrenergic blockers

Beta-adrenergic blockers reduce the response to catecholamines and sympathetic nerve stimulation by inhibiting beta receptors in the myocardium. They protect the myocardium, lowering the workload of the heart and lowering myocardial oxygen demand, lowering the chance of recurrent infarction.

ANSWER NUMBER 07.41

Solution of the Question - C. Arrhythmias

The most prevalent consequence of a MI is arrhythmias, which are produced by oxygen deprivation in the myocardium.

ANSWER NUMBER 07.42

Solution of the Question - B. Heart failure

The failure of the heart to pump is indicated by elevated venous pressure, which manifests as jugular vein distention.

ANSWER NUMBER 07.43

Solution of the Question - C. Raised 30 degrees

With the head of the bed tilted between 15 and 30 degrees, jugular venous pressure is measured with a centimeter ruler to determine the vertical distance between the sternal angle and the point of greatest pulsation.

ANSWER NUMBER 07.44

Solution of the Question - A. Apical pulse

Before delivering digoxin, an apical pulse is required to precisely determine the client's heart rate. The most precise spot in the body is the apical pulse.

ANSWER NUMBER 07.45

Solution of the Question - A. Digoxin

The visual disturbance known as the green halo indication is one of the most prominent indicators of digoxin intoxication.

ANSWER NUMBER 07.46

Solution of the Question - A. Crackles

Lung crackles are a common symptom of left-sided heart failure. Fluid backing up into the pulmonary system causes these sounds. The heart's left ventricle isn't pumping enough blood around the body anymore. Blood builds up in the pulmonary veins as a result (the blood vessels that carry blood away from the lungs). Shortness of breath, difficulty breathing, or coughing are common symptoms, especially after strenuous exertion. The most prevalent type of heart failure is left-sided heart failure.

ANSWER NUMBER 07.47

Solution of the Question - D. Right-sided heart failure

The sacral area is the most appropriate area of the body to assess dependent edema in a bedridden client. Right-sided heart failure causes sacral, or dependent, edema.

ANSWER NUMBER 07.48

Solution of the Question - C. Oliguria

After right-sided heart failure, the liver's insufficient deactivation of aldosterone promotes fluid retention, which produces oliguria. Oliguria is a late symptom of heart failure that appears in people who have a significantly reduced cardiac output due to substantially diminished LV function.

ANSWER NUMBER 07.49

Solution of the Question - D. Inotropic agents

Inotropic drugs are used to increase the force of the heart's contractions, resulting in increased ventricular contractility and, as a result, increased cardiac output.

ANSWER NUMBER 07.50

Solution of the Question - B. Tachycardia

Tachycardia and enhanced contractility are caused by sympathetic nervous system stimulation. The right stellate ganglion releases norepinephrine, which increases heart rate and shortens atrioventricular conduction via the sinus and atrioventricular nodes.

ANSWER NUMBER 07.51

Solution of the Question - D. Right-sided heart failure

Secondary consequences of right-sided heart failure include weight gain, nausea, and a decrease in urine production. The heart's right ventricle is too weak to pump enough blood to the lungs in this case. Blood builds up in the veins as a result of this (the blood vessels that carry blood from the organs and tissue back to the heart). Increased pressure inside the veins might cause fluid to leak out and into the surrounding tissue. This causes fluid to accumulate in the legs, or less usually, the vaginal area, organs, or the abdomen (belly).

ANSWER NUMBER 07.52

Solution of the Question - A. Atherosclerosis

75 percent of all abdominal aortic aneurysms are caused by atherosclerosis. Plaques build up on the vessel's wall, weakening it and producing an aneurysm. AAA is assumed to be an aortic degenerative process, the source of which is unknown. Because these alterations are noticed in the aneurysm at the time of surgery, it is frequently attributed to atherosclerosis.

ANSWER NUMBER 07.53

Solution of the Question - B. Distal to the renal arteries

Because the aorta distal to the renal arteries is not surrounded by stable structures, it is more prone to aneurysm than the proximal region of the aorta.

ANSWER NUMBER 07.54

Solution of the Question - A. Abdominal aortic aneurysm

A pulsing mass in the belly is unusual and usually indicates an outpouching in a weakened vessel, such as in an abdominal aortic aneurysm. However, for a skinny person, the discovery may be typical.

ANSWER NUMBER 07.55

Solution of the Question - A. Abdominal pain

The disturbance of normal circulation in the abdominal region causes abdominal pain in a client with an abdominal aortic aneurysm. Before the rupture, patients may have modest back, flank, abdominal, or groin discomfort. Isolated groin pain is an especially deceptive symptom. Retroperitoneal enlargement and pressure on the right or left femoral nerve cause this. This symptom can appear without any other signs or symptoms, thus a high level of suspicion is required to make the diagnosis.

ANSWER NUMBER 07.56

Solution of the Question - D. Lower back pain

The growth of an aneurysm causes lower back pain. The pressure in the abdominal cavity is applied by the expansion, and the discomfort is transferred to the lower back.

ANSWER NUMBER 07.57

Solution of the Question - B. Arteriogram

An arteriogram illustrates the vasculature correctly and immediately, vividly delineating the vessels and any anomalies.

ANSWER NUMBER 07.58

Solution of the Question - B. Aneurysm rupture

Aneurysm rupture is a life-threatening emergency that the nurse caring for this type of client is most concerned about. The aortic wall's layers can also split (aortic dissection). The pain in the chest, back, or abdomen is acute and ripping. The most serious risk linked with an aortic aneurysm is the possibility of rupture. Internal bleeding and/or a stroke can be life-threatening if an aortic aneurysm ruptures.

ANSWER NUMBER 07.59

Solution of the Question - C. Media

A damaged media is a common component in all forms of aneurysms. Because the medium has more smooth muscle and less elastic fibers, it is more capable of both constriction and dilation of the blood vessels.

ANSWER NUMBER 07.60

Solution of the Question - C. Middle lower abdomen to the left of the midline

Because the aorta is straight to the left of the umbilicus, any other area should not be palpated. Just above and to the left of the umbilicus, the aortic pulse can be felt. By placing both hands palms down on the patient's belly and one index finger on either side of the aorta, the breadth of the aorta can be determined. Each systole should separate the fingers.

ANSWER NUMBER 07.61

Solution of the Question - B. HPN

Hypertension puts constant strain on the vessel walls, weakening them and causing an aneurysm. Because hypertension is more common in people who are overweight or obese, have less physical activity, smoke, or eat a poor diet, the link between hypertension and AAA could be muddled by other risk factors.

ANSWER NUMBER 07.62

Solution of the Question - A. Bruit

Partial arterial occlusion is indicated by a bruit, a vascular sound that sounds like a heart murmur. Auscultation for abdominal or femoral bruits, in addition to abdominal palpation, may be effective for clinical identification of AAA. Auscultation is done along the aortic and femoral arteries' path. However, the absence of a bruit does not rule out the possibility of an aneurysm.

ANSWER NUMBER 07.63

Solution of the Question - B. Severe lower back pain, decreased BP, decreased RBC, increased WBC

Aneurysm rupture caused by pressure applied to the abdomen cavity is indicated by severe lower back discomfort. The pain is persistent when an aneurysm ruptures since it can't be relieved until the aneurysm is repaired. Due to the loss of blood, blood pressure drops. Because the vasculature is disrupted and blood volume is lost when an aneurysm ruptures, blood pressure does not rise. The RBC count has declined – not increased – for the same reason. As cells migrate to the injury site, the number of white blood cells (WBCs) rises.

ANSWER NUMBER 07.64

Solution of the Question - C. Retroperitoneal rupture at the repair site

Blood accumulates in the retroperitoneal space, resulting in a hematoma in the perineal area. Leakage at the repair site is the most prevalent cause of this rupture.

ANSWER NUMBER 07.65

Solution of the Question - C. Marfan's syndrome

The elastic fibers of the aortic media degenerate as a result of Marfan's syndrome. As a result, people who have the condition are more prone to have an aortic aneurysm. Marfan syndrome (MFS) is a group of illnesses characterized by a heritable connective tissue genetic abnormality that is passed down in an autosomal dominant pattern. The FBN1 gene on chromosome 15, which codes for the connective tissue protein fibrillin, has been identified as the source of the abnormality. Abnormalities in this protein produce a variety of clinical issues, the most common of which are musculoskeletal, cardiac, and visual system issues.

ANSWER NUMBER 07.66

Solution of the Question - D. Surgical intervention

When a blood vessel ruptures, surgery is the only way to heal it. Aneurysm surgery techniques have been standardized for a long time. A modest frontotemporal craniotomy centered over the pterion can reach 95 percent of aneurysms. Different surgical methods are required only in rare circumstances, such as aneurysms of the distal anterior cerebral artery and the lower vertebrobasilar trunk.

ANSWER NUMBER 07.67

Solution of the Question - A. Cardiomyopathy

Cardiomyopathy isn't always linked to an underlying cardiac condition like atherosclerosis. In the majority of cases, the cause is unknown.

ANSWER NUMBER 07.68

Solution of the Question - A. Dilated

Cardiac dilatation and heart failure can occur during the last month of pregnancy or the first few months following birth, for reasons that are unknown. The disease could be the outcome of an undiagnosed cardiomyopathy previous to pregnancy.

ANSWER NUMBER 07.69

Solution of the Question - C. Hypertrophic

Hypertrophy of the ventricular septum – not the ventricle chambers – is visible in hypertrophic cardiomyopathy. Hypertrophic cardiomyopathy (HCM) is a type of cardiovascular illness caused by a genetic mutation. It's characterized by an increase in left ventricular wall thickness that isn't primarily due to excessive loading. A mutation in the cardiac sarcomere protein genes causes this condition, which is usually passed down as an autosomal dominant trait.

ANSWER NUMBER 07.70

Solution of the Question - A. Heart failure

Heart failure is the most prevalent complication of cardiomyopathy because the structure and function of the heart muscle are impaired. When the heart muscle is weak (systolic failure) or stiff and unable to relax normally, heart failure can result (diastolic failure). One of the many reasons of heart failure is cardiomyopathy, which means "disease of the heart muscle."

ANSWER NUMBER 07.71

Solution of the Question - A. Cardiomegaly

An enlarged heart muscle is referred to as cardiomegaly. Dilated hypertrophy, fibrosis, and contractile dysfunction are the most important pathophysiological alterations that contribute to cardiomegaly. Hypertrophic or dilated cardiomyopathy can be caused by contractile dysfunction and aberrant myocardium remodeling. In cardiomyocytes, mechanical stretching, circulating neurohormones, and oxidative stress are all important triggers for inflammatory cytokines and MAP kinase signaling. Changes in structural proteins and proteins that govern excitation-contraction are caused by signal transduction. Mutations in dilated cardiomyopathy cause a decrease in sarcomere contraction force and a decrease in sarcomere content. Hypertrophic cardiomyopathy mutations cause hyperdynamic contractility, poor relaxation, and excessive energy consumption at the molecular level.

ANSWER NUMBER 07.72

Solution of the Question - D. Restrictive

These are some of the most common signs and symptoms of heart failure. Heart failure is a pathophysiologic situation in which the heart fails to pump blood at a rate commensurate with the needs of the metabolizing tissues due to an impairment of cardiac function (detectable or not), or can only do so with an elevated diastolic filling pressure.

ANSWER NUMBER 07.73

Solution of the Question - B. Hypertrophic

Because the size of the ventricle remains basically unaltered, hypertrophic cardiomyopathy has no effect on cardiac output. The following are three possible explanations for the mitral valve's systolic anterior motion: (1) Because of the valve's abnormal location and septal hypertrophy altering the orientation of the papillary muscles, the mitral valve is pulled against the septum; (2) the mitral valve is pushed against the septum because of its abnormal position in the outflow tract; (3) the mitral valve is drawn toward the septum because of the lower pressure that occurs as blood is ejected at high velocity through a narrowed outflow tract (Venturi effect).

ANSWER NUMBER 07.74

Solution of the Question - D. Failure of the ventricle to eject all the blood during systole

After atrial contraction, increased resistance to ventricular filling causes an S4. This higher resistance is linked to a decrease in ventricle compliance.

ANSWER NUMBER 07.75

Solution of the Question - B. Beta-adrenergic blockers

Beta-adrenergic blockers increase myocardial filling and cardiac output by lowering heart rate and contractility, which are main goals in the therapy of cardiomyopathy.

Answer – Set 8

ANSWER NUMBER 08.01

Solution of the Question - C. The client with chest pain and a history of angina

Because chest pain could signal a myocardial infarction, the client with chest pain should be evaluated first. Despite significant advancements in therapy, acute MI still has a 5-to-30% mortality rate, with the majority of deaths occurring before reaching the hospital. Furthermore, there is an additional death rate of 5% to 12% within the first year after a MI. The severity of cardiac muscle injury and ejection fraction determine the overall prognosis.

ANSWER NUMBER 08.02

Solution of the Question - B. Three times per day with meals

For best results, pancreatic enzymes should be taken with meals. These enzymes help the body absorb the nutrition it requires. Regular pancreatic enzymes, fat-soluble vitamins (A, D, E, K), mucolytics, bronchodilators, antibiotics, and anti-inflammatory medications are all part of CF patients' long-term supportive therapy.

ANSWER NUMBER 08.03

Solution of the Question - C. The lens focuses light rays on the retina.

Light passes through the pupil and is focused on the retina by the lens. The lens is a curved component in the eye that bends and focuses light for the retina, allowing you to view images clearly. A clear disk beneath the iris, the crystalline lens, is flexible and changes form to let you view objects at different distances.

ANSWER NUMBER 08.04

Solution of the Question - C. Constrict the pupils

Miotic eye drops restrict the pupil, allowing aqueous fluid to drain from the Schlemm Canal. Pilocarpine is a muscarinic acetylcholine agonist that can help with acute angle closure glaucoma and radiation-induced xerostomia. Although it is not a first-line treatment for glaucoma, it can be used as a supplement in the form of ophthalmic drops.

ANSWER NUMBER 08.05

Solution of the Question - A. Allow 5 minutes between the two medications.

Allow 5 minutes between eye drops if you're using them both. A doctor may give antibiotic eye drops to treat bacterial eye infections. They function by destroying the bacteria (microscopic organisms) that caused the infection in the first place.

ANSWER NUMBER 08.06

Solution of the Question - B. Violet

Violets, blues, and green will most likely be difficult to discern for color blind clients. Protanopia and deuteranopia are the most prevalent kinds, both of which are caused by the loss of function of one of the cones, resulting in dichromic vision. Protanopia is a condition in which the L cones (red) are lost, leaving only green-blue vision. Deuteranopia is a condition in which the M cones (green) are lost, leaving only red-blue vision.

ANSWER NUMBER 08.07

Solution of the Question - D. Monitor his pulse rate

A pacemaker patient should be taught how to count and record his pulse rate. Pacemakers are electronic pulse generators that create pulses with a duration of 0.5 to 25 milliseconds and a voltage output of 0.1 to 15 volts at a frequency of up to 300 times per minute. Whether the device is temporary or permanent, the cardiologist or pacemaker technologist will be able to examine and control the pacing rate, pulse width, and voltage.

ANSWER NUMBER 08.08

Solution of the Question - A. 1900

After around 7 p.m., or 1900, clients who are being retrained for bladder control should be taught to withhold fluids. If you go to the bathroom too often "just in case," you may aggravate your overactive bladder symptoms by training your bladder to send a signal that you need to urinate even if there is only a small amount of urine in it.

ANSWER NUMBER 08.09

Solution of the Question - D. Drink a glass of cranberry juice every day.

Cranberry juice is more alkaline and is expelled in acidic urine when digested by the body. In acidic urine, bacteria cannot thrive. In a 2003 study of 324 women, it was discovered that drinking freshly squeezed, 100 percent juice, particularly berry juice, as well as fermented dairy items like yogurt, was linked to a lower risk of UTI.

ANSWER NUMBER 08.10

Solution of the Question - C. "I will eat a snack around three o'clock each afternoon."

Because NPH insulin peaks in 8–12 hours, a food should be served then. It is on the World Health Organization's list of essential medicines (WHO). NPH insulin has been licensed by the FDA for the treatment of type 1 and type 2 diabetes in adults and children. It is the most extensively used basal insulin that mimics the physiological action of basal insulin. Despite fasting, such as between meals and overnight, basal insulin maintains a steady supply of insulin in the body that is required for glucose homeostasis.

ANSWER NUMBER 08.11

Solution of the Question - B. Chest tubes serve as a method of draining blood and serous fluid and assist in re-inflating the lungs.

The purpose of chest tubes is to re-inflate the lungs and remove the serous fluid. A chest tube is used by doctors to create negative pressure in the chest cavity and allow the lung to expand again. It helps to clear the intrathoracic space of air (pneumothorax), blood (hemothorax), fluid (pleural effusion or hydrothorax), chyle (chylothorax), or purulence (empyema).

ANSWER NUMBER 08.12

Solution of the Question - D. Mother's desire to breastfeed

Breastfeeding success is determined by a variety of circumstances, but the most reliable cause for success is the desire and readiness to continue breastfeeding until the newborn and mother have adjusted. Breastfeeding is an essential element of a baby's development. Breastfeeding or lactation ensures the baby's complete nutritional and emotional dependence on the mother. The mother-child dyad must have a strong emotional relationship in order to successfully extend nursing.

ANSWER NUMBER 08.13

Solution of the Question - C. The presence of green-tinged amniotic fluid

Meconium staining is indicated by green-tinged amniotic fluid. This discovery implies that the fetus is in distress. The fluid in the amniotic sac should be clear or straw-colored with little vernix particles. The passage of meconium is indicated by a brown or green discoloration of the fluid. Meconium can be present in the infant's oropharynx during delivery because the fetus eats amniotic fluid while in the womb. If meconium-stained amniotic fluid is discovered during birth, a newborn resuscitation team should be contacted right away.

ANSWER NUMBER 08.14

Solution of the Question - C. Duration is measured by timing from the beginning of one contraction to the end of the same contraction.

The length of a contraction is measured from the start to the finish of the same contraction. The duration of a contraction is measured from the time you first feel it until it stops. In most cases, this time is expressed in seconds.

ANSWER NUMBER 08.15

Solution of the Question - B. Fetal bradycardia

Decelerations in the client taking Pitocin should be watched. While delivering oxytocin, it's critical to keep track of the patient's fluid intake and output, as well as the frequency of uterine contractions, patient blood pressure, and the unborn fetus' heart rate.

ANSWER NUMBER 08.16

Solution of the Question - D. Fetal development depends on adequate insulin regulation.

Appropriate diet and insulin management are essential for fetal development. During pregnancy, significant changes in maternal metabolism guarantee a constant supply of nutrients to the fetus. The fetus's main source of energy is glucose. Increases in maternal insulin sensitivity allow for the storage of energy and nutrients during early pregnancy.

ANSWER NUMBER 08.17

Solution of the Question - A. Providing a calm environment

To prevent seizure activity, a quiet environment is required. Seizures can be triggered by any stimuli. Establish strategies to reduce the likelihood of seizures, such as keeping the room dark and quiet, limiting visitors, planning and coordinating care, and encouraging relaxation. Reduces the effects of environmental stimuli that can irritate the cerebrum and produce convulsions.

ANSWER NUMBER 08.18

Solution of the Question - A. Down syndrome

The 42-year-old customer is at risk of prenatal defects such Down syndrome and other genetic abnormalities. Chromosome abnormalities are more likely. Certain genetic disorders, such as Down syndrome, are more common among babies born to older moms.

ANSWER NUMBER 08.19

Solution of the Question - C. Dinoprostone (Prostin E.)

Induction of labor will be performed on the client who has had a missed abortion. Prostaglandin E is a prostaglandin that softens the cervix. Prostaglandin E2 (PGE2), also known as dinoprostone, is a naturally occurring substance that promotes labor while also being implicated in the inflammatory process. The FDA has approved prostaglandin E2 for cervical ripening in the induction of labor in patients who have a medical reason to do so.

ANSWER NUMBER 08.20

Solution of the Question - A. Continue the infusion of magnesium sulfate while monitoring the client's blood pressure

Blood pressure and urine production are both within typical ranges for the client. Deep tendon reflexes are reduced, which is the only difference from normal. The nurse should continue to check the magnesium level and monitor the blood pressure. The therapeutic range is between 4.8 and 9.6 mg/dL. Magnesium levels should be checked every 6 to 8 hours in the serum or clinically by monitoring patellar reflexes or urine output.

ANSWER NUMBER 08.21

Solution of the Question - C. Affected parents have a one in four chance of passing on the defective gene.

Autosomal recessive disorders can be passed down through the generations. If both parents pass the trait on to their children, the youngster will inherit two faulty genes as well as the condition. The trait can also be passed down from parents to their children. Each chromosome in patients with autosomal recessive (AR) illnesses has a disease allele. The pattern of individuals affected by an AR disease can be tracked through a family to establish who is a carrier and who is at risk of becoming afflicted.

ANSWER NUMBER 08.22

Solution of the Question - D. To detect neurological defects

The screening test alpha fetoprotein is used to detect neural tube disorders such as spina bifida. The embryonic yolk sac and the fetal liver produce the plasma protein alpha-fetoprotein (AFP). AFP levels in serum, amniotic fluid, and urine are used to screen for congenital impairments, chromosomal abnormalities, and a variety of other adult-onset cancers and diseases.

ANSWER NUMBER 08.23

Solution of the Question - B. Regulation of thyroid medication is more difficult because the thyroid gland increases in size during pregnancy.

The thyroid gland triples in size during pregnancy. Thyroid medication regulation becomes more complicated as a result of this. The maternal body's metabolic needs rise during pregnancy, resulting in alterations in thyroid physiology. Thyroid function tests are altered as a result of these alterations in thyroid physiology.

ANSWER NUMBER 08.24

Solution of the Question - C. Cyanosis of the feet and hands

Acrocyanosis is cyanosis of the feet and hands. This is a typical 1 minute after birth finding. Acrocyanosis is characterized by a blueish coloring around the lips and extremities, with the rest of the body remaining pink. It's a harmless finding that occurs frequently in healthy babies in the first few days of life due to peripheral vasoconstriction. This is taken care of as part of standard newborn care. Pulse oximetry and screening for congenital heart disease are part of normal neonatal care (CHD).

ANSWER NUMBER 08.25

Solution of the Question - A. Supplemental oxygen

Heat, hydration, oxygen, and pain treatment are given to sickle cell crisis patients. Some people with sickle cell disease may benefit from the extra oxygen provided by oxygen treatment. However, because high amounts of oxygen are known to limit the development of new red blood cells, the use of oxygen treatment in sickle cell disease remains contentious. As a result, oxygen therapy is only indicated when oxygen levels fall below a critical level.

ANSWER NUMBER 08.26

Solution of the Question - A. Increasing fluid intake

The client should be taught to drink enough of fluids and not to void prior to the ultrasonography. Drink plenty of water and wait until after the scan to go to the bathroom - this may be required before a scan of the unborn baby or the pelvic area. The ultrasonography examination requires a full bladder. 90 minutes before the exam, empty the bladder, then drink one 8-ounce glass of liquids (water, milk, coffee, etc.) around an hour before the exam.

ANSWER NUMBER 08.27

Solution of the Question - D. 24 pounds

By the age of one year, the infant should have tripled his birth weight. Weight gain decreases a little between six months and a year. By the age of five to six months, most babies have doubled their birth weight, and by the age of a year, they have tripled it. A baby girl's average weight at one year is around 19 pounds 10 ounces (8.9 kg), whereas a boy's average weight is roughly 21 pounds 3 ounces (9.6 kg).

ANSWER NUMBER 08.28

Solution of the Question - B. Measures the activity of the fetus

A nonstress test is used to assess the fetus's periodic movement. The prenatal non-stress test, or NST, is a technique for assessing fetal well-being prior to the commencement of labor. As part or component of the biophysical profile, a prenatal non-stress test is used in overall antepartum surveillance with ultrasonography. The most important component of the non-stress test is the existence of fetal movements and fetal heart rate acceleration.

ANSWER NUMBER 08.29

Solution of the Question - D. The urethral meatus opens on the underside of the penis.

The urethral meatus is on the underside of the penis in hypospadias, a congenital anomaly in which the urethral meatus is on the underside of the penis. Hypospadias is a male external genital deformity that occurs at birth. It is defined by aberrant development of the urethral fold and the ventral foreskin of the penis, resulting in incorrect urethral opening location.

ANSWER NUMBER 08.30

Solution of the Question - A. Alteration in coping related to pain

Due to the intensity of the contractions, the client loses concentration throughout transition. Examine vaginal show, cervical dilatation, effacement, fetal station, and fetal descent for the nature and amount of vaginal show. In the nullipara, cervical dilation should be around 1.2 cm/hr, and in the multipara, 1.5 cm/hr; vaginal show increases with fetal descent. The degree of dilation and contractile pattern influence medication selection and timing.

ANSWER NUMBER 08.31

Solution of the Question - C. Antivirals

Chickenpox is Varicella. Antiviral medicines are used to treat the herpes virus. Adults tend to have a more severe infection, thus antiviral medicines (acyclovir or valacyclovir) are recommended if begun within 24 to 48 hours of rash onset. When given to children within 24 hours of the onset of the rash, acyclovir reduces symptoms by one day, but it has little effect on complication rates and is not indicated for people with normal immune function.

ANSWER NUMBER 08.32

Solution of the Question - B. Ampicillin

There is no reason to use an antibiotic like ampicillin. Penicillins were once quite successful against S. aureus; but, in the past, S. aureus was able to develop resistance to them by creating a penicillin hydrolyzing enzyme called penicillinase. Ampicillin was produced as a result of subsequent efforts to overcome this problem and extend the antibacterial coverage of penicillins. It's also acid-resistant, allowing it to be taken orally.

ANSWER NUMBER 08.33

Solution of the Question - B. Take prescribed anti-inflammatory medications with meals.

To avoid stomach distress, anti-inflammatory medications should be taken with meals. As soon as rheumatoid arthritis is diagnosed, disease-modifying anti-rheumatic medications (DMARDs) are started. Methotrexate, leflunomide, sulfasalazine, and hydroxychloroquine are examples of traditional or conventional DMARDs. TNF (tumor necrosis factor) DMARDs include Adalimumab, Etanercept, Infliximab, Golilumab, and Certolizumab. Tocilizumab (interleukin-6 inhibitor), Abatacept (inhibits T-cell costimulation), and Rituximab are non-TNF inhibitors (anti-B cell).

ANSWER NUMBER 08.34

Solution of the Question - D. Morphine 8 mg IM q 4 hours PRN pain

234

Morphine is not recommended for people who have gallbladder illness or pancreatitis since it causes Sphincter of Oddi spasms. Another key contraindication is GI blockage. Many people consider it a contraindication to give opioids to those who have a history of substance abuse, especially if the patient has abused opioids before.

ANSWER NUMBER 08.35

Solution of the Question - B. Hallucinogenic drugs induce a state of altered perception.

Hallucinations are a side effect of hallucinogenic substances. To prevent the client from injuring himself during withdrawal, the client must be monitored at all times. Adverse effects are very subjective, with a great deal of variation and unpredictability. One patient may report vivid hallucinations, images, and sensations, as well as greater awareness and euphoria as a result of mind expansion. A "good trip" is a term used to describe a favorable range of effects.

ANSWER NUMBER 08.36

Solution of the Question - C. Careful assessment of vital signs.

A vital sign examination is always the first nurse intervention for a patient who arrives in the ED in distress. This reveals the amount of the physical damage and serves as a starting point for future evaluation and treatment. During the initial anginal episode, check vital signs every 5 minutes. Because of sympathetic activation, blood pressure may rise at first, then decline if cardiac output is reduced. Tachycardia can also arise as a result of sympathetic stimulation, and it can be sustained as a compensatory reaction if cardiac output drops.

ANSWER NUMBER 08.37

Solution of the Question - C. The patient may discontinue the prescribed course of oral antibiotics once the symptoms have completely resolved.

It is crucial that patients who are being discharged from the hospital take their prescriptions exactly as prescribed. To avoid incomplete eradication of the organism and recurrence of infection, antibiotics must be used for the entire course, even if symptoms have subsided. Antibiotics should be taken exactly as prescribed. Just because you're feeling better doesn't mean you should stop taking your medicine. The customer must finish the entire course of antibiotics.

ANSWER NUMBER 08.38

Solution of the Question - C. If possible, keep the other bed in the room unassigned to provide privacy and comfort to the family.

It is most important for nursing staff to establish a culturally sensitive environment as much as feasible within the hospital routine while a family member is dying. It is important in Vietnamese culture for the dying to be surrounded by loved ones rather being left alone. Traditional foods and rituals are supposed to help people transition to the next life more easily. Allowing the family privacy for this traditional behavior whenever possible is excellent for them and the patient.

ANSWER NUMBER 08.39

Solution of the Question - A. A one-week postoperative coronary bypass patient, who is being evaluated for placement of a pacemaker prior to discharge.

When organizing assignments, the charge nurse must consider the talents of the staff as well as the needs of the patients. The labor and delivery nurse who isn't familiar with cardiac patients' needs should be assigned to those with the least urgent needs. A patient who is one week post-op and on the verge of release will almost certainly require routine care.

ANSWER NUMBER 08.40

Solution of the Question - B. Glucagon treats hypoglycemia resulting from insulin overdose.

Insulin overdose in an unresponsive patient is treated with glucagon. Patients with low levels of consciousness cannot safely absorb the oral carbohydrates required to elevate blood sugar without risking aspiration, and gaining IV access in the diabetic population can be difficult, preventing prompt IV glucose administration.

ANSWER NUMBER 08.41

Solution of the Question - A. Sudden weight gain

The accumulation of fluid causes weight gain, which is an early indication of congestive heart failure. Renal fluid retention, renin-angiotensin-mediated vasoconstriction, and sympathetic overactivity are all important. Excessive fluid retention raises cardiac output by raising end diastolic volume (preload), but it also causes pulmonary and systemic congestion symptoms.

ANSWER NUMBER 08.42

Solution of the Question - B. 4 mcg/mL

Dilantin has a therapeutic serum level of 10–20 mcg/mL. A level of 4 mcg/mL is considered subtherapeutic and could be due to patient noncompliance or accelerated medication metabolism. To guarantee that phenytoin dosages are delivered at therapeutic levels, therapeutic drug monitoring is required.

ANSWER NUMBER 08.43

Solution of the Question - D. Hepatic damage

Even modestly high dosages of acetaminophen can induce substantial liver damage, which can lead to death. Immediate examination of liver function is recommended, with N-acetylcysteine delivery as an antidote being considered. Acetaminophen is rapidly absorbed from the GI system, reaching therapeutic levels in 30 minutes to 2 hours. Unless there are additional circumstances that could delay stomach emptying, such as a co-ingestion of a gastric motility-slowing drug or if the acetaminophen is in an extended-release form, overdose levels peak at 4 hours.

ANSWER NUMBER 08.44

Solution of the Question - B. Monitor respiratory rate

Morphine sulfate inhibits breathing and respiratory reflexes like coughing. To avoid respiratory compromise, patients should be checked for these effects on a frequent basis. Respiratory depression is one of the more dangerous side effects of opiate usage, and it's especially crucial to keep an eye on in postoperative patients.

ANSWER NUMBER 08.45

Solution of the Question - C. X-ray the leg.

An x-ray should be taken after triage to rule out fractures. Follow-up and serial X-rays should be reviewed. Determines the amount of activity and the need for modifications in or further therapy by providing visual proof of appropriate alignment or the start of callus formation and healing.

ANSWER NUMBER 08.46

Solution of the Question - C. A patient with a history of ventricular tachycardia and syncopal episodes.

To stop ventricular tachycardia and ventricular fibrillation, an automated internal cardioverter-defibrillator provides an electric shock to the heart. In a patient with substantial ventricular symptoms, such as tachycardia resulting in syncope, this is required. Secondary indications are when a patient has already experienced and survived cardiac arrest owing to ventricular fibrillation/ventricular tachycardia, or main indications are when a patient is at high risk of sudden cardiac death due to VF/VT but has never experienced one.

ANSWER NUMBER 08.47

Solution of the Question - B. The patient has a pacemaker.

The implanted pacemaker will interfere with the MRI scanner's magnetic fields and may be disabled as a result. MRI scanners' powerful static magnetic fields (B0) can attract and accelerate ferromagnetic objects into the machine's core, turning them into deadly missiles. This magnetic field has the potential to dislodge implants and interfere with the operation of devices like pacemakers and pumps.

ANSWER NUMBER 08.48

Solution of the Question - B. The patient suddenly complains of chest pain and shortness of breath.

Chest pain, shortness of breath, and extreme anxiety are common pulmonary embolism symptoms. The doctor should be notified right away. A thrombus that originates elsewhere disrupts the flow of blood in the pulmonary artery or its branches, resulting in pulmonary embolism (PE). The most common symptom is chest pain, which is caused by pleural irritation produced by distant emboli producing pulmonary infarction. Chest pain in central PE can be caused by underlying right ventricular (RV) ischemia, which must be distinguished from an acute coronary syndrome or an aortic dissection.

ANSWER NUMBER 08.49

Solution of the Question - C. The patient will be admitted to the surgical unit and resection will be scheduled.

An abdominal aortic aneurysm that is quickly expanding poses a substantial risk of rupture and should be removed as soon as possible. AAA is a life-threatening disorder that necessitates monitoring or treatment, depending on the size of the aneurysm and/or symptomatology. AAA might be discovered by chance or through a rupture. An arterial aneurysm is defined as a permanent localized dilation of the vessel of at least 150 percent as compared to the neighboring artery's relative normal diameter.

ANSWER NUMBER 08.50

Solution of the Question - D. Check for signs of bleeding, including examination of urine and stool for blood.

A platelet count of 25,000/microliter indicates severe thrombocytopenia and should urge the use of bleeding measures, such as checking urine and stool for signs of bleeding. Platelet count, prothrombin time/international normalized ratio (PT/INR), activated partial thromboplastin time (aPTT), fibrinogen, bleeding time, fibrin breakdown products, vitamin K, activated coagulation time (ACT).

ANSWER NUMBER 08.51

Solution of the Question - C. We will bring in fresh flowers to brighten the room.

During induction chemotherapy, the leukemia patient's immune system is significantly damaged, putting him or her at danger of infection. Microbes can be carried by fresh flowers, fruit, and plants, so they should be avoided. Before and after each care activity, teach correct hand washing with antibacterial soap. Cross-contamination is reduced through hand washing and hand hygiene. Note: Methicillin-resistant Staphylococcus aureus (MRSA) is most typically spread by direct contact with health-care workers who are unable to wash their hands between client interactions.

ANSWER NUMBER 08.52

Solution of the Question - A. 3-10 years

At the age of four, the incidence of ALL reaches its peak (range 3-10). After the mid-teen years, it is infrequent. Every year, roughly 4000 persons in the United States are diagnosed with it, the majority of them are under the age of 18. It is the most frequent type of childhood cancer. Between the ages of two and ten, children are most likely to be diagnosed.

ANSWER NUMBER 08.53

Solution of the Question - B. Night sweats and fatigue

Night sweats, tiredness, weakness, and tachycardia are all symptoms of Hodgkin's disease. Hodgkin lymphoma (HL) is an uncommon monoclonal lymphoid tumor with a high cure rate. It was previously known as Hodgkin's disease. This disease category has been separated into two distinct categories based on biological and clinical studies: classical Hodgkin lymphoma and nodular lymphocyte-predominant Hodgkin lymphoma (NLP-HL).

ANSWER NUMBER 08.54

Solution of the Question - A. Reed-Sternberg cells

If Reed-Sternberg cells are detected on pathologic inspection of the removed lymph node, a conclusive diagnosis of Hodgkin's disease is made. Hodgkin lymphomas are distinguished by four characteristics. They most commonly develop in the cervical lymph nodes; the disease is more common in young adults; there are scattered large mononuclear Hodgkin and multinucleated cells (Reed-Sternberg) intermixed in a background of non-neoplastic inflammatory cells; and, finally, T lymphocytes are frequently seen surrounding the characteristic neoplastic cells.

ANSWER NUMBER 08.55

Solution of the Question - C. Stay with the patient and focus on slow, deep breathing for relaxation.

The most effective way to reduce anxiety and tension is to breathe slowly and deeply. It increases calm and relaxation by lowering carbon dioxide levels in the brain. During panic attacks, stay with the sufferer. Use concise, straightforward instructions. Encourage the client to do relaxation methods such deep breathing, progressive muscular relaxation, guided visualization, and meditation.

ANSWER NUMBER 08.56

Solution of the Question - C. Bowel control is usually achieved before bladder control, and the average age for completion of toilet training varies widely from 24 to 36 months.

Bowel control is often learned before bladder control in toddlers, with boys requiring longer to complete toilet training than girls. The readiness of a youngster to begin toilet training varies. Starting before the age of two (24 months) is not recommended. Between the ages of 18 months and 2.5 years, a child's readiness skills and physical growth are required.

ANSWER NUMBER 08.57

Solution of the Question - C. Give only a bottle of water at bedtime.

Due to the risk of dental decay, babies and toddlers should not fall asleep with bottles containing liquid other than simple water. Wean one ounce at a time over the course of a night. Assume the youngster drinks three 4 oz bottles every night. On night one, take the last bottle and lower it by an ounce. Reduce bottle 2 by 1 oz. on night 2. Reduce Bottle #1 by 1 oz. on night 3. Substitute a bottle of water when a bottle is down to 2 oz. Remove the bottle after this step. If the infant sleeps through a feeding, don't wake them up–this is the purpose.

ANSWER NUMBER 08.58

Solution of the Question - B. Allow the infant to cry for 5 minutes before responding if she wakes during the night as she may fall back asleep.

Infants under the age of six months may find it difficult to sleep for lengthy periods of time because their stomachs are too small to retain enough food to get them through the night. Allowing babies to put themselves back to sleep after awakening during the night may be beneficial after 6 months, but not before 6 months. Most newborns are biologically capable of sleeping through the night by 6 months of age and do not require nocturnal feedings. However, 25 percent to 50 percent of people wake up in the middle of the night. When it comes to nighttime waking, the most important thing to remember is that all babies wake up four to six times during the night. Self-soothers (babies who can soothe themselves back to sleep) awaken momentarily and then go back to sleep.

ANSWER NUMBER 08.59

Solution of the Question - A, B, and C

If the patient is comfortable and the bowels move regularly, a daily bowel movement is not required. Moderate exercise, such as walking, and plenty of water are both beneficial to gut health. A high-fiber diet is also beneficial. Examine your regular elimination pattern, including stool frequency and consistency. It's critical to understand what's "normal" for each patient. Stool transit might occur anywhere from twice everyday to once every third or fourth day. Constipation is often characterized by dry and firm stools.

ANSWER NUMBER 08.60

Solution of the Question - C. A negative antistreptolysin O titer.

An untreated group A B hemolytic Streptococcus infection in the previous 2-6 weeks causes rheumatic fever, which is validated by a positive antistreptolysin O titer. Streptococcal antibodies directed against streptococcal lysin O are detected using the ASO test. A high titer indicates that you have had a past streptococcal infection. It is frequently higher after a pharyngeal infection than after a cutaneous infection, but the ADB is usually higher regardless of the infection site.

ANSWER NUMBER 08.61

Solution of the Question - D. Check blood pressure.

Pulmonary edema, which can induce severe hypertension, can develop in a patient with congestive heart failure and dyspnea. As a result, the initial step should be to take the patient's blood pressure. Keep an eye on your blood pressure and central venous pressure (CVP). Hypertension and an increased CVP indicate an excess of fluid in the body and may indicate the onset of pulmonary congestion, or HF.

ANSWER NUMBER 08.62

Solution of the Question - C. "Headaches are a frequent side effect of nitroglycerine because it causes vasodilation."

Nitroglycerin is a powerful vasodilator that frequently causes side effects such headaches, dizziness, and hypotension. Headaches can be intense, throbbing, and long-lasting, and they can happen right after you use it. Many of these side effects are caused by nitroglycerin's hypotensive effects. Patients may experience dizziness, weakness, palpitations, and vertigo as a result of orthostatic hypotension. Patients with preload-dependent diseases may experience severe hypotension.

ANSWER NUMBER 08.63

Solution of the Question - A. The symptoms may be the result of anemia caused by chemotherapy.

The patient is likely to be experiencing side effects three months following surgery and chemotherapy, which commonly include anemia due to bone marrow suppression. Cancer chemotherapy might have short-term or long-term adverse effects, therefore it's important to keep track of them. It would necessitate multidisciplinary monitoring since certain patient groups may be more susceptible to problems. Exercise, better sleep quality, and behavioral therapy like relaxation can all help with weariness.

ANSWER NUMBER 08.64

Solution of the Question - C. The patient should use iron cookware to prepare foods, such as dark green, leafy vegetables and legumes, which are high in iron.

Hemoglobin levels in the normal range are 11.5-15.0. This vegetarian patient has a slight anemia problem. The iron content of food is raised when it is cooked in iron cookware. Anemia is defined as hemoglobin levels that are less than two standard deviations below the mean for the patient's age and gender. The molecule of hemoglobin requires iron to function properly. Iron deficiency is the most prevalent cause of anemia worldwide, resulting in microcytic and hypochromic red cells on the peripheral smear.

ANSWER NUMBER 08.65

Solution of the Question - D. A nurse should remain in the room during the first 15 minutes of infusion.

The first 15 minutes of infusion are when a transfusion reaction is most likely to occur, and a nurse should be present at this time. The nurse stays with the client for up to 5 minutes, assessing signs and symptoms and monitoring vital signs. To double-check blood product and patient identity prior to transfusion, meticulous patient identification verification begins with type and crossmatch sample collection and labeling.

ANSWER NUMBER 08.66

Solution of the Question - C. A patient with abdominal and chest pain following a large, spicy meal.

Emergency triage entails a fast assessment of the patient to determine which patients require additional evaluation and care. Trauma, chest pain, respiratory distress, and abrupt neurological abnormalities are always prioritized. While the patient with chest pain in the question may have recently eaten a spicy meal and be experiencing heartburn, he could also be suffering from an acute myocardial infarction and require immediate medical attention.

ANSWER NUMBER 08.67

Solution of the Question - C. Hypoactive bowel sounds

Calcium levels in the blood should be between 8.5 and 10 mg/dL. The patient is deficient in calcium. Hypocalcemia is indicated by increased stomach motility, which results in hyperactive (not hypoactive) bowel noises, abdominal discomfort, and diarrhea. When the total serum calcium concentration is less than 8.8 mg/dl, hypocalcemia is present. The illness can be acquired or inherited, and it can manifest in a variety of ways, ranging from asymptomatic to life-threatening. Hypocalcemia is a common occurrence in hospitalized patients, and it is usually minor in character, requiring only supportive care.

ANSWER NUMBER 08.68

Solution of the Question - A. pH 7.52, PCO2 54 mmHg.

The loss of hydrochloric acid in stomach fluid puts a patient on nasogastric suction at danger of metabolic alkalosis. Only response A (pH 7.52, PCO2 54 mm Hg) represents alkalosis among the options. pH levels should be between 7.35-7.45. The usual range for CO2 levels is 35 to 45 mmHg. HCO3 levels should be between 22 and 26 mmol/L. The patient is more acidotic if the value is lower. The more base in the blood sample, the higher the pH.

ANSWER NUMBER 08.69

Solution of the Question - A. Draw a blood sample for prothrombin (PT) and international normalized ratio (INR) level.

Coumadin works by preventing blood from clotting. The next step is to establish the patient's anticoagulation status and bleeding risk by checking the PT and INR. Patients who are taking warfarin should be closely monitored to ensure the medication's safety and efficacy. Periodic blood testing is advised to determine the patient's prothrombin time (PT) and international normalized ratio (INR).

ANSWER NUMBER 08.70

Solution of the Question - A and B

Option A: A complete blood count (CBC) includes the measurement of hemoglobin levels in the blood. Hemoglobin concentrations in men range from 13.5-18.0 grams per deciliter, whereas women's concentrations range from 11.5-16.0 grams per deciliter. The mean corpuscular volume of erythrocytes is also measured by CBC (MCV).

Option B: Levels of total cholesterol of less than 200 mg/dL are deemed normal. Serum is used to determine cholesterol levels. A non-fasting lipid test can be performed at any time without the need to fast; a fasting lipid test necessitates a 12-hour fast with the exception of water. Serum is used to determine total and HDL cholesterol levels.

ANSWER NUMBER 08.71

Solution of the Question - C. Nonsteroidal anti-inflammatory drugs are the first choice in treatment.

For juvenile idiopathic arthritis, nonsteroidal anti-inflammatory medications (NSAIDs) are an important first-line treatment (formerly known as juvenile rheumatoid arthritis). The therapeutic anti-inflammatory benefits of NSAIDs take 3-4 weeks to manifest. For all subtypes, nonsteroidal anti-inflammatory medications (NSAIDs) are the backbone of initial symptomatic treatment. With current aggressive treatment, such as methotrexate and biologics, the usage of NSAIDs in JIA has reduced over time.

ANSWER NUMBER 08.72

Solution of the Question - B. A blood culture is drawn.

Because antibiotics may interfere with the identification of the causal organism, they must be started after the blood culture is drawn. The cornerstone of osteomyelitis treatment is long-term antibiotic therapy. If possible, the results of culture and sensitivity should guide antibiotic treatment, but in the absence of this information, empiric antibiotics should be started.

ANSWER NUMBER 08.73

ANSWER NUMBER 08.74

Solution of the Question - A, B and D.

Cerebral palsy is characterized by delayed developmental milestones, hence regular assessment and treatments are critical. Children may experience ocular and speech difficulties as a result of upper motor neuron injury. Parent support groups assist families in sharing and coping with their problems.

Option A: Encourage age-appropriate play and other activities that support gross and fine motor development, sensory development, and cognitive development, such as allowing the child to place green balls in the left basket and red balls in the right basket. These activities promote a child's growth and development while also providing stimulation.

Option B: Become familiar with the demands of the patient and pay attention to nonverbal cues. The nurse should schedule enough time to attend to all of the patient's needs. In the case of a communication deficit, care measures may take longer to complete. Provide a another mode of communication. If speech is problematic, the client can express themselves via alternative formats such as flash cards, whiteboards, hand signs, or a picture board.

Option D: Encourage the parent to share how their child's illness has affected their family. Evaluate the family's ability to cope. This will establish how much help and direction the family will require. Educate the family on the various skills required to manage the child's care (for example, physical rehabilitation and adequate nutrition).

ANSWER NUMBER 08.75

Solution of the Question - A. Duchenne's is an X-linked recessive disorder, so daughters have a 50% chance of being carriers and sons a 50% chance of developing the disease.

The recessive Duchenne gene is found on one of a female carrier's two X chromosomes. DMD is caused by a mutation in the dystrophin gene, which is found on chromosome Xp21. It is inherited as an X-linked recessive condition; however, new mutations account for about 30% of cases. Female carriers do not display signs of muscle weakness, but symptomatic female carriers have been reported. Female carriers in the range of 2.5 percent to 20% may be impacted. The Lyon hypothesis states that the normal X chromosome becomes inactive, allowing the X chromosome with the mutation to express.

Answer - Set 9

ANSWER NUMBER 09.01

Solution of the Question - A, B, & C.

The skilled nursing assistant would know how to adjust the patient and reapply compression boots, as well as remind the patient to complete the actions he was taught.

ANSWER NUMBER 09.02

Solution of the Question - A. Position the patient sitting up in bed before you feed her.

Aspiration is less likely when the patient is in a seated position.

ANSWER NUMBER 09.03

Solution of the Question - B. Infuse ceftriaxone (Rocephin) 2000 mg IV to treat the infection.

Because untreated bacterial meningitis has a near-100 percent fatality rate, prompt antibiotic treatment is critical.

ANSWER NUMBER 09.04

Solution of the Question - A. The student enters the room without putting on a mask and gown.

Because meningococcal meningitis is transferred by contact with respiratory secretions, wearing a mask and gown is needed to prevent the infection from spreading to other patients or staff members. Other acts may or may not be appropriate, but they might not necessitate immediate involvement.

ANSWER NUMBER 09.05

Solution of the Question - B & E

LPN curriculum and scope of practice include the administration of non-high-risk drugs. An LPN/LVN who observes the initial seizure activity can collect data regarding the seizure activity. If a patient begins to seize, an LPN/LVN would immediately contact the supervising RN.

ANSWER NUMBER 09.06

Solution of the Question - C. Turn the patient to the side and protect the airway.

Protecting the airway is the most important thing to do during a generalized tonic-clonic seizure.

ANSWER NUMBER 09.07

Solution of the Question - B. The white blood cell count is 2300/mm3.

Phenytoin has a dangerous side effect called leukopenia, which necessitates stopping the medicine.

ANSWER NUMBER 09.08

Solution of the Question - D. A 63-year-old with multiple sclerosis who has an oral temperature of 101.80 F and flank pain.

Because of the influence on bladder function, urinary tract infections are a common consequence in patients with multiple sclerosis. This patient's raised temperature and reduced breath sounds point to pyelonephritis. The doctor should be notified right away so that antibiotic medication can begin right once.

ANSWER NUMBER 09.09

Solution of the Question - A, C, and E

Taking pulse and blood pressure measures is part of NA's education and scope of practice. NAs can also reinforce past training or skills provided by the RN or other disciplines, such as speech or physical therapy.

ANSWER NUMBER 09.10

Solution of the Question - A. Check for improvement in resident memory after medication therapy is initiated.

Checking for therapeutic and harmful effects of drugs is part of LPN education and team leader responsibilities. Changes in the residents' memory would be reported to the RN supervisor, who is in charge of managing each resident's care plan.

ANSWER NUMBER 09.11

Solution of the Question - B. Caregiver Role Strain related to continuous need for providing care

The husband's comments about not getting enough sleep and being concerned about whether the patient is getting the right drugs back up this diagnosis.

ANSWER NUMBER 09.12

Solution of the Question - A. The patient does not recognize family members.

This patient's inability to recognize a family member is a new neurologic deficiency, indicating an increase in intracranial pressure (ICP). This change should be immediately notified to the physician so that treatment can begin.

ANSWER NUMBER 09.13

Solution of the Question - B. Transfer to radiology for a CT scan.

According to the patient's history and assessment results, he may have a chronic subdural hematoma. The most important goal is to get a quick diagnosis and get the patient to surgery so the hematoma may be removed.

ANSWER NUMBER 09.14

Solution of the Question - C. A 46-year-old patient who was admitted 48 hours ago with bacterial meningitis and has an antibiotic dose due.

Of the patients listed, this one is the most stable. The administration of IV antibiotics would be familiar to an RN from the medical unit.

ANSWER NUMBER 09.15

Solution of the Question - A. Acute pain related to biologic and chemical factors

Pain management is the top priority for interdisciplinary care for patients with migraine headaches.

ANSWER NUMBER 09.16

Solution of the Question - C. Loose, bloody

Normal bowel function and soft-formed feces do not often appear until the seventh day after surgery. The amount of water absorbed is proportional to the consistency of the feces.

ANSWER NUMBER 09.17

Solution of the Question - A. On the client's right side

The client is visually impaired on the left side. Only the right side of the client will be visible. Homonymous hemianopsia is a condition in which a person can only perceive one side of the visual world of each eye, either right or left. It's possible that the person is unaware that the visual loss affects both eyes, not just one. The left side of each eye's visual world is lost when the right side of the brain is injured.

ANSWER NUMBER 09.18

Solution of the Question - C. Check respirations, stabilize the spine and check the circulation

The priority would be to check the airway, and a neck injury should be suspected. Normal oxygenation and ventilation within the body, as well as enough respiratory effort, are both required for normal physiological processes to operate without metabolic disruption.

ANSWER NUMBER 09.19

Solution of the Question - D. Decreasing venous return through vasodilation.

Because nitroglycerin causes vasodilation and reduces venous return, the heart does not have to work as hard.

ANSWER NUMBER 09.20

Solution of the Question - A. Call for help and note the time.

The nurse should contact for assistance as soon as possible after determining that the client is unconscious rather than sleeping. This can be done by phoning the operator from the client's phone and telling the operator the hospital code for cardiac arrest and the client's room number, or by pressing the emergency call button if the phone is not available. It's crucial to keep track of the time throughout a cardiac arrest operation.

ANSWER NUMBER 09.21

Solution of the Question - C. Make sure that the client takes food and medications at prescribed intervals.

Food and pharmacological therapy can either avoid the accumulation of hydrochloric acid or neutralize and buffer it if it happens.

ANSWER NUMBER 09.22

Solution of the Question - B. Continue treatment as ordered.

The PTT is used to monitor the effects of heparin; the therapeutic level is 1.5 to 2 times that of the normal level.

ANSWER NUMBER 09.23

Solution of the Question - B. In the operating room

In the operation room, the stoma drainage bag is used. Ileostomy drainage comprises digestive enzyme-rich discharges that are particularly irritating to the skin. The skin is immediately protected from the impacts of these enzymes. Even if just for a brief period, skin exposed to these enzymes becomes reddish, irritated, and excoriated.

ANSWER NUMBER 09.24

Solution of the Question - B. Flat on back

The client is kept in a flat supine posture for approximately 4 to 12 hours postoperatively to minimize the complication of a painful spinal headache that can linger for several days. The seepage of CSF fluid from the puncture site is thought to be the source of headaches. The pressures in the cerebral spinal fluid are equalized by maintaining the client flat, which prevents damage to the neurons.

ANSWER NUMBER 09.25

Solution of the Question - C. The client is oriented when aroused from sleep and goes back to sleep immediately.

This research shows that people's consciousness is dwindling.

ANSWER NUMBER 09.26

Solution of the Question - A. Altered mental status and dehydration

Due to a weakened immune response, elderly clients may initially present with simply altered mental status and dehydration.

ANSWER NUMBER 09.27

Solution of the Question - B. Chills, fever, night sweats, and hemoptysis

Chills, fever, nocturnal sweats, and hemoptysis are common signs and symptoms.

ANSWER NUMBER 09.28

Solution of the Question - A. Acute asthma

Acute asthma is the most likely diagnosis based on the client's history and symptoms.

ANSWER NUMBER 09.29

Solution of the Question - B. Respiratory arrest

If taken in large quantities, narcotics can cause respiratory arrest.

ANSWER NUMBER 09.30

Solution of the Question - D. Decreased vital capacity

A typical physiologic alteration that includes decreased elastic rebound of the lungs, fewer functioning capillaries in the alveoli, and a rise in residual volume is vital capacity reduction.

ANSWER NUMBER 09.31

Solution of the Question - C. Presence of premature ventricular contractions (PVCs) on a cardiac monitor.

Lidocaine infusions are often used to treat patients with arrhythmias that have not responded to oral medicine and who have PVCs evident on a cardiac monitor.

ANSWER NUMBER 09.32

Solution of the Question - B. Avoid foods high in vitamin K.

Vitamin K can interact with anticoagulation, hence the client should avoid ingesting significant doses of the vitamin.

ANSWER NUMBER 09.33

Solution of the Question - C. Clipping the hair in the area.

Hair can be an infection cause and should be clipped away.

ANSWER NUMBER 09.34

Solution of the Question - A. Bone fracture

A prominent complication of osteoporosis is bone fracture, which occurs when the loss of calcium and phosphate causes the bones to become more fragile.

ANSWER NUMBER 09.35

Solution of the Question - C. Changes from previous examinations.

Women are told to inspect themselves to see if there have been any changes in their breasts.

ANSWER NUMBER 09.36

Solution of the Question - C. Balance the client's periods of activity and rest.

A hyperthyroid client should be urged to alternate times of exercise and rest. Many hyperthyroid patients are hyperactive and complain of being overheated.

ANSWER NUMBER 09.37

Solution of the Question - B. Increase his activity level.

The client should be encouraged to improve his degree of physical exercise.

ANSWER NUMBER 09.38

Solution of the Question - A. Laminectomy

When rotating a client who has had spinal surgery, such as a laminectomy, the spinal column must be log rolled to keep it straight.

ANSWER NUMBER 09.39

Solution of the Question - D. Avoiding straining during bowel movement or bending at the waist.

Because these actions increase intraocular pressure, the client should avoid straining, carrying large things, and coughing violently.

ANSWER NUMBER 09.40

Solution of the Question - D. Before age 20.

Men between the ages of 20 and 30 are more likely to get testicular cancer. Before the age of 20, a male client should be taught how to undertake testicular self-examination, preferably when he is in his teens.

ANSWER NUMBER 09.41

Solution of the Question - B. Place a saline-soaked sterile dressing on the wound.

To prevent tissue drying and infection, the nurse should apply saline-soaked sterile cloths to the exposed wound first.

ANSWER NUMBER 09.42

Solution of the Question - A. Progressively deeper breaths followed by shallower breaths with apneic periods.

Cheyne-Stokes breathing is characterized by deeper breaths followed by shallower breaths during apneic periods.

ANSWER NUMBER 09.43

Solution of the Question - B. Fine crackles

Fluid in the alveoli causes fine crackles, which are typical in patients with heart failure.

ANSWER NUMBER 09.44

Solution of the Question - B. The airways are so swollen that no air cannot get through.

Because the airways are so enlarged that air can't get through during an acute episode, wheezing may stop and breath sounds become inaudible.

ANSWER NUMBER 09.45

Solution of the Question - D. Place the client on his side, remove dangerous objects, and protect his head.

Place the client on his side, remove harmful objects, and protect his head from injury while he is having an active seizure.

ANSWER NUMBER 09.46

Solution of the Question - B. Kinked or obstructed chest tube

A common cause of a tension pneumothorax is kinking and obstruction of the chest tube.

ANSWER NUMBER 09.47

Solution of the Question - D. Stay with him but not intervene at this time.

If the client coughs, he should be able to dislodge or completely obstruct the object. If the client is standing and a total obstruction occurs, the nurse should conduct the abdominal thrust maneuver.

ANSWER NUMBER 09.48

Solution of the Question - B. Current health promotion activities

Recognizing a person's favorable health indicators is quite beneficial.

ANSWER NUMBER 09.49

Solution of the Question - C. Place the client in a side-lying position, with the head of the bed lowered.

To avoid aspiration, the client should be placed in a side-lying position with the head of the bed lowered. To eliminate collected secretions, a small amount of toothpaste should be applied and the mouth swabbed or suctioned.

ANSWER NUMBER 09.50

Solution of the Question - C. Pneumonia

Pneumonia is characterized by a fever, a strong cough, and pleuritic chest pain.

ANSWER NUMBER 09.51

Solution of the Question - C. A 43-year-old homeless man with a history of alcoholism

Clients who are economically deprived, malnourished, and have a weakened immune system, such as those who have a history of drinking, are at an extraordinarily high risk of contracting tuberculosis.

ANSWER NUMBER 09.52

Solution of the Question - C. To determine the extent of lesions

The existence of lesions in the lungs will be visible on a chest X-ray if they are large enough.

ANSWER NUMBER 09.53

Solution of the Question - B. Bronchodilators

Because bronchoconstriction is the source of restricted airflow, bronchodilators are the primary line of treatment for asthma.

ANSWER NUMBER 09.54

Solution of the Question - C. Chronic obstructive bronchitis

The client is most likely suffering from chronic obstructive bronchitis as a result of his extensive smoking history and symptoms.

ANSWER NUMBER 09.55

Solution of the Question - A. The patient is under local anesthesia during the procedure

Antibiotics, cytotoxic medicines, and corticosteroids are given to the patient before the procedure to assist avoid infection and rejection of the transplanted cells. The patient is put under general anesthesia for the transplant.

ANSWER NUMBER 09.56

Solution of the Question - D. Raise the side rails

A bewildered patient is at risk of falling out of bed. The nurse's first step should be to raise the side rails to protect the patient's safety.

ANSWER NUMBER 09.57

Solution of the Question - A. Crowd red blood cells

Anemia is caused by the overproduction of white blood cells, which pushes out the production of red blood cells.

ANSWER NUMBER 09.58

Solution of the Question - B. Leukocytosis

Increased production of leukocytes and lymphocytes, resulting in leukocytosis, and proliferation of these cells inside the bone marrow, spleen, and liver characterize Chronic Lymphocytic Leukemia (CLL).

ANSWER NUMBER 09.59

Solution of the Question - A. Explain the risks of not having the surgery.

Explaining the risks of not having the procedure is the best first reaction.

ANSWER NUMBER 09.60

Solution of the Question - D. The 75-year-old client who was admitted 1 hour ago with new-onset atrial fibrillation and is receiving L.V. diltiazem (Cardizem).

The client with atrial fibrillation, who is on L.V. medication and must be closely monitored, has the greatest risk of becoming unstable.

ANSWER NUMBER 09.61

Solution of the Question - C. Cocaine

The nurse should query the client about her cocaine use because of her age and unfavorable medical history. Cocaine causes coronary artery spasm and increases myocardial oxygen consumption, resulting in tachycardia, ventricular fibrillation, myocardial ischemia, and myocardial infarction.

ANSWER NUMBER 09.62

Solution of the Question - B. Nonmobile mass with irregular edges

Breast cancer tumors are hard, fixed, and irregularly shaped with uneven borders.

ANSWER NUMBER 09.63

Solution of the Question - C. Radiation

External or intravaginal radiation therapy is the most common treatment for vaginal cancer.

ANSWER NUMBER 09.64

Solution of the Question - B. Carcinoma in situ, no abnormal regional lymph nodes, and no evidence of distant metastasis

TIS, N0, M0 means cancer in situ, no abnormal regional lymph nodes, and no distant metastases.

ANSWER NUMBER 09.65

Solution of the Question - D. "Keep the stoma moist."

Because a dry stoma might become irritated, the nurse should instruct the client to keep the stoma wet, such as by spreading a thin coating of petroleum jelly around the borders.

ANSWER NUMBER 09.66

Solution of the Question - B. Lung cancer

In both men and women, lung cancer is the most lethal type of cancer.

ANSWER NUMBER 09.67

Solution of the Question - A. Miosis, partial eyelid ptosis, and anhidrosis on the affected side of the face.

Horner's syndrome is characterized by miosis, partial eyelid ptosis, and anhidrosis on the affected side of the face when a lung tumor invades the ribs and affects the sympathetic nerve ganglia.

ANSWER NUMBER 09.68

Solution of the Question - A. Prostate-specific antigen, which is used to screen for prostate cancer.

Prostate-specific antigen (PSA) is a test that is used to detect prostate cancer.

ANSWER NUMBER 09.69

Solution of the Question - D. "Remain supine for the time specified by the physician."

The nurse should tell the client to lie down for the amount of time prescribed by the doctor.

ANSWER NUMBER 09.70

Solution of the Question - C. Sigmoidoscopy

Sigmoidoscopy and proctoscopy, which are used to visualize the lower GI tract, help detect two-thirds of all colorectal malignancies.

ANSWER NUMBER 09.71

Solution of the Question - B. A fixed nodular mass with dimpling of the overlying skin

During the late stages of breast cancer, a fixed nodular mass with dimpling of the underlying skin is prevalent.

ANSWER NUMBER 09.72

Solution of the Question - A. Liver

One of the five most prevalent cancer metastatic sites is the liver. The lymph nodes, lung, bone, and brain are the others.

ANSWER NUMBER 09.73

Solution of the Question - D. The client wears a watch and wedding band.

The client should not wear any metal things, such as jewelry, during an MRI since the powerful magnetic field can tug on them, causing damage to the client and bystanders (if they fly off).

ANSWER NUMBER 09.74

Solution of the Question - C. The recommended daily allowance of calcium may be found in a wide variety of foods.

Women in their premenopausal years need 1,000 mg of calcium every day. Women after menopause take 1,500 mg per day. It's usually possible to get the required daily need from foods, though it's not always the case.

ANSWER NUMBER 09.75

Solution of the Question - C. Joint flexion of less than 50%

Because of technical difficulties in inserting the instrument into the joint to examine it properly, arthroscopy is not recommended in patients with joint flexion of less than 50%. Skin and wound infections are other contraindications to this surgery.

Answer - Set 10

ANSWER NUMBER 10.01

Solution of the Question - B. Exertional Dyspnea

Mitral regurgitation (MR) is a condition in which blood flow from the left ventricle (LV) to the left atrium is abnormally reversed (LA). Exertional dyspnea is caused by weight gain due to fluid retention and increasing heart failure in patients with mitral regurgitation. The patient will typically experience severe dyspnea at rest, which is aggravated in the supine position, as well as a cough with clear or pink, frothy sputum.

ANSWER NUMBER 10.02

Solution of the Question - D. Right or left costovertebral angle

An irregular reversal of blood flow from the left ventricle (LV) to the left atrium (LA) is known as mitral regurgitation (MR) (LA). Exertional dyspnea occurs in patients with mitral regurgitation due to weight increase from fluid retention and increasing heart failure. The patient will usually have severe dyspnea at rest, which is aggravated in the supine position, as well as a cough with clear or pink, frothy sputum.

ANSWER NUMBER 10.03

Solution of the Question - A. Blood pressure

Blood pressure, which is an indirect representation of cardiac output, is the best way to evaluate perfusion. Uncontrolled high blood pressure can narrow, weaken, or stiffen the arteries surrounding the kidneys over time. These arteries are unable to carry enough blood to the renal tissue due to their impairment. Kidney arteries that have been damaged do not filter blood effectively. The blood is filtered by little, finger-like nephrons in the kidneys.

ANSWER NUMBER 10.04

Solution of the Question - C. Myoclonic seizure

A myoclonic seizure is defined by sudden, uncontrollable jerking movements of one or more muscle groups. Rapid, short, jerky, or shock-like movements involving a muscle or group of muscles are referred to as myoclonus. Myoclonus is the quickest and most brief of all the hyperkinetic movement disorders. Positive myoclonus is induced by a rapid muscle contraction, whereas "negative myoclonus" is caused by a transient reduction of muscular tone, as in asterixis.

ANSWER NUMBER 10.05

Solution of the Question - D. Nicotine (Nicotrol)

Nicotine (Nicotrol) is used to treat nicotine withdrawal syndrome in controlled and decreasing doses. Nicotine replacement treatment (NRT) is for people who want to quit smoking but don't want to go cold turkey because it can create withdrawal symptoms and cravings. Nicotine withdrawal happens when a person abruptly stops smoking cigarettes. Because the body still gets nicotine from another safer method, using NRT helps to reduce the motivation to smoke cigarettes.

ANSWER NUMBER 10.06

Solution of the Question - D. Episodic vasospastic disorder of the small arteries

Vasospasms of the tiny cutaneous arteries in the fingers and toes characterize Raynaud's illness. Blood flow is restricted in Raynaud's syndrome due to cold weather and emotional stress. There is vasoconstriction of the digital arteries and cutaneous arterioles in Raynaud syndrome.

ANSWER NUMBER 10.07

Solution of the Question - A. More accurate

Urine testing is an indirect indicator that can be influenced by kidney function, but blood glucose testing is a more direct and accurate indicator. The capillary blood glucose test is inferior to accurate blood glucose measurement. This, however, is contingent on the laboratory satisfying industry standards.

ANSWER NUMBER 10.08

Solution of the Question - C. 2.0 L

A liter of liquids weighs approximately 2.2 pounds. A weight decrease of 4.5 pounds is to 2 liters. Diuresis is required for a range of non-edematous and edematous disorders that necessitate the removal of excess water when the body improperly sequesters fluid in the third space as edema.

ANSWER NUMBER 10.09

Solution of the Question - A. Osmosis

Osmosis is the transfer of fluid from a low-solute-concentration area to a higher-solute-concentration area. Osmosis (Greek for "push") is the net passage of water across a semipermeable membrane in physiology. Water will tend to migrate from a high-concentration area to a low-concentration area over this membrane. It's vital to note that perfect osmosis simply requires pure water to pass through the membrane, with no solute particles passing through the semipermeable membrane.

ANSWER NUMBER 10.10

Solution of the Question - D. Forearm weakness

Crutch pressure on the axillae can induce radial nerve damage, which might manifest as forearm muscular weakness. Users of axilla crutches who rest their weight on the shoulder rest develop crutch palsy. The radial and ulnar nerves can be paralyzed due to strain on the brachial plexus. Crutch palsy can be avoided by providing more padding to the shoulder rest.

ANSWER NUMBER 10.11

Solution of the Question - B. Using suppositories or enemas

Clients who are neutropenic are susceptible to infection, particularly bacterial infections of the gastrointestinal and respiratory tract. An improperly administered enema can cause tissue injury in your rectum/colon, bowel perforation, and infections if the instrument is not sterile.

ANSWER NUMBER 10.12

Solution of the Question - C. Semi-fowlers position

The spilled stomach contents will be located in the lower region of the abdominal cavity in the semi-fowlers position. Fluid resuscitation should begin as soon as the diagnosis is confirmed. A nasogastric tube is inserted to decompress the stomach, and a Foley catheter is inserted to monitor urine output.

ANSWER NUMBER 10.13

Solution of the Question - C. Position client laterally with the neck extended

The airway is not obstructed when the client is positioned laterally with the neck extended, allowing for secretion drainage and oxygen and carbon dioxide exchange. During respiratory distress, this position promotes oxygenation by allowing for maximum chest expansion. Allowing the client to slip down causes the abdomen to pressure the diaphragm, perhaps causing respiratory problems.

ANSWER NUMBER 10.14

Solution of the Question - B. Check the system for air leaks

Excessive bubbling signals an air leak that must be repaired in order for the lungs to expand. By clamping the thoracic catheter just distal to the outflow from the chest, you can determine the position of the air leak (patient- or system-centered). When the catheter is constricted at the insertion site and the bubbling stops, the leak is patient-centered (at insertion site or within the patient).

ANSWER NUMBER 10.15

Solution of the Question - C. I can eat shredded wheat cereal

Wheat cereal contains a modest amount of sodium. Sodium regulates fluid balance in the body and keeps blood volume and pressure in check. Too much sodium in the diet can elevate blood pressure and promote fluid retention, which can lead to leg and foot edema and other health problems.

ANSWER NUMBER 10.16

Solution of the Question - A. Pressure in the portal vein

Cirrhotic liver enlargement impinges on the portal system, resulting in increased hydrostatic pressure and ascites. Vasodilation occurs when portal pressure rises above a crucial threshold and circulating nitric oxide levels rise. The plasma levels of vasoconstrictor sodium-retentive hormones rise when the state of vasodilation worsens, renal function degrades, and ascitic fluid develops, leading in hepatic decompensation.

ANSWER NUMBER 10.17

Solution of the Question - C. Airway

The priority is to check for an open airway. The anesthetic may have altered the swallowing reflex, or the inflammation may have closed up on the airway, resulting in poor air exchange. The throat may feel itchy for several days after the numbness wears off. In 1 to 2 hours after the test, the cough reflex will recover. After that, the client is free to eat and drink as usual.

ANSWER NUMBER 10.18

Solution of the Question - A. Systolic blood pressure less than 90 mm Hg

A systolic blood pressure of less than 90 mm Hg is one of the most common indications and symptoms of hypovolemic shock. In hypovolemic shock, the initial changes in vital signs are an increase in diastolic blood pressure and a narrower pulse pressure. Systolic blood pressure decreases when volume status decreases. As a result, oxygen transport to important organs can no longer keep up with demand.

ANSWER NUMBER 10.19

Solution of the Question - D. Aspirin-containing medications should not be taken 14 days before surgery

To reduce the risk of bleeding, aspirin-containing drugs should not be used 14 days before to surgery. Impaired coagulation might lead to difficulties after surgery. Patients should be questioned about a history of excessive bruising or bleeding, the use of coagulation-altering medicines, supplements, or vitamins, and a history of previous thrombotic episodes. Preoperatively, any medicine, vitamin, or supplement that affects coagulation may need to be stopped.

ANSWER NUMBER 10.20

Solution of the Question - A. Regular insulin

Anaerobic metabolism is caused by the body's inability to utilise circulating glucose, resulting in metabolic acidosis. Insulin administration corrects the issue. The discovery of insulin, together with antibiotics, has resulted in a 90% reduction in DKA mortality, down to 1%. The standard of therapy is continuous intravenous insulin infusion. The administration of a 0.1 U/kg bolus followed by a 0.1 U/kg/h infusion has been advised in previous treatment protocols.

ANSWER NUMBER 10.21

Solution of the Question - D. Spinach and mangoes

Antioxidants such as beta-carotene and vitamin E aid to prevent oxidation. Wheat germ, corn, almonds, seeds, olives, spinach, asparagus, and other green leafy vegetables are all high in vitamin E. Dark green vegetables, carrots, mangoes, and tomatoes are all good sources of beta-carotene.

ANSWER NUMBER 10.22

Solution of the Question - A. Rest in a sitting position

Gravity aids digestion by preventing stomach contents from refluxing into the esophagus. Instruct students to stay upright for at least 2 hours after meals and to avoid eating three hours before bedtime. Helps to regulate reflux and reduces esophageal discomfort caused by reflux.

ANSWER NUMBER 10.23

Solution of the Question - B. Abdominal distention

Abdominal distension that is accompanied by pain could be a sign of perforation, a complication that could result in peritonitis. Perforation of the bowel occurs in less than 0.3 percent of cases, and infection is uncommon. Complications are usually discovered within the first 24 hours of the operation. Fever, tachycardia, stomach pain, or discomfort are all signs of perforation.

ANSWER NUMBER 10.24

Solution of the Question - D. "Most people can tolerate regular diet after this type of surgery"

Although it may take 4 to 6 months to consume anything, most people are able to eat everything they want. To avoid nausea, vomiting, and constipation following surgery, start with clear drinks (soup, Jell-O, juices, popsicles, and carbonated beverages.) After that, transition to a regular low-fat diet. Instead of fewer larger meals, eat smaller meals more frequently.

ANSWER NUMBER 10.25

Solution of the Question - D. Clay-colored stools

Hepatic blockage is indicated by clay-colored feces. Nausea, vomiting, right upper quadrant stomach discomfort, malaise, anorexia, myalgia, lethargy, and fever are common symptoms of an acute HAV infection. Within a week, patients may experience dark urine and pale feces, as well as jaundice, icteric (yellow-tinged) sclera, and pruritus.

ANSWER NUMBER 10.26

Solution of the Question - D. Streptomycin

Streptomycin is an aminoglycoside, and aminoglycosides frequently cause damage to the eighth cranial nerve (ototoxicity). Streptomycin toxicity is typically assumed to be characterized by ototoxicity and vestibular dysfunction. Ototoxicity can result in deafness in extreme circumstances, thus use caution when taking streptomycin with other potentially ototoxic medications. Vestibular damage commonly develops during treatment and is usually irreversible.

ANSWER NUMBER 10.27

Solution of the Question - D. Helicobacter pylori infection

Helicobacter pylori, a gram-negative bacteria, is the most common cause of peptic ulcers. H. pylorus is a gram-negative bacillus that lives in the epithelial cells of the stomach. 90 percent of duodenal ulcers and 70 percent to 90 percent of stomach ulcers are caused by this bacterium. H. pylori infection is more common in persons with a lower socioeconomic status, and it is often acquired as a child. The bacterium contains a wide range of virulence characteristics that allow it to cling to the stomach mucosa and inflame it. Hypochlorhydria or achlorhydria develops as a result, resulting in stomach ulcers.

ANSWER NUMBER 10.28

Solution of the Question - D. Dark brown

Gastric drainage is generally brown 12 to 24 hours after subtotal gastrectomy, indicating digested food. Examine the color, quantity, and odor of your stomach discharge, noting any changes or the presence of clots or bright blood. The discharge appears brilliant crimson at first. Over the first 2 to 3 days, it turns black, then clear or greenish-yellow. A change in color, amount, or odor could suggest a problem such bleeding, intestinal obstruction, or infection.

ANSWER NUMBER 10.29

Solution of the Question - C. Watching TV

Because watching TV does not require the eye to move rapidly and does not cause an increase in intraocular pressure, it is acceptable. It is suggested that the patient rest their eyes and take a nap when they come home. Most people can watch television or stare at a computer screen for a short length of time many hours after surgery. Because cataract surgery is only done on one eye at a time, the patient may experience vision imbalances until the second eye is worked on (typically 1–4 weeks later).

ANSWER NUMBER 10.30

Solution of the Question - A. Fracture

Pain, deformity, shortening of the extremity, crepitus, and swelling are all common indications and symptoms of a fracture. Pain, deformity, swelling, and a potentially bleeding wound are all indications of these injuries. It's worth noting that the wound could not be right above the fracture. To determine whether a possible nerve or vascular injury is connected with the fracture, the mobility and neurovascular state of all afflicted limbs should be examined.

ANSWER NUMBER 10.31

Solution of the Question - C. Placing the tip of the dropper on the edge of the ear canal.

The dropper must not come into contact with any object or part of the client's ear. Allow no contact between the dropper tip and the ear, fingers, or any other surface. It's possible that it'll pick up bacteria or other germs that could cause an ear infection.

ANSWER NUMBER 10.32

Solution of the Question - A. Absence of drainage from the ileostomy for 6 or more hours

A sudden decrease in drainage or the onset of significant stomach pain should be reported to a doctor right once because it could indicate the development of an obstruction. After surgery, the ileostomy may not function for a brief amount of time. This isn't normally a concern, but if the stoma isn't used for more than 6 hours and the patient has cramps or nausea, he could have an obstruction.

ANSWER NUMBER 10.33

Solution of the Question - B. Peritonitis

Peritonitis, perforation, and abscess formation are all complications of acute appendicitis. Diffuse peritonitis and sepsis are also serious complications, which can lead to substantial morbidity and death. After appendectomies, problems such as postoperative abscesses, hematomas, and wound complications are common. Bacteroides may grow if the wound becomes infected. If too much of the appendiceal stump is left following an appendectomy, "recurrent" appendicitis might develop.

ANSWER NUMBER 10.34

Solution of the Question - D. Pneumonia

A client with acute pancreatitis is more likely to have respiratory problems. The literature has discussed the link between Mycoplasma pneumoniae infection and acute pancreatitis. Mardh et al. reported four adult cases of acute pancreatitis after pneumonia caused by MP in 1973; in three of the patients, the pancreatitis developed in the third week after the commencement of cough, by which time the respiratory symptoms had almost vanished.

ANSWER NUMBER 10.35

Solution of the Question - B. Yellow sclera

The normal flow of bile is obstructed by inflammation and blockage in the liver. Excess bilirubin causes yellowing of the skin and sclera, as well as black, foamy urine. The urine darkens after 3 to 10 days, followed by jaundice. Despite worsening jaundice, patients often experience a remission of systemic symptoms, and they feel better. The liver is frequently engorged and painful, yet the liver's border is soft and smooth. In 15 to 20% of patients, mild splenomegaly develops. Within 1 to 2 weeks, jaundice commonly peaks.

ANSWER NUMBER 10.36

Solution of the Question - C. Steroids

Glucocorticoids (steroids) are used to treat edema because of their anti-inflammatory properties. Corticosteroids exert their effects in a variety of ways. They have anti-inflammatory and immunosuppressive effects, as well as metabolic effects on protein and carbohydrate, water and electrolyte effects, central nervous system effects, and blood cell effects.

ANSWER NUMBER 10.37

Solution of the Question - A. Increase the flow of normal saline

To keep the line patent and maintain blood volume, the blood must be stopped immediately and regular saline given. Stopping the transfusion, leaving the IV in place, intravenous fluids with normal saline, keeping urine output more than 100 mL/hour, diuretics, and cardiorespiratory support as needed are all options for treatment. A hemolytic workup should also be completed, which includes sending donor blood and tubing to the blood bank, as well as post-transfusion labs (see list below).

ANSWER NUMBER 10.38

Solution of the Question - B. Positive ELISA and western blot tests

These tests establish the existence of HIV antibodies, which are produced when the human immunodeficiency virus is present (HIV). When acute or early HIV infection is suspected, the most sensitive screening immunoassay available (preferably, a combination antigen/antibody immunoassay) is used in conjunction with an HIV virologic (viral load) test. The viral load test based on RT-PCR is preferred. In most cases, a positive HIV virologic test implies HIV infection.

ANSWER NUMBER 10.39

Solution of the Question - D. Cottage cheese

Cottage cheese has about 225 calories, 27 grams of protein, 9 grams of fat, 30 milligrams of cholesterol, and 6 grams of carbohydrate per cup. Proteins with high biological value (HBV) have appropriate amounts of critical amino acids. Proteins derived from animals have a higher biological value than proteins derived from plants. Meat, poultry, fish, eggs, milk, cheese, and yogurt are all animal sources of protein that have high biological value proteins.

ANSWER NUMBER 10.40

Solution of the Question - A. Flapping hand tremors

The irritation of the nerves caused by an increase in uremic waste products induces flapping hand tremors. Although hepatic illnesses are the most common cause of asterixis, other conditions such as azotemia and respiratory sickness can also cause it. Asterixis is a motor control condition defined by an inability to actively hold a stance and resulting irregular myoclonic lapses of posture that affect different portions of the body in different ways.

ANSWER NUMBER 10.41

Solution of the Question - B. Distention of the lower abdomen

This signifies that the bladder is swollen and palpable due to urine. The examination should include an abdominal examination (searching for palpable bladder/loin discomfort) and an examination of the external genitalia in the elective situation (meatal stenosis or phimosis). Benign prostatic hyperplasia (BPH) is a common cause of lower urinary tract symptoms in men and refers to the nonmalignant expansion or hyperplasia of prostate tissue.

ANSWER NUMBER 10.42

Solution of the Question - C. Elevate the scrotum using a soft support

Elevation improves lymphatic drainage, which helps to reduce edema and pain. The penis should then be positioned high on the lower abdomen to prevent any postoperative downward curvature. After the sterile dressing is removed, scrotal support or tight mesh underwear can be used.

ANSWER NUMBER 10.43

Solution of the Question - B. Myocardial damage

Myoglobin detection is a diagnostic method for determining if cardiac injury has occurred. In the emergency room, myoglobin, an oxygen-carrying protein found in cardiac muscle and striated skeletal muscle, offers an appealing alternative to CPK and LDH for detecting acute myocardial infarction. Myoglobin levels in the serum can rise as quickly as one hour following myocardial cell death, with peak levels reaching four to six hours later.

ANSWER NUMBER 10.44

Solution of the Question - D. Pulmonary

Because there is no valve to prevent retrograde flow into the pulmonary vein when mitral stenosis is present, the left atrium has trouble emptying its contents into the left ventricle, putting the pulmonary circulation under pressure. Blood flow from the left atrium to the left ventricle is obstructed by mitral valve regions of less than 2 square centimeters. A pressure gradient is created across the mitral valve as a result of this. The left ventricle requires the atrial kick to fill with blood when the gradient across the mitral valve increases.

ANSWER NUMBER 10.45

Solution of the Question - A. Ineffective health maintenance

The objective for a hypertensive client is to control their blood pressure. Pain, a lack of volume, and compromised skin integrity are common in hypertensive patients. The fact that hypertension is asymptomatic makes it difficult to manage. Monitor and keep track of your blood pressure. For the initial evaluation, measure both arms and thighs three times, 3–5 minutes apart, while the patient is at rest, sitting, and standing. Use the proper cuff size and method.

ANSWER NUMBER 10.46

Solution of the Question - C. Headache

Nitroglycerin frequently causes adverse effects such as headache, hypotension, and dizziness due to its extensive vasodilating properties. Headaches can be intense, throbbing, and long-lasting, and they can happen right after you use it. Increased intracranial pressures can be caused by vasodilation and venous pooling, which can produce chronic, throbbing headaches, as well as confusion, fever, vertigo, nausea, vomiting, and visual abnormalities.

ANSWER NUMBER 10.47

Solution of the Question - A. High levels of low-density lipid (LDL) cholesterol

An increase in LDL cholesterol concentration has been identified as a risk factor for atherosclerosis development. LDL cholesterol is accumulated in the blood vessel walls rather than being broken down by the liver. LDL particles are captured by proteoglycans when they leave the circulation and enter the artery intima, where they aggregate and are changed. While the exact alterations of LDL are unknown, oxidative modification, which results in oxidized LDL, looks to be a promising possibility.

ANSWER NUMBER 10.48

Solution of the Question - D. Potential alteration in renal perfusion

There may be a change in renal perfusion, as evidenced by decreased urine output. Renal artery embolism, prolonged hypotension, or prolonged aortic cross-clamping after surgery could all be factors in the altered renal perfusion. In patients at high risk for open surgery, the risks of intervention or surgical therapy should be weighed against the advantages of repair, and in certain circumstances, no intervention may be necessary. Patients should be well-informed about their alternatives, repair risks, and postoperative consequences.

ANSWER NUMBER 10.49

Solution of the Question - A. Dairy products

Dairy products and meats are good sources of vitamin B12. Vitamin B12, which is spontaneously generated by the ruminal bacteria and transmitted to milk, is particularly abundant in ruminant products. Dairy products maintain a large portion of the vitamin B12 naturally present in milk, and some processing circumstances, such as in Swiss-type cheeses, may even add to the basal level by producing vitamin B12 from propionic bacteria.

ANSWER NUMBER 10.50

Solution of the Question - C. Bleeding tendencies

Aplastic anemia reduces the synthesis of RBCs, white blood cells, and platelets in the bone marrow. Bruising and bleeding tendencies are a concern for the client. Aplastic anemia is a syndrome of persistent primary hematopoietic failure caused by damage, with decreased or nonexistent hematopoietic precursors in the bone marrow and pancytopenia as a result.

ANSWER NUMBER 10.51

Solution of the Question - B. Vital signs

An elective surgery is scheduled ahead of time to allow for the necessary preparations. The vital signs are the final check that must be performed before the client leaves the room in order to ensure continuity of treatment and assessment.

ANSWER NUMBER 10.52

Solution of the Question - A. 4 to 12 years

Acute Lymphocytic Leukemia (ALL) is most common in children under the age of four. After the age of 15, it is unusual. Every year, roughly 4000 persons in the United States are diagnosed with it, the majority of them are under the age of 18. It is the most frequent type of childhood cancer. Between the ages of two and ten, children are most likely to be diagnosed.

ANSWER NUMBER 10.53

Solution of the Question - D. Gastric distension

Gastric distention is not a symptom of Acute Lymphocytic Leukemia (ALL). It does infiltrate the central nervous system, and meningeal irritation causes headaches and vomiting in patients. After treatment, the primary care physician and nurse practitioner may be in charge of follow-up and reporting to the interprofessional team. Because these individuals are prone to infections, coagulation dyscrasias, and recurrence, they must be closely monitored.

ANSWER NUMBER 10.54

Solution of the Question - B. Administering Coumadin

Oral anticoagulants like Coumadin haven't been found to help with disseminated intravascular coagulation (DIC). Patients with hemorrhagic tendencies (e.g., active GI ulceration, patients bleeding from the GI, respiratory, or GU tracts; a cerebral aneurysm; central nervous system (CNS) hemorrhage; dissecting aortic aneurysm; spinal puncture, and other diagnostic or therapeutic procedures with the potential for significant bleeding) should not take warfarin.

ANSWER NUMBER 10.55

Solution of the Question - A. Urine output greater than 30ml/hr

Urine output is the most sensitive indicator of a patient's responsiveness to hypovolemic shock therapy. Urine output should be between 30 and 35 mL/hr on a regular basis. Hypovolemic shock can result from salt and fluid losses in the kidneys. Sodium and water are normally excreted in a manner that corresponds to consumption. Excessive renal salt and volume loss can occur as a result of diuretic medication and osmotic diuresis caused by hyperglycemia. Furthermore, there are other tubular and interstitial disorders that induce severe salt-wasting nephropathy that are beyond the scope of this article.

ANSWER NUMBER 10.56

Solution of the Question - C. Hoarseness

Early indications of laryngeal cancer differ depending on where the tumor is located. Because hoarseness that lasts longer than two weeks is one of the most common warning signals, it should be evaluated. Patients are usually men who have used tobacco in the past or currently. Due to vocal cord immobility or fixation, hoarseness is a common early sign of glottic malignancies, with swallowing difficulty and transferred ear pain indicating advanced disease.

ANSWER NUMBER 10.57

Solution of the Question - C. Decreases the production of autoantibodies that attack the acetylcholine receptors.

Steroids suppress the immune system, which reduces the generation of antibodies that assault acetylcholine receptors at the neuromuscular junction. Immunotherapy is used to upregulate or downregulate the immune system to achieve a therapeutic effect in immunologically mediated disorders such as immunodeficiencies, hypersensitivity reactions, autoimmune diseases, tissue and organ transplantation, malignancies, inflammatory disorders, infectious diseases, and any other disease where immunotherapy can improve the quality of life and length of life.

ANSWER NUMBER 10.58

Solution of the Question - C. Urine output hourly

Because it increases the intravascular volume that must be filtered and expelled by the kidney, the osmotic diuretic mannitol is contraindicated in the presence of poor renal function or heart failure. Urine output should also be monitored; if urine production does not increase following mannitol delivery, the mannitol should be stopped and the patient evaluated for probable renal or genitourinary disorders.

ANSWER NUMBER 10.59

Solution of the Question - A. Accurate dose delivery

These devices are more accurate because they are simple to use, and they help young people stick to their insulin regimes because the drug may be given discreetly. Most insulin analog vials, cartridges, and prefilled pens must be thrown after 28 days if they have been used. As a result, many people who use a 10-ml vial find up squandering insulin or using it past the suggested discard date. Patients who use a 3-ml prefilled pen or a reusable pen with a 3-ml insulin cartridge rarely have this difficulty.

ANSWER NUMBER 10.60

Solution of the Question - C. Prolonged reperfusion of the toes after blanching

The vascular perfusion of the toes may be reduced due to damage to blood vessels, indicating a loss of blood supply to the extremities. A decrease in arterial input will occur if the intracompartmental pressure exceeds the arterial pressure. Ischemia is caused by a decrease in tissue oxygenation caused by a reduction in venous outflow and arterial inflow. If the oxygenation deficit becomes severe enough, permanent necrosis may result.

ANSWER NUMBER 10.61

Solution of the Question - D. Elevate the leg when sitting for long periods of time.

Elevation will aid in the control of edema, which is common.

ANSWER NUMBER 10.62

Solution of the Question - B. Ears

Because uric acid has a low solubility, it tends to precipitate and deposit in places where blood flow is low, such as cartilaginous tissue like the ears. Patients with prolonged hyperuricemia may develop tophi, which are nodules formed by subcutaneous urate depositions. Joints, ears, finger pads, tendons, and bursae are all common places for tophi to appear.

ANSWER NUMBER 10.63

Solution of the Question - B. Palms of the hand

To protect the axilla's nerves, the client's weight should be supported by the palms. This is the most common method. The injured leg, as well as the left and right crutches, are advanced, while the unaffected leg maintains the body weight. The unaffected leg is then advanced. Each type of crutch has its own set of hand grips. They act as a vital link between the crutch and the person using it. Depending on the crutch, hand grips have always been adjustable in the up, down, forward, and back positions.

ANSWER NUMBER 10.64

Solution of the Question - A. Active joint flexion and extension

Exudates in the joints are mobilized by active workouts such as alternating extension, flexion, abduction, and adduction, which reduce stiffness and pain. The value of exercise in supporting joint health in people with RA is critical, especially because joint disease is the most apparent and unchanging aspect of the disease pathology.

ANSWER NUMBER 10.65

Solution of the Question - C. Assess the client's feet for sensation and circulation

If you notice changes in your sensation or circulation, it's a sign that your spinal cord is damaged; if this happens, call your doctor right once. Examine the lower extremities and feet (lumbar) as well as the hands and arms for movement and feeling (cervical). Although sensory impairment is usually evident, worsening and alterations may represent the formation or resolution of spinal cord edema and inflammation of the tissues as a result of surgical manipulation damage to the motor nerve roots.

ANSWER NUMBER 10.66

Solution of the Question - A. Hypovolemia

Fluid retained during the oliguric phase is expelled during the diuretic phase, which can amount to 3 to 5 liters per day. Hypovolemia might ensue, and fluids should be replenished. The diuretic stage normally lasts 1-2 weeks, although it can last up to a month. As the kidney continues to heal, an increase in urine production is noticed, and uremia begins to fade.

ANSWER NUMBER 10.67

Solution of the Question - C. Glucose

CSF contains elements that are comparable to those found in blood plasma. To establish whether a bodily fluid is mucus or CSF, it is tested for glucose content. Glucose is normally present in CSF. CSF glucose cannot be given a real normal range. In a healthy adult, CSF glucose is roughly two-thirds of the blood glucose measured in the previous two to four hours. As serum glucose levels rise, this ratio drops. Regardless of serum glucose levels, CSF glucose levels rarely exceed 300 mg per dL (16.7 mmol per L).

ANSWER NUMBER 10.68

Solution of the Question - B. Head trauma

In adults, trauma is one of the leading causes of brain injury and seizure activity. Neoplasms, drug and alcohol withdrawal, and vascular illness are all common causes of seizure activity in adults. Alcohol and narcotics, head injuries, and epilepsy are all common reasons of emergency room admissions after seizures.

ANSWER NUMBER 10.69

Solution of the Question - A. Pupil size and papillary response

To detect changes surrounding the cranial nerves, it's critical to keep an eye on pupil size and pupillary response. The oculomotor (III) cranial nerve controls pupil reactions, which can be used to determine whether the brain stem is intact. The balance of parasympathetic and sympathetic innervation determines pupil size and equalization. The combined function of the optic (II) and oculomotor (III) cranial nerves is reflected in the response to light.

ANSWER NUMBER 10.70

Solution of the Question - C. "Keep active, use stress reduction strategies, and avoid fatigue".

Because it is crucial to strengthen the immune system while remaining active, the nurse's most constructive approach is to urge the client with multiple sclerosis to be active, employ stress reduction measures, and prevent weariness. Participation in fitness or exercise organizations, as well as the Multiple Sclerosis Society, is recommended. Can assist the patient in remaining motivated to be active within the limitations of his or her disability or condition. To suit the patient's needs and prevent discouragement or worry, group activities must be carefully chosen.

ANSWER NUMBER 10.71

Solution of the Question - D. Restlessness

Hypoxia can be detected early on by restlessness. When an unconscious client becomes restless, the nurse should suspect hypoxia. Organ function begins to decline when oxygen delivery is severely impeded. With mild hypoxia, neurologic symptoms include restlessness, headache, and disorientation. Alternate mentation and coma can develop in severe cases, and if not treated promptly, can result in death.

ANSWER NUMBER 10.72

Solution of the Question - B. Atonic

The bladder becomes entirely atonic in spinal shock and will continue to fill until the patient is catheterized. Motor and sensory reflexes, such as the bulbocavernosus reflex and the anal wink reflex, should be included in a thorough spinal evaluation. Not only do skeletal muscles lose motor function and strength, but so do internal organs including the colon and bladder. Constipation and urine retention result from this decrease.

ANSWER NUMBER 10.73

Solution of the Question - A. Progression stage

The transition from a preneoplastic state or low degree of malignancy to a fast-growing tumor that cannot be reversed is referred to as the progression stage. The expression of the malignant phenotype and the tendency of malignant cells to acquire increasingly aggressive traits over time make up tumor development. Metastasis may also involve tumor cells' ability to secrete proteases that facilitate penetration beyond the primary tumor's local site. The proclivity for genomic instability and uncontrolled development is a significant feature of the malignant phenotype.

ANSWER NUMBER 10.74

Solution of the Question - D. Intensity

Intensity is the most essential predictor of pain severity and is crucial for therapy evaluation. The degree of pain as evaluated by the patient or the impact pain has on function are both factors in determining the severity of pain. Intensity can be measured using a variety of scales, which will be discussed further below. Changes in everyday activities, activity level, and work-related obligations may all have an impact on function. Sleep, mood, hunger, and social interactions can all be affected by pain.

ANSWER NUMBER 10.75

Solution of the Question - B. Daily baths with fragrant soap

Fragrant soap is extremely drying to the skin, resulting in pruritus. Overheating, hot baths, and soaps, shower and bath products are all variables that can cause skin dryness. Emollients can be used to moisturize dry skin during washing, bathing, or showering.

Answer - Set 11

ANSWER NUMBER 11.01

Solution of the Question - D. Gouty arthritis

Gouty arthritis is a metabolic condition that causes urate deposits and joint discomfort, particularly in the feet and legs. In septic or traumatic arthritis, urea deposits do not form.

ANSWER NUMBER 11.02

Solution of the Question - B. 30 ml/hour

An infusion of 25,000 units of heparin in 500 milliliters of saline solution provides 50 units of heparin per milliliter. 50 units multiplied by X (the unknown quantity) equals 1,500 units/hour, with X equaling 30 ml/hour.

ANSWER NUMBER 11.03

Solution of the Question - B. Loss of muscle contraction decreasing venous return

The loss of muscular contraction in clients with hemiplegia or hemiparesis reduces venous return and might induce edema in the afflicted extremity.

ANSWER NUMBER 11.04

Solution of the Question - B. It appears on the distal interphalangeal joint.

Both men and women have Heberden's nodes on the distal interphalangeal joint.

ANSWER NUMBER 11.05

Solution of the Question - B. Osteoarthritis is a localized disease; rheumatoid arthritis is systemic

Rheumatoid arthritis is a systemic disease, whereas osteoarthritis is a localized condition.

ANSWER NUMBER 11.06

Solution of the Question - C. The cane should be used on the unaffected side

On the unaffected side, a cane should be utilized. A client with osteoarthritis should be encouraged to utilize a cane, walker, or other assistive equipment to ambulate as needed; this relieves weight and stress on joints.

ANSWER NUMBER 11.07

Solution of the Question - A. 9 U regular insulin and 21 U neutral protamine Hagedorn (NPH).

A 70/30 insulin formulation consists of 70% NPH and 30% normal insulin. As a result, a proper substitution necessitates combining 21 units of NPH with 9 units of normal insulin.

ANSWER NUMBER 11.08

Solution of the Question - C. Colchicines

Gout is a joint inflammatory condition caused by urate crystal deposits in the joints (particularly in the great toe). Colchicine is prescribed by the doctor to help diminish these deposits and so minimize joint inflammation.

ANSWER NUMBER 11.09

Solution of the Question - A. Adrenal cortex

The client's hypertension is caused by excessive aldosterone secretion in the adrenal cortex. This hormone operates on the renal tubule, promoting sodium reabsorption and potassium and hydrogen ion excretion.

ANSWER NUMBER 11.10

Solution of the Question - C. They debride the wound and promote healing by secondary intention

Wet-to-dry dressings are best for this client because they clean the foot ulcer by debriding exudate and necrotic tissue, which promotes secondary healing.

ANSWER NUMBER 11.11

Solution of the Question - A. Hyperkalemia

Due to decreased aldosterone secretion, the client has hyperkalemia in adrenal insufficiency.

ANSWER NUMBER 11.12

Solution of the Question - C. Restricting fluids.

The nurse should limit fluids in a client with SIADH to decrease water retention.

ANSWER NUMBER 11.13

Solution of the Question - D. Glycosylated hemoglobin level.

Glycosylated hemoglobin levels provide information on blood glucose levels throughout the previous three months because some glucose in the bloodstream attaches to some hemoglobin and stays attached for the 120-day lifespan of red blood cells.

ANSWER NUMBER 11.14

Solution of the Question - C. 4:00 pm

NPH is an intermediate-acting insulin that reaches its peak 8 to 12 hours after injection. The client is most at risk for hypoglycemia from 3 p.m. to 7 p.m. because the nurse gave NPH insulin at 7 a.m.

ANSWER NUMBER 11.15

Solution of the Question - A. Glucocorticoids and androgens

The cortex and medulla are the two divisions of the adrenal glands. Glucocorticoids, mineralocorticoids, and androgens are the three types of hormones produced by the cortex.

ANSWER NUMBER 11.16

Solution of the Question - A. Hypocalcemia

If the parathyroid glands were mistakenly removed during thyroid surgery, hypocalcemia could result. Hypocalcemia symptoms and signs may not appear for up to 7 days after surgery. Thyroid surgery does not induce anomalies in serum sodium, potassium, or magnesium.

ANSWER NUMBER 11.17

Solution of the Question - D. Carcinoembryonic antigen level

The level of carcinoembryonic antigen is higher in clients who smoke. As a result, it can't be utilized as a general cancer indicator. It is, nevertheless, useful in monitoring cancer treatment since, if treatment is successful, the level usually returns to normal within a month.

ANSWER NUMBER 11.18

Solution of the Question - B. Dyspnea, tachycardia, and pallor

Dyspnea, tachycardia, and pallor, as well as weariness, listlessness, irritability, and headache, are all symptoms of iron deficiency anemia.

ANSWER NUMBER 11.19

Solution of the Question - D. "I'll need to have a C-section if I become pregnant and have a baby."

When the mother is HIV-positive, a Cesarean section is not required.

ANSWER NUMBER 11.20

Solution of the Question - C. "Avoid sharing such articles as toothbrushes and razors."

In the blood, the human immunodeficiency virus (HIV), which causes AIDS, is most concentrated. As a result, the client should not share personal items that may be blood-contaminated with other family members, such as toothbrushes and razors.

ANSWER NUMBER 11.21

Solution of the Question - B. Pallor, tachycardia, and a sore tongue

Pernicious anemia is characterized by paleness, tachycardia, and a painful tongue. Anorexia, weight loss, a smooth, meaty red tongue, a wide pulse pressure, palpitations, angina, weakness, weariness, and paresthesia of the hands and feet are some of the other clinical signs.

ANSWER NUMBER 11.22

Solution of the Question - B. Administer epinephrine, as prescribed, and prepare to intubate the client if necessary.

To treat anaphylactic shock, the nurse should first provide epinephrine, a powerful bronchodilator, as directed by the doctor.

ANSWER NUMBER 11.23

Solution of the Question - D. Bilateral hearing loss.

Long-term use of aspirin and other salicylates can result in a 30 to 40 decibel hearing loss on both sides. This side effect usually goes away within two weeks of stopping the therapy.

ANSWER NUMBER 11.24

Solution of the Question - D. Lymphocyte

The lymphocyte is responsible for adaptive immunity, which involves the identification of a foreign antigen and the creation of memory cells to combat it. B and T cells mediate adaptive immunity, which can be acquired actively or passively.

ANSWER NUMBER 11.25

Solution of the Question - A. Moisture replacement.

Sjogren's syndrome is an autoimmune condition that causes the skin, GI tract, ears, nose, and vaginal lubrication to gradually deteriorate. The mainstay of therapy is moisture replacement.

ANSWER NUMBER 11.26

Solution of the Question - C. Stool for Clostridium difficile test.

C. difficile infection, which causes "horse barn" smelling diarrhea, is a danger for immunocompromised patients, such as those taking chemotherapy. A correct diagnosis, which involves a stool test, is the first step toward successful therapy.

ANSWER NUMBER 11.27

Solution of the Question - D. Western blot test with ELISA.

Antibodies to HIV, which form roughly 2 to 12 weeks after HIV exposure and indicate infection, are used to detect HIV infection. When used in conjunction with the ELISA, the Western blot test (electrophoresis of antibody proteins) is more than 98 percent accurate in detecting HIV antibodies. When used alone, it isn't very specific.

ANSWER NUMBER 11.28

Solution of the Question - C. Abnormally low hematocrit (HCT) and hemoglobin (Hb) levels.

Low HCT and Hb levels before surgery indicate that the patient may need a blood transfusion. If the HCT and Hb levels drop after surgery due to blood loss, the need for a transfusion becomes more likely.

ANSWER NUMBER 11.29

Solution of the Question - A. Platelet count, prothrombin time, and partial thromboplastin time

The results of prothrombin time, platelet count, thrombin time, partial thromboplastin time, and fibrinogen level laboratory tests, as well as client history and other evaluation variables, are used to diagnose DIC.

ANSWER NUMBER 11.30

Solution of the Question - D. Strawberries

Berries, peanuts, Brazil nuts, cashews, shellfish, and eggs are common dietary allergies.

ANSWER NUMBER 11.31

Solution of the Question - B. A client with a cast on the right leg who states, "I have a funny feeling in my right leg."

It could be a sign of neurovascular impairment, necessitating rapid medical attention.

ANSWER NUMBER 11.32

Solution of the Question - D. A 62-year-old who had an abdominal-perineal resection three days ago; client complains of chills.

The client is at risk for peritonitis; subsequent symptoms and infection should be investigated.

ANSWER NUMBER 11.33

Solution of the Question - C. The client spontaneously flexes his wrist when the blood pressure is obtained.

Hypocalcemia is indicated by carpal spasms.

ANSWER NUMBER 11.34

Solution of the Question - D. Use comfort measures and pillows to position the client.

A non-pharmacological form of pain management is to use comfort measures and cushions to position the client.

ANSWER NUMBER 11.35

Solution of the Question - B. Warm the dialysate solution.

Dialysis with cold dialysate causes more discomfort. Warm the solution in a warmer or heating pad to body temperature; do not use a microwave oven.

ANSWER NUMBER 11.36

Solution of the Question - C. The client holds the cane with his left hand, moves the cane forward followed by the right leg, and then moves the left leg.

The cane provides support and weight-bearing assistance for the weaker right leg.

ANSWER NUMBER 11.37

Solution of the Question - A. Ask the woman's family to provide personal items such as photos or mementos.

Visual stimulation is provided via photos and souvenirs, which helps to alleviate sensory loss.

ANSWER NUMBER 11.38

Solution of the Question - B. The client lifts the walker, moves it forward 10 inches, and then takes several small steps forward.

A walker must be taken up and positioned on all four legs.

ANSWER NUMBER 11.39

Solution of the Question - B. Decreased visual, auditory, and gustatory abilities.

Normal functioning is hampered by gradual loss of vision, hearing, and taste.

ANSWER NUMBER 11.40

Solution of the Question - A. Encourage the client to perform pursed-lip breathing.

Pursed lip breathing helps the client manage the rate and depth of their breathing and prevents the lung unit from collapsing.

ANSWER NUMBER 11.41

Solution of the Question - C. Hypertension

Acute rejection is characterized by hypertension, fever, and pain over the grafted kidney.

ANSWER NUMBER 11.42

Solution of the Question - A. Pain

ANSWER NUMBER 11.43

Solution of the Question - D. Decrease the size and vascularity of the thyroid gland.

Lugol's solution contains iodine, which helps to reduce the vascularity of the thyroid gland, lowering the risk of hemorrhage after surgery.

ANSWER NUMBER 11.44

Solution of the Question - A. Liver Disease

Because of a diminished ability to create glycogen (glycogenesis) and form glucose from glycogen, the client with liver illness has a reduced ability to metabolize carbs.

ANSWER NUMBER 11.45

Solution of the Question - C. Leukopenia

Leukopenia, or a decrease in white blood cells, is a side effect of chemotherapy that occurs as a result of myelosuppression.

ANSWER NUMBER 11.46

Solution of the Question - C. Avoid foods that in the past caused flatus.

Foods that troubled a person before surgery will continue to bother them after surgery.

ANSWER NUMBER 11.47

Solution of the Question - B. Keep the irrigating container less than 18 inches above the stoma."

This height allows the solution to flow slowly and with little effort, preventing excessive peristalsis from forming right once.

ANSWER NUMBER 11.48

Solution of the Question - A. Administer Kayexalate

A potassium exchange resin called kayexalate allows sodium to be exchanged for potassium in the intestine, lowering serum potassium levels.

ANSWER NUMBER 11.49

Solution of the Question - B. 28 gtt/min

Multiply the amount to be infused (2000 ml) by the drop factor (10) and divide the result by the time in minutes to get the correct flow rate (12 hours x 60 minutes)

ANSWER NUMBER 11.50

Solution of the Question - D. Upper trunk

The percentage assigned to each burned part of the body using the rule of nines is: 9% for the head and neck, 9% for the right upper extremities, 9% for the left upper extremity, 18% for the anterior trunk, 18% for the posterior trunk, 18% for the right lower extremity, 18% for the left lower extremity, and 1% for the perineum.

ANSWER NUMBER 11.51

Solution of the Question - C. Bleeding from ears

A comprehensive examination by the nurse is required, as it may indicate changes in cerebral function, high intracranial pressures, fractures, and bleeding. Ear bleeding is caused only by basal skull fractures, which can easily lead to increased intracranial pressure and brain herniation.

ANSWER NUMBER 11.52

Solution of the Question - D. may engage in contact sports

The nurse should counsel the client to stay away from contact sports. This will prevent injury to the pacemaker generator's location.

ANSWER NUMBER 11.53

Solution of the Question - A. Oxygen at 1-2L/min is given to maintain the hypoxic stimulus for breathing.

COPD promotes CO_2 retention in the medulla, making it unresponsive to CO_2 stimulation for breathing. The client's hypoxic status then serves as a breathing stimulus. The client's hypoxic drive will be maintained if oxygen is given at low concentrations.

ANSWER NUMBER 11.54

Solution of the Question - B. Facilitate ventilation of the left lung.

Because just a partial pneumonectomy is performed, the client must be positioned on the opposite unoperated side to stimulate expansion of the remaining left lung.

ANSWER NUMBER 11.55

Solution of the Question - A. Food and fluids will be withheld for at least 2 hours.

The doctors spray anesthetic in the back of the throat before the bronchoscopy to reduce the gag reflex and therefore make the bronchoscope insertion easier. Giving food and drink to the client after the procedure without first testing for the recovery of the gag reflex can cause aspiration. After two hours, the gag reflex normally returns.

ANSWER NUMBER 11.56

Solution of the Question - C. Hyperkalemia.

A common consequence of acute renal failure is hyperkalemia. If quick action is not done to reverse it, it is life-threatening. By transporting potassium into the cells and thereby lowering serum potassium levels, glucose and normal insulin, along with sodium bicarbonate if necessary, can temporarily prevent cardiac arrest.

ANSWER NUMBER 11.57

Solution of the Question - A. This condition puts her at a higher risk for cervical cancer; therefore, she should have a Papanicolaou (Pap) smear annually.

Condylomata acuminata puts women at risk for cervix and vulva cancer. Annual Pap smears are essential for early detection. There is no permanent cure for condylomata acuminata because it is a virus.

ANSWER NUMBER 11.58

Solution of the Question - A. The left kidney usually is slightly higher than the right one.

In most cases, the left kidney is slightly higher than the right. Each kidney has an adrenal gland on top of it.

ANSWER NUMBER 11.59

Solution of the Question - C. Blood urea nitrogen (BUN) 100 mg/dl and serum creatinine 6.5 mg/dl.

BUN levels should be between 8 and 23 mg/dl, while serum creatinine should be between 0.7 and 1.5 mg/dl. Option C's test results are excessively high, indicating CRF and the kidneys' reduced ability to eliminate nonprotein nitrogen waste from the bloodstream.

ANSWER NUMBER 11.60

Solution of the Question - D. Alteration in the size, shape, and organization of differentiated cells

A change in the size, shape, or arrangement of differentiated cells is referred to as dysplasia.

ANSWER NUMBER 11.61

Solution of the Question - D. Kaposi's sarcoma

The most frequent malignancy linked to AIDS is Kaposi's sarcoma.

ANSWER NUMBER 11.62

Solution of the Question - C. To prevent cerebrospinal fluid (CSF) leakage

The most frequent malignancy linked to AIDS is Kaposi's sarcoma.

ANSWER NUMBER 11.63

Solution of the Question - A. Auscultate bowel sounds.

If the nausea is accompanied by abdominal distention, the nurse must first listen for bowel noises. If there are no bowel noises, the nurse should suspect gastric or small intestinal dilatation, which should be reported to the doctor.

ANSWER NUMBER 11.64

Solution of the Question - B. Lying on the left side with knees bent

The client should be positioned on his or her left side with knees bent for a colonoscopy.

ANSWER NUMBER 11.65

Solution of the Question - A. Blood supply to the stoma has been interrupted

When the ileum is transported through the abdominal wall to the surface skin, an ileostomy stoma occurs, establishing an artificial hole for waste evacuation. The stoma should be cherry red, indicating that arterial perfusion is sufficient.

A dusky stoma indicates a reduction in perfusion, which could be caused by a disruption in the stoma's blood supply, resulting in tissue injury or necrosis.

ANSWER NUMBER 11.66

Solution of the Question - A. Applying knee splints.

Knee splints keep the joints in a functional position, preventing leg contractures.

ANSWER NUMBER 11.67

Solution of the Question - B. Urine output of 20 ml/hour.

In a client with burns, a urine production of less than 40 mL/hour indicates a fluid volume deficit.

ANSWER NUMBER 11.68

Solution of the Question - A. Turn him frequently.

Frequent position adjustments, which relieve pressure on the skin and underlying tissues, are the most significant intervention for preventing pressure ulcers. Capillaries become blocked if pressure is not relieved, limiting circulation and oxygenation of the tissues, resulting in cell death and ulcer formation.

ANSWER NUMBER 11.69

Solution of the Question - C. In long, even, outward, and downward strokes in the direction of hair growth

When applying a topical medication, the nurse should start at the midline and work in the direction of hair development, using long, even, outward, and downward strokes. Follicle irritation and skin inflammation are less likely with this application technique.

ANSWER NUMBER 11.70

Solution of the Question - A. Beta-adrenergic blockers

Beta-adrenergic blockers reduce the response to catecholamines and sympathetic nerve stimulation by inhibiting beta receptors in the myocardium. They serve to protect the myocardium by lowering myocardial oxygen demand, lowering the chance of recurrent infarction.

ANSWER NUMBER 11.71

Solution of the Question - C. Raised 30 degrees

With the head of the bed tilted between 15 and 30 degrees, jugular venous pressure is measured with a centimeter ruler to determine the vertical distance between the sternal angle and the point of greatest pulsation.

ANSWER NUMBER 11.72

Solution of the Question - D. Inotropic agents

Inotropic drugs are used to increase the force of the heart's contractions, resulting in increased ventricular contractility and, as a result, increased cardiac output.

ANSWER NUMBER 11.73

Solution of the Question - B. Less than 30% of calories from fat

Fat should account for fewer than 30% of daily calories for a customer with low blood HDL and high serum LDL levels.

ANSWER NUMBER 11.74

Solution of the Question - C. The emergency department nurse calls up the latest electrocardiogram results to check the client's progress

Because the emergency room nurse is no longer involved in the client's care, she has no legal claim to information about his current state.

ANSWER NUMBER 11.75

Solution of the Question - B. Check endotracheal tube placement.

As soon as the client comes in the emergency department, the placement of the ET tube should be confirmed. After the airway has been secured, an end-tidal carbon dioxide monitor and pulse oximetry should be used to check oxygenation and ventilation.

Answer - Set 12

ANSWER NUMBER 12.01

Solution of the Question - A. Elevated serum calcium

The calcium level in the blood is controlled by the parathyroid glands. The serum calcium level will be raised in hyperparathyroidism. In the context of hypercalcemia, a normal PTH is regarded inappropriate and is nonetheless indicative of PTH-dependent hypercalcemia. PTH levels in patients with PTH-independent hypercalcemia should be very low. In a patient with persistent hypercalcemia and an increased serum level of parathyroid hormone, a full clinical evaluation along with normal laboratory and radiologic investigations should be adequate to make the diagnosis of primary hyperparathyroidism.

ANSWER NUMBER 12.02

Solution of the Question - D. A restricted sodium diet.

To avoid excessive fluid loss, a patient with Addison's disease requires adequate dietary salt. Don't cut back on salt in your diet. During hot and humid conditions, or after exercise, the client may need to add more salt to his food to replenish salt lost via sweating. Salt replacements should not be used.

ANSWER NUMBER 12.03

Solution of the Question - C. Hypoglycemia

Hypoglycemia is likely to be present in a diabetic patient who is unable to eat after surgery. The actual treatment recommendations for a given patient should be tailored, based on the patient's diabetes classification, usual diabetes regimen, glycemic control, surgical procedure nature and extent, and available expertise.

ANSWER NUMBER 12.04

Solution of the Question - A. Bowel perforation

The most serious consequence of fiberoptic colonoscopy is bowel perforation. Progressive abdominal pain, fever, chills, and tachycardia are all warning indications of developing peritonitis. Intestinal perforation occurs when the mucosa of the bowel wall is insulted or injured as a result of a breach of the closed system. This exposes the peritoneal cavity's structures to stomach contents. Patients experiencing stomach pain and distension should be checked for this condition, especially if they have a relevant medical history, as a delayed diagnosis can result in life-threatening infections such as peritonitis.

ANSWER NUMBER 12.05

Solution of the Question - A, B, and C

Coagulation tests look at prothrombin time, partial thromboplastin time, and platelet count.

Option A: Except for factor VII (tissue factor) and factor XIII, PTT examines the function of all coagulation factors (fibrin stabilizing factor). PTT is extensively used in clinical practice to evaluate patient response to unfractionated heparin infusions, to target therapeutic anticoagulation, and as part of a "coagulation screen" to assist diagnose bleeding or clotting abnormalities.

Option B: The prothrombin time (PT) is one of numerous blood tests used in clinical practice to assess a patient's coagulation status. PT is used to assess the extrinsic and common coagulation pathways, detecting inadequacies of factors II, V, VII, and X, as well as low fibrinogen concentrations.

Option C: Clinicians can analyze the bleeding time, which is the period between breaking the vasculature and forming an effective platelet plug, to monitor platelet function. This period may be prolonged in diseases such as uremia, in which the platelet count is normal but the platelet function is compromised.

ANSWER NUMBER 12.06

Solution of the Question - D. The right side of the sternum just below the clavicle and left of the precordium.

As suggested by the anatomic placement of the heart, one gel pad should be put to the right of the sternum, just below the collarbone, and the other to the left of the precordium. The paddles are put over the pads to defibrillate. The sternal paddle should be placed "just to the right of the upper sternal border below the collarbone," and the apical paddle should be "to the left of the nipple with the center of the electrode in the mid-axillary line," according to ILCOR recommendations.

ANSWER NUMBER 12.07

Solution of the Question - D. All of the above.

The statements are all correct. Most gastrointestinal and genitourinary disorders can be diagnosed with an abdominal examination, which can also reveal abnormalities in other organ systems. The necessity for thorough radiological examinations is reduced by a well-performed abdominal examination, which also plays an important role in patient care.

ANSWER NUMBER 12.08

Solution of the Question - A. Irrigate the eye repeatedly with normal saline solution.

Emergency treatment following a chemical splash to the eye includes immediate irrigation with normal saline. The irrigation should be continued for at least 10 minutes. Immediate irrigation with copious amounts of an isotonic solution is the mainstay of treatment for chemical burns. Never use any substance to neutralize chemical exposure as the exothermic reaction can lead to secondary thermal injuries. Irrigation should continue until the pH of the eye is between 7.0 to 7.4 and remains within this range for at least 30 minutes after the irrigation has been discontinued.

ANSWER NUMBER 12.09

Solution of the Question - D. Temperature of 101.8 F (38.7° C).

The risk of neurovascular problems and the development of infection should be the primary focus of post-surgical nursing assessment after hip replacement. A postoperative temperature of 101.8° F (38.7° C) is greater than the low grade that should be expected and should be cause for worry. The THA postoperative wound complication spectrum includes cellulitis, superficial dehiscence, and/or delayed wound healing, as well as deep infections that end in full-thickness necrosis. Deep infections necessitate trips to the operating room for irrigation, debridement (incision and drainage), and, depending on the infection's time, THA component explanation.

ANSWER NUMBER 12.10

Solution of the Question - B. Restrain the patient's limbs.

Nursing efforts during a witnessed seizure should be focused on ensuring the patient's safety and halting the seizure. Because forceful muscle contractions can cause harm, restraining the limbs is not recommended. When the bed is in the lowest position, use and pad side rails, or set the bed against the wall and pad the floor if rails are not available or acceptable.

ANSWER NUMBER 12.11

Solution of the Question - B. An increase in hematocrit.

Epoetin is a type of erythropoietin that increases hematocrit by stimulating the synthesis of red blood cells. Patients who are anemic, often as a result of chemotherapy, are given epoetin. Epoetin alfa is a 165-amino-acid glycoprotein produced using recombinant DNA technology that possesses biological properties similar to endogenous erythropoietin. Erythropoietin increases the synthesis of red blood cells in the body. It's a hormone made in the kidney that helps erythroid progenitors in the bone marrow differentiate.

ANSWER NUMBER 12.12

Solution of the Question - B, C, D & E

Polycythemia vera is a disorder in which the bone marrow creates an excessive number of red blood cells. The hematocrit and viscosity of the blood both rise as a result of this. Headaches, dizziness, tinnitus, and vision abnormalities are all possible side effects. Increased blood pressure and a longer clotting time are two cardiovascular consequences.

Option B: Patients with bleeding and thrombotic problems account for 1% of all cases. Epistaxis, gum bleeding, and gastrointestinal (GI) bleeding are all examples of bleeding episodes. Deep venous thrombosis (DVT), pulmonary embolism (PE), Budd-Chiari syndrome, splanchnic vein thrombosis, stroke, and arterial thrombosis are all examples of thrombotic occurrences.

Option C: Polycythemia vera's overproduction of red blood cells and high hematocrit levels can contribute to systemic hypertension; high hematocrit levels have been observed to interfere with nitric oxide's vasodilatory effects. Polycythemia treatment, which may include phlebotomy, can help to reduce systemic hypertension and the physiological effects of having a high red blood cell count.

Option D: Because polycythemia vera is a myeloproliferative condition, it is characterized by an autonomic rise in the proliferation of all hematopoietic cells, with erythropoiesis being the most prevalent. Increased blood viscosity causes microcirculation to be disrupted, resulting in headaches with clinical symptoms.

Option E: The symptoms are caused by hyperviscosity and thrombosis, which obstructs oxygen delivery. Fatigue, headaches, dizziness, tinnitus, visual problems, and insomnia are examples of physical ailments.

ANSWER NUMBER 12.13

Solution of the Question - A. Observe for evidence of spontaneous bleeding.

Platelet counts of less than 30,000 per microliter can produce petechiae and bruising, especially in the extremities. When the count goes below 15,000, there is a risk of spontaneous bleeding into the brain and other internal organs. The blood clotting cascade is a complex mechanism that requires both intrinsic and extrinsic elements to function properly. Clotting ability can be impaired by a variety of factors. These lab tests reveal crucial information about the patient's coagulation status and bleeding risk. The laboratory values that will be monitored will be determined by the patient's clinical condition.

ANSWER NUMBER 12.14

Solution of the Question - A, B, & D

Weight gain, fluid retention with hypertension, Cushingoid characteristics, a low serum albumin, and a decreased inflammatory response are all side effects of corticosteroids. Patients are urged to eat a low-sodium, high-protein, vitamin, and mineral-rich diet.

Option A: Corticosteroid use has been linked to hypertension, hyperglycemia, and obesity, with evidence for hyperlipidemia being mixed. Mineralocorticoid action, which varies by corticosteroid, causes free water and sodium retention while potassium is excreted.

Option B: Patients receiving corticosteroids via any method of administration may develop Cushing syndrome. Excess cortisol causes weight gain and adiposity redistribution (dorsocervical fat pad, also known as "buffalo hump," facial fat rise, also known as "moon facies," and truncal obesity). These characteristics could emerge as early as the first year.

Option D: The degree of prednisolone plasma protein binding and serum albumin concentration had a significant relationship. In vitro, azathioprine had no effect on prednisolone plasma binding. Prednisolone's plasma half-life was extended in two of the three patients with chronic liver disease who were investigated. When compared to equivalent doses of prednisone or prednisolone in subjects without liver disease, these factors, combined with low serum albumin concentrations, are associated with higher levels of circulating unbound prednisolone, resulting in very different levels of biologically active corticosteroids.

ANSWER NUMBER 12.15

Solution of the Question - B. Change gloves immediately after use.

The neutropenic patient is at risk of infection. By changing gloves as soon as possible after use, patients are protected against infections picked up on hospital surfaces. This pollution can have devastating consequences for an immunocompromised patient. When providing direct care, use gloves and clean your hands once you've disposed of them properly.

ANSWER NUMBER 12.16

Solution of the Question - D. Immunization provides acquired immunity from some specific diseases.

Immunization is available to protect against some diseases, but not all. Immunity is "acquired" when antibodies are generated in response to a specific disease. Live vaccines are more effective than killed vaccines because they retain more antigens from the microorganisms. Toxoids that cause tetanus and diphtheria, on the other hand, are the most effective bacterial vaccines because they are based on inactivated exotoxins that stimulate considerable antibody development. Subunit vaccines for hepatitis B, meningococcal, and Haemophilus influenzae B are effective when conjugated to carrier proteins such tetanus toxoid.

ANSWER NUMBER 12.17

Solution of the Question - B. Maintain a patent airway.

It's possible that the patient is having an anaphylactic reaction. The importance of airway management cannot be overstated. Examine the patient thoroughly for airway patency or any signs of impending airway loss. Due to the significant risk of perioral edema, stridor, and angioedema, getting a definitive airway is critical. As swelling continues, delaying intubation may diminish the likelihood of a successful intubation, increasing the danger of a surgical airway.

ANSWER NUMBER 12.18

Solution of the Question - A, B, D & E

CNS stimulant drugs, which increase attention and improve concentration, are widely used to treat ADHD in children. Insomnia, irritability, and a loss of appetite are common in children. Dextroamphetamine and levoamphetamine are often used in ADHD treatment, as well as pure dextroamphetamine and lisdexamfetamine.

Option No. 1: One of the most prevalent negative effects of ADHD stimulants is a loss of appetite. Approximately 20% of patients with ADHD who were treated with stimulants experienced a lack of appetite, according to research. Weight loss and digestive issues are also very prevalent.

Option B: One of the most common side effects of stimulant drugs is insomnia or a delayed SOL of more than 30 minutes. This is not to be confused with nighttime resistance, which occurs when a youngster refuses to go to bed. According to parent reports or side effects scales completed by parents, insomnia is a common adverse effect of all stimulant drugs.

Option D: Immediate psychological consequences of stimulant ingestion include feelings of euphoria, enthusiasm, heightened alertness, and increased motor activity. Stimulants can also decrease food intake, shorten sleep time, and boost socializing. Stimulants may also help people perform better on psychomotor activities. Excessive doses might cause restlessness and agitation, and high levels can cause stereotypic behavior.

ANSWER NUMBER 12.19

Solution of the Question - D. Tardive dyskinesia

In a patient receiving haloperidol, abnormal facial movements and tongue protrusion are most likely attributable to tardive dyskinesia, an antipsychotic side effect. Tardive dyskinesia is a term used to describe a collection of iatrogenic movement disorders induced by dopamine receptor inhibition. Acathisia, dystonia, buccolingual stereotypy, myoclonus, chorea, tics, and other aberrant involuntary movements are all common movement disorders produced by long-term use of conventional antipsychotics.

ANSWER NUMBER 12.20

Solution of the Question - B. Confusion

In diabetes mellitus, hypoglycemia produces confusion and signals the need for carbs. Neuroglycopenic signs and symptoms are those that occur as a result of glucose deficiency in the central nervous system (CNS). If not treated right once, these symptoms can include behavioral abnormalities, confusion, exhaustion, seizure, coma, and even death.

ANSWER NUMBER 12.21

Solution of the Question - C. The tumor extended beyond the kidney but was completely resected.

The tumor expands beyond the kidney in stage II, but it is totally removed. A tumor that has developed outside the kidney to some extent, such as into adjacent fatty tissue, is classified as Stage II. The tumor is usually entirely removed during surgery, and the regional lymph nodes are negative. This stage is present in around 20% of all Wilms tumors.

ANSWER NUMBER 12.22

Solution of the Question - A, B, C & E

Acute glomerulonephritis is marked by a high urine specific gravity due to oliguria, as well as a dark "tea-colored" urine due to a large volume of red blood cells. Symptoms such as edema and hypertension develop as the glomerular filtration rate (GFR) decreases, owing to the subsequent salt and water retention induced by the activation of the renin-angiotensin-aldosterone system.

Option A: Glomerulonephritis and pyelonephritis produce a decrease in urine volume and a drop in specific gravity. Damage to the tubules of the kidney reduces the kidney's ability to reabsorb water in several disorders. As a result, the urine is still watery.

Option B: Acute glomerulonephritis affects about half of the population. If symptoms do arise, the first signs are tissue swelling (edema) caused by fluid retention, as well as low blood pressure.

Option C: When the kidneys fail, the concentration and accumulation of chemicals in the urine increases, resulting in a deeper color that might be brown, red, or purple. A defective protein or sugar, a high concentration of red and white blood cells, and a large number of tube-shaped particles known as cellular casts are all contributing to the color shift.

Option E: Patients with edema, hypertension, and oliguria frequently come with a mix of edema, hypertension, and oliguria, while having a normal physical examination and blood pressure. Symptoms of fluid overload, such as periorbital and/or pedal edema, should be looked for by the doctor.

ANSWER NUMBER 12.23

Solution of the Question - B. Prior infection with group A Streptococcus within the past 10-14 days.

The immunological response to a previous upper respiratory infection with group A Streptococcus is the most common cause of acute glomerulonephritis. PSGN usually appears 1 to 2 weeks after a streptococcal throat infection or 6 weeks after a streptococcal skin infection in youngsters. The surface M protein and opacity factor, both of which are known to be nephrogenic and to cause PSGN, have been used to subtype Group A Streptococcus (GAS).

ANSWER NUMBER 12.24

Solution of the Question - C. No treatment is necessary; the fluid is reabsorbing normally.

A hydrocele is a fluid buildup in the scrotum caused by a patent tunica vaginalis. The transparent fluid is visible when the scrotum is illuminated with a pocket light. The fluid is reabsorbed in the majority of cases within the first few months of life, and no treatment is required.

ANSWER NUMBER 12.25

Solution of the Question - A. Inadequate tissue perfusion leading to nerve damage.

Nerve injury is common in patients with peripheral vascular disease due to insufficient tissue perfusion. When blood flow distal to the blockage is sufficiently degraded, intermittent claudication occurs, resulting in fixed oxygen supply that is unable to match oxygen demand. Critical limb ischemia, which is defined as limb pain at rest or impending limb loss, is the most severe form of PAD.

ANSWER NUMBER 12.26

Solution of the Question - B. Contaminated food

Hepatitis A is the only form that spreads through contaminated food via the fecal-oral pathway. In developing countries with weak socioeconomic conditions and poor sanitation and hygiene standards, endemic rates are high. Childhood exposure is common in these underdeveloped countries. The prevalence of HAV in a population is linked to socioeconomic factors like as income, housing density, sanitation, and water quality.

ANSWER NUMBER 12.27

Solution of the Question - A. A history of hepatitis C five years previously.

Hepatitis C is a viral infection that causes liver inflammation and is transferred by bodily fluids such as blood. Due to the increased risk of infection in the recipient, patients with hepatitis C should not donate blood for transfusion. Parenteral, perinatal, and sexual transmission are all possible, with the most prevalent form of transmission being the sharing of contaminated needles among IV drug users. People who require regular blood transfusions and organ transplantation from contaminated donors are also high-risk categories.

ANSWER NUMBER 12.28

Solution of the Question - A. naproxen sodium (Naprosyn)

The nonsteroidal anti-inflammatory medicine naproxen sodium can cause inflammation of the upper gastrointestinal system. As a result, it's not recommended for people who have gastritis. Inhibition of COX-1 and COX-2 reduces prostaglandin generation in the stomach mucosa. Because prostaglandins maintain mucosal integrity, decreasing production results in decreased tissue protection. COX-1, on the other hand, appears to have a greater impact on the integrity of the mucosa; as a result, selective COX-2 inhibitors like Celecoxib have less of an impact on stomach tissue.

ANSWER NUMBER 12.29

Solution of the Question - D. The patient should limit fatty foods.

Cholecystitis, or gallbladder inflammation, is most usually caused by gallstones, which can prevent bile (essential for fat absorption) from entering the intestines. To avoid gallbladder discomfort, patients should limit dietary fat by avoiding fatty meats, fried foods, and creamy desserts.

ANSWER NUMBER 12.30

Solution of the Question - D. Air hunger

Air hunger, anxiety, and agitation are common symptoms of pulmonary edema. Shortness of breath is the most common symptom, which can be severe (within minutes to hours) or progressive (between hours to days), depending on the etiology of pulmonary edema.

ANSWER NUMBER 12.31

Solution of the Question - D. Change the dressing and document the clean appearance of the wound site.

Normal healing is indicated by a moderate amount of serous leakage from a recent surgical site. Serous drainage is fluid, transparent, and thin. During the natural inflammatory healing period, the body produces serous leakage as a normal response.

ANSWER NUMBER 12.32

Solution of the Question - C. Severe pain in the right lower arm.

Inadequate perfusion to the right lower arm as a result of a closed cast might result in neurovascular deterioration and significant discomfort, necessitating cast removal soon away. The venous outflow is reduced when the compartmental pressure rises. This raises venous pressure and, as a result, venous capillary pressure. A decrease in arterial input will occur if the intracompartmental pressure exceeds the arterial pressure. Ischemia is caused by a decrease in tissue oxygenation caused by a reduction in venous outflow and arterial inflow.

ANSWER NUMBER 12.33

Solution of the Question - A. Increased physical activity and daily exercise will help decrease discomfort associated with the condition.

Physical activity and everyday exercise can assist people with osteoarthritis improve their mobility and reduce their pain. Multiple studies have indicated that exercise programs that mix aerobic and resistance training can reduce pain and improve physical function, and physicians should encourage patients to do so on a regular basis.

ANSWER NUMBER 12.34

Solution of the Question - D. A patient on bed rest who must maintain a supine position.

Because alendronate can have serious gastrointestinal adverse effects, including as esophageal irritation, it should not be used if a patient is confined to a supine position. To enhance absorption, take it first thing in the morning with 8 ounces of water on an empty stomach. After receiving the medication, the patient should not eat or drink for 30 minutes and should not lie down.

ANSWER NUMBER 12.35

Solution of the Question - C. Prophylactic antibiotic therapy prior to anticipated exposure to ticks.

Antibiotics are not recommended as a preventative measure for Lyme disease. Antibiotics are only used when symptoms arise as a result of a tick bite. The type of treatment depends on the patient's age and the stage of the disease. Doxycycline is prescribed for 10 days for patients older than 8 years old with early, localized illness. To avoid tooth discoloration caused by tetracycline use in young children, patients under the age of eight should get amoxicillin or cefuroxime for 14 days.

ANSWER NUMBER 12.36

Solution of the Question - B. The area proximal to the insertion site is reddened, warm, and painful.

An IV site that is red, warm, painful and swollen indicates that phlebitis has developed and the line should be discontinued and restarted at another site. Phlebitis is inflammation of a vein. It is usually associated with acidic or alkaline solutions or solutions that have a high osmolarity. Phlebitis can also occur as a result of vein trauma during insertion, use of an inappropriate I.V. catheter size for the vein, or prolonged use of the same I.V. site.

ANSWER NUMBER 12.37

Solution of the Question - D. Fluid overload

Fluid overload occurs when the amount of fluid infused in a short period of time exceeds the vascular system's capacity, resulting in fluid leakage into the lungs. As in the case of the patient, symptoms include dyspnea, fast breathing, and discomfort. Any four of the following symptoms occur within 6 hours of a blood transfusion: immediate respiratory distress, tachycardia, elevated blood pressure (BP), acute or progressive pulmonary edema, and evidence of a positive fluid balance.

ANSWER NUMBER 12.38

Solution of the Question - B, C, D & E.

Following amniotomy, uterine contractions usually become stronger and more closely spaced. The FHR is evaluated right after the procedure and constantly monitored to detect any changes that could suggest cord compression. The surgery itself is painless, and the amniotic fluid is quickly expelled.

ANSWER NUMBER 12.39

Solution of the Question - D. Keep the baby quiet and swaddled, and place the bassinet in a dimly lit area.

To help metabolize the bilirubin, an infant released home with hyperbilirubinemia (newborn jaundice) should be placed in a sunny rather than poorly lit location with skin exposed. On the basis of risk factors and the blood bilirubin level on the nomogram, phototherapy is initiated. Bilirubin absorbs light best in the blue-green region (460 to 490 nm) and is secreted in the bile or transformed into lumirubin and expelled in the urine. During phototherapy, the newborn's eyes must be covered and the maximum amount of body surface area exposed to the light must be covered.

ANSWER NUMBER 12.40

Solution of the Question - A. The infant should be restrained in an infant car seat, properly secured in the back seat in a rear-facing position.

All newborns under the age of one year who weigh less than 20 pounds should be buckled into a rear-facing infant car seat in the back seat. Rear-facing car seats for newborns are likely the least contentious; rear-facing car seats are more effective than forward-facing car seats in preventing serious injury to infants in automobile accidents. When compared to children in forward-facing safety seats, children aged 24 months were 1.76 times less likely to be seriously wounded in all types of car incidents.

ANSWER NUMBER 12.41

Solution of the Question - C. Decreased pain

The loop diuretic furosemide has little effect on pain. Furosemide has been licensed by the Food and Drug Administration (FDA) for the treatment of volume overload and edema caused by congestive heart failure exacerbation, liver failure, or renal failure, including the nephrotic syndrome.

ANSWER NUMBER 12.42

Solution of the Question - A. Obesity

Obesity is a major risk factor for coronary artery disease that can be mitigated with a healthier diet and weight loss. When a person's body mass index (BMI) is between 25 and 29.8 kg/m2, they are considered overweight, and when their BMI is greater than or equal to 30 kg/m2, they are considered obese. Overweight and obesity both raise the risk of ASCVD when compared to a healthy weight. The BMI should be calculated annually, and lifestyle changes, such as calorie restriction and weight loss, should be made based on the BMI values.

ANSWER NUMBER 12.43

Solution of the Question - B. History of cerebral hemorrhage.

Because tPA increases the risk of bleeding, a history of cerebral hemorrhage is a contraindication. There are two types of bleeding that can occur as a result of alteplase therapy. Intracranial hemorrhage (0.4 percent to 15.4%), retroperitoneal bleeding (less than 1%), gastrointestinal (GI) bleeding (5%), genitourinary bleeding (4%), and pulmonary bleeding are all examples of internal bleeding. Invaded or disturbed sites, such as venous cutdowns, arterial punctures, and recent surgical intervention sites, are the most common locations for surface bleeding.

ANSWER NUMBER 12.44

Solution of the Question - C. Prevents DVT (deep vein thrombosis).

To avoid deep vein thrombosis, all hospitalized patients should exercise. In the lower extremities, muscular contraction enhances venous return and prevents hemostasis. Encourage the patient to engage in physical exercise that is appropriate for his or her energy level. Helps to foster a sense of independence while remaining realistic about one's limitations. Walking 20 feet down the hall or through the home, then gradually progressing outside the house, conserving energy for the return trip.

ANSWER NUMBER 12.45

Solution of the Question - D. Confusion

Cardiogenic shock inhibits the heart muscle's pumping function, resulting in reduced blood flow to the body's organs. As a result, there is a reduction in brain function and confusion. Cardiogenic shock is a type of heart failure characterized by decreased cardiac output, which causes end-organ hypoperfusion and tissue hypoxia.

ANSWER NUMBER 12.46

Solution of the Question - A. Family history of heart disease

A family history of heart disease is a hereditary risk factor that cannot be changed by changing one's lifestyle. It's been proven that having a first-degree relative with heart disease raises your risk. The etiology of ASCVD is complex. Hypercholesterolemia (LDL-cholesterol), hypertension, diabetes mellitus, cigarette smoking, age (males over 45 years and females over 55 years), male gender, and a strong family history are the most common risk factors (male relative younger than 55 years and female relative younger than 65 years).

ANSWER NUMBER 12.47

Solution of the Question - A, C, D, & E.

Claudication is the pain a patient with peripheral vascular disease feels when the demand for oxygen in the leg muscles exceeds the supply. This is most common during activity, when muscular tissue demand increases, and is usually reduced after rest. Cramping, weakness, and discomfort occur as the tissue becomes hypoxic.

Option A: Intermittent claudication (IC) is skeletal muscle pain in the lower extremities that occurs during exercise. Insufficient oxygen delivery to meet the metabolic requirements of the skeletal muscles causes IC.

Option C: Intermittent claudication is distinguished by the repeatability of muscle soreness. The pain is frequently triggered by physical exertion and goes away after a short period of relaxation. Inadequate blood flow is the primary cause of pain.

Option D: These patients' physical examinations may reveal signs of arterial insufficiency. It's possible that the affected limb will feel chilly and have slowed pulses. The femoral, popliteal, dorsalis pedis, and posterior tibial artery pulses should all be checked during the physical examination.

Option E: Structured walking programs are more effective than pharmacologic therapy alone in increasing pain-free walking distance. It's worth noting that continuing to smoke while receiving walking therapy limits these patients' progress.

ANSWER NUMBER 12.48

Solution of the Question - C. Avoid crossing the legs.

Crossing the legs should be avoided by patients with peripheral vascular disease because it can obstruct blood flow. To enhance peripheral blood flow, place the client's legs in a dependent position in regard to the heart. If you're unsure about the nature of the client's peripheral vascular difficulties, put him in a neutral, flat, supine position.

ANSWER NUMBER 12.49

Solution of the Question - C. A young woman

Raynaud's illness is most common in young women, and it's often linked to rheumatic diseases like lupus and rheumatoid arthritis. Different etiologies are linked to secondary Raynaud phenomenon. Scleroderma, systemic lupus erythematosus, Sjogren syndrome, and antiphospholipid syndrome are the most common connective tissue illnesses.

ANSWER NUMBER 12.50

Solution of the Question - B. Pulmonary embolism due to deep vein thrombosis (DVT).

Pulmonary embolism is the most common cause of rapid onset shortness of breath and chest discomfort in a hospitalized patient on prolonged bed rest. Both pregnancy and extended inactivity raise the risk of clot development in the legs' deep veins. After that, the clots can break free and migrate to the lungs. Lower extremity DVTs are the most common cause of pulmonary embolisms. As a result, the risk factors for pulmonary embolism (PE) and DVT are the same. Virchow's triad of hypercoagulability, venous stasis, and endothelial injury provides an understanding of these risk factors.

ANSWER NUMBER 12.51

Solution of the Question - B. Cerebral hemorrhage

When treating a stroke victim with thrombolytic therapy to dissolve a suspected clot, cerebral bleeding is a considerable concern. Treatment success necessitates starting it as soon as feasible, frequently before the etiology of the stroke has been discovered. Bleeding is the most common side effect of thrombolytic therapy, and it can happen in a puncture site or anyplace else in the body. The most serious danger is intracranial bleeding or hemorrhagic stroke.

ANSWER NUMBER 12.52

Solution of the Question - A. Torticollis, with shortening of the sternocleidomastoid muscle.

The sternocleidomastoid muscle contracts in torticollis, reducing neck range of motion and causing the chin to point to the opposite side. Torticollis, also known as twisted neck (tortum collum) or "torti colli," is a severe head and neck posture characterized by aberrant slope and rotation. Flexion, extension, and right or left tilt are some of the possible presentation positions. Horizontal torticollis, vertical torticollis, oblique torticollis, and torsion are some of the terms used to describe these conditions.

ANSWER NUMBER 12.53

Solution of the Question - C. The student experiences pain in the inferior aspect of the knee.

When the infrapatellar ligament of the quadriceps muscle presses on the tibial tubercle, causing pain and swelling in the inferior side of the knee, it is known as Osgood-Schlatter disease. Activities that involve repeated use of the quadriceps, such as track and soccer, are common causes of Osgood-Schlatter disease.

ANSWER NUMBER 12.54

Solution of the Question - D. Scoliosis

A typical teenage exam should include a check for scoliosis, which is a lateral deviation of the spine. It's determined by bending the teen's waist with arms dangling and looking for lateral curvature and unequal rib level. Female teenagers are more likely to develop scoliosis. A screening evaluation is usually conducted by a school organization, a sports coach, or a pediatrician. X-ray imaging is part of the right formal examination.

ANSWER NUMBER 12.55

Solution of the Question - C. Self-blame for the injury to the child

A parent at risk of abusive behavior has a tendency to blame the child or others for the hurt they have sustained. Parents may see their child as a miniature version of themselves. The lack of self-esteem and poor self-image of the parents may have an impact on the child. The child is made a scapegoat for the parents' emotions of failure and inadequacy.

ANSWER NUMBER 12.56

Solution of the Question - B. Repeated vomiting.

Increased pressure within the skull produced by bleeding or swelling can harm fragile brain tissue and be life threatening. Because the vomit center within the medulla is triggered, repeated vomiting can be an early symptom of hypertension. If a patient exhibits the following signs and symptoms: headaches, vomiting, and altered mental status ranging from drowsiness to coma, clinical suspicion for intracranial hypertension should be raised.

ANSWER NUMBER 12.57

Solution of the Question - A. Small blue-white spots are visible on the oral mucosa.

Koplik's spots, which appear as little blue-white dots on the oral mucosa, are a symptom of measles infection. The disease's characteristic Koplik spots, which emerge two to three days before the rash and fade on the third day, are found in the buccal mucosa at the height of the second molar.

ANSWER NUMBER 12.58

Solution of the Question - C. Petechiae occur on the soft palate.

The presence of Petechiae on the soft palate is a sign of rubella infection. Rubella infection after birth can be asymptomatic in 25 percent to 50 percent of patients, particularly in young infants. A prodromal disease with low-grade fever, malaise, anorexia, headaches, sore throat, and adenopathy follows the incubation phase, which lasts 14 to 21 days.

ANSWER NUMBER 12.59

Solution of the Question - B. The dose is too low.

The pediatric dose of diphenhydramine is 5 mg/kg/day (5 X 30 = 150 mg/day) for this child, who weighs 30 kg. As a result, the recommended daily intake is 150 mg. Diphenhydramine is a first-generation antihistamine that is used to treat and prevent dystonias, sleeplessness, itch, urticaria, vertigo, and motion sickness. It is accessible as an over-the-counter medicine.

ANSWER NUMBER 12.60

Solution of the Question - D. Normally, the testes descend by one year of age.

By the age of one year, the testes should have descended. When the environment is chilly or the cremasteric reflex is triggered, it is usual for the testes to retract into the inguinal canal in young newborns. About 3% of full-term male infants and 30% of preterm male children are born without one or both testicles. By the third month of life, approximately 80% of cryptorchid testes have descended. This puts the genuine incidence at roughly 1%.

ANSWER NUMBER 12.61

Solution of the Question - B. Crackles

Fluid builds up in the capillary network of the lungs as a result of left-sided heart failure. At the end of inspiration, fluid enters alveolar gaps, causing crackling sounds. Crackling noises in the lungs can be caused by pulmonary edema. Pulmonary edema is common in people with congestive heart failure (CHF). CHF develops when the heart is unable to adequately pump blood. This generates a blood backup, which raises blood pressure and causes fluid to pool in the lungs' air sacs.

ANSWER NUMBER 12.62

Solution of the Question - B. Prevents shock and relieves pain

Morphine is a central nervous system depressant that is used to treat pain from myocardial infarction, as well as to reduce anxiety and prevent cardiogenic shock. The FDA has approved morphine sulfate for the treatment of moderate to severe pain, which can be acute or chronic. Morphine is a regularly used pain reliever that provides significant relief to those suffering from pain.

ANSWER NUMBER 12.63

Solution of the Question - D. Visual disturbances such as seeing yellow spots

The symptoms of digitalis poisoning include seeing yellow dots and having colored vision. Visual alterations, particularly those involving colors, such as seeing a yellow hue, are more well-known and seen in digitalis poisoning. Photophobia, photopsia, and decreased visual acuity are some of the other visual issues.

ANSWER NUMBER 12.64

Solution of the Question - C. Prevents sleep disturbances during night

When diuretics are taken in the morning, the client will need to void less frequently during the day and less frequently at night. When someone takes furosemide, either orally or intravenously, their sodium excretion in the urine increases. The first dose of furosemide generates considerable sodium excretion and diuresis within the first 3 to 6 hours in a patient with extracellular volume expansion who has never been exposed to the medicine.

ANSWER NUMBER 12.65

Solution of the Question - B. Increase cardiac output

Increased cardiac output is the primary goal of therapy for a patient with pulmonary edema or heart failure. Pulmonary edema is a medical emergency that necessitates rapid treatment. Preload reduction minimizes fluid transudation into the lung interstitium and alveoli by lowering pulmonary capillary hydrostatic pressure. Afterload reduction raises cardiac output and improves renal perfusion, allowing diuresis in fluid-overloaded patients.

ANSWER NUMBER 12.66

Solution of the Question - C. Extension of the extremities after a stimulus

Decerebrate posturing is the extension of the extremities in response to a stimulus, which can happen as a result of an upper brain stem damage. Adduction and internal rotation of the shoulder, extension of the elbows with pronation of the forearm, and flexion of the fingers are all examples of decerebrate posture.

ANSWER NUMBER 12.67

Solution of the Question - C. Abdominal cramps

Abdominal pains and nausea are the most common Cascara Sagrada (Laxative) adverse effects. When consumed for less than one week, Cascara sagrada is probably safe for most adults. Constipation and stomach cramps are two common side effects.

ANSWER NUMBER 12.68

Solution of the Question - D. Obtaining infusion pump for the medication

For accurate drug control, an intravenous nitroglycerin infusion necessitates the use of a pump. Nitroglycerin is most typically administered via intravenous (IV) methods in emergency rooms and intensive care units (ICU). It is given as a 5% dextrose in water drip and is used when sublingual nitroglycerin has failed to offer symptomatic relief or when immediate and continuous symptom alleviation is required. Its effect, once delivered, necessitates close monitoring, as detailed below.

ANSWER NUMBER 12.69

Solution of the Question - A. Able to perform self-care activities without pain

Clients are able to provide care without chest pain by the second day of hospitalization after suffering a Myocardial Infarction. Instruct the patient to report pain as soon as possible. Provide a tranquil atmosphere, relaxing activities, and comfort measures. Approach the patient with confidence and calmness. Reduces external stimuli, which can exacerbate anxiety and heart strain, limit coping capacities, and make it more difficult to respond to the current situation.

ANSWER NUMBER 12.70

Solution of the Question - B. Use hand roll and extend the left upper extremity on a pillow to prevent contractions

A right-sided brain attack will affect the left side of the body. On admission, begin active or passive ROM to all extremities (including splinted). Encourage quadriceps/glutes exercises, squeezing a rubber ball, and finger and leg/foot extension. Reduces muscle atrophy, improves circulation, and aids in the prevention of contractures. If the underlying condition is bleeding, it lowers the likelihood of hypercalciuria and osteoporosis.

ANSWER NUMBER 12.71

Solution of the Question - A. Hourly urine output

Urine output must be measured every hour after nephrectomy. This is done to assess the remaining kidney's functionality as well as to discover renal failure early. The health care team will monitor the client's blood pressure, electrolytes, and fluid balance immediately after surgery. The kidneys have a role in several of these bodily activities. During the recovery, the client will most likely have a urinary catheter (tube to drain urine) in the bladder for a short period.

ANSWER NUMBER 12.72

Solution of the Question - B. To visualize the disease process in the coronary arteries.

Cardiac catheterization can be used to measure the artery lumen. The narrowing of the coronary arteries is the most common cause of angina. Catheterization of the left heart can be used for both diagnostic and therapeutic purposes. It is used to measure cardiac hemodynamics and valvular abnormalities, but its primary diagnostic use is to diagnose coronary artery disease. In today's world, left heart catheterization, particularly selective coronary angiography, is the gold standard technique for detecting coronary artery disease.

ANSWER NUMBER 12.73

Solution of the Question - C. Frequently monitor the client's apical pulse and blood pressure.

The blood pressure is checked to see whether there is any hypotension, which could suggest shock or hemorrhage. The apical pulse is used to detect cardiac irritability-related arrhythmias. A nurse is appointed to keep track of vital signs throughout the treatment. The nurse is also responsible for verifying that the access site is not bleeding and that the distal extremity pulses remain intact after the procedure.

ANSWER NUMBER 12.74

Solution of the Question - A. Protamine Sulfate

In a client who has had open heart surgery, protamine sulfate is given to avoid persistent bleeding. Protamine is a drug that works to reverse and neutralize heparin's anticoagulant effects. Heparin-induced anticoagulation is neutralized by protamine, a particular antagonist. Protamine is a polycationic low-molecular-weight protein discovered in salmon sperm that is also available in a recombinant form. It is extremely alkaline (almost two-thirds of the amino acid makeup is arginine).

ANSWER NUMBER 12.75

Solution of the Question - C. Manual toothbrush

The use of an electric toothbrush, irrigation device, or dental floss can cause gum bleeding, which allows bacteria to enter the body and raises the risk of endocarditis. In the moderate-risk category of patients, effective oral hygiene and infection management can reduce the occurrence of endocarditis and eliminate the need for antibiotic prophylaxis for endocarditis.

CONCLUSION

Everyone who graduates from nursing school deserves to pass the NCLEX, and you are no particular case! You have effectively demonstrated your potential as a nurse by graduating from nursing school. You accomplished more than complete your coursework. You have shown that you are resilient, creative, caring, and intelligent. Your flexibility, commitment, and want to successfully finish nursing school is more impressive than passing the NCLEX. Presently, you must transition from nursing student to nurse. The NCLEX is your final obstacle to earning the option to practice as a licensed, proficient nurse.

Passing the National Council Licensure Examination (NCLEX) test is a significant milestone for many nurses, which assists them with demonstrating their qualifications and seeking after open nursing positions. Yet, if you're hoping to take the NCLEX test, it's critical to create and practice solid test-taking procedures to assist you with succeeding during the examination. In this book, I talk about the NCLEX test and list different systems to help you prepare and take the NCLEX exam.

BIBLIOGRAPHY

NCLEX-RN Practice Questions Set 8 (75 Questions). (2021, 12 13). Retrieved from stuvia: https://www.stuvia.com/en-us/doc/1450786/nclex-rn-practice-questions-set-8-75-questions

Nguyen, K. (18 February 2021). *NCLEX-RN Study Guide! Complete Review of NCLEX Examination Concepts Ultimate Trainer & Test Prep Book To Help Pass The Test!* . USA: House of Lords LLC. Retrieved from https://www.amazon.ae/NCLEX-RN-Complete-Examination-Concepts-Ultimate/dp/1617045187#detailBullets_feature_div

Rnpedia. (2020, 10 19). *Medical Surgical Nursing Practice Test Part 2 (Practice Mode)- Rnpedia*. Retrieved from ProProfs: https://www.proprofs.com/quiz-school/story.php?title=medical-surgical-nursing-practice-test-part-2_2

unknown. (n.d.). *What is the NCLEX-RN®?* Retrieved from Kaptest: https://www.kaptest.com/nclex/what-is-the-nclex-rn

Vera, M. (2019, 10 6). *NCLEX Practice Questions Test Bank for Free (2022 Update)*. Retrieved from Nurse Labs: https://nurseslabs.com/nclex-practice-questions/

Printed in the United States
by Baker & Taylor Publisher Services